Time
Pathology

Current Concepts in Gastrointestinal Pathology

Guest Editors

JOHN HART, MD
AMY E. NOFFSINGER, MD

SURGICAL PATHOLOGY CLINICS

surgpath.theclinics.com

Consulting Editor
JOHN R. GOLDBLUM, MD

June 2010 • Volume 3 • Number 2

SAUNDERS an imprint of ELSEVIER, Inc.

W.B. SAUNDERS COMPANY
A Division of Elsevier Inc.

1600 John F. Kennedy Boulevard • Suite 1800 • Philadelphia, Pennsylvania 19103-2899

http://www.theclinics.com

SURGICAL PATHOLOGY CLINICS Volume 3, Number 2
June 2010 ISSN 1875-9181, ISBN-13: 978-1-4377-0550-8

Editor: Joanne Husovski
Developmental Editor: Donald Mumford

Surgical Pathology Clinics (ISSN 1875-9181) is published quarterly by Elsevier Inc., 360 Park Avenue South, New York, NY 10010. Months of issue are March, June, September, and December. Business and Editorial Office: Elsevier Inc., 1600 John F. Kennedy Blvd., Ste. 1800, Philadelphia, PA 19103-2899. Accounting and Circulation Offices: Elsevier Inc., 3251 Riverport Lane, Maryland Heights, MO 63043. Periodicals postage paid at New York, NY and at additional mailing offices. Subscription prices are $159.00 per year (US individuals), $199.00 per year (US institutions), $80.00 per year (US students/residents), $199.00 per year (Canadian individuals), $225.00 per year (Canadian Institutions), $199.00 per year (foreign individuals), $225.00 per year (foreign institutions), and $99.00 per year (international & Canadian students/residents). Foreign air speed delivery is included in all *Clinics'* subscription prices. All prices are subject to change without notice. **POSTMASTER:** Send address changes to *Surgical Pathology Clinics*, Elsevier, 3251 Riverport Lane, Maryland Heights, MO 63043. Customer Service: 1-800-654-2452 (US). From outside the United States, call 1-314-453-7041. Fax: 1-314-453-5170. E-mail: JournalsCustomerServiceusa@elsevier.com (for print support) and JournalsOnlineSupport-usa@elsevier.com (for online support).

Reprints. For copies of 100 or more, of articles in this publication, please contact the Commercial Reprints Department, Elsevier Inc., 360 Park Avenue South, New York, NY 10010-1710. Tel. (212) 633-3812; Fax: (212) 462-1935; email: reprints@elsevier.com.

Printed in the United States of America.

Contributors

CONSULTING EDITOR

JOHN R. GOLDBLUM, MD
Chairman, Department of Anatomic Pathology,
Professor of Pathology, Cleveland Clinics
Lerner College of Medicine, Cleveland Clinic,
Cleveland, Ohio

GUEST EDITORS

JOHN HART, MD
Professor of Pathology, Department
of Pathology, University of Chicago
Medical Center, Chicago, Illinois

AMY E. NOFFSINGER, MD
Professor, Department of Pathology,
University of Cincinnati College of Medicine,
Cincinnati, Ohio

AUTHORS

MITUAL AMIN, MD
Department of Anatomic Pathology, William
Beaumont Hospital, Royal Oak, Michigan

KAMRAN BADIZADEGAN, MD
Gastrointestinal Pathology Service, James
Homer Wright Pathology Laboratories,
Massachusetts General Hospital; Department
of Pathology, Harvard Medical School, Boston;
Harvard-MIT Division of Health Sciences and
Technology, Cambridge, Massachusetts

KENNETH P. BATTS, MD
Staff Pathologist, Department of Pathology and
Laboratory Medicine, Abbott Northwestern
Hospital and Virginia Piper Cancer Institute,
Minneapolis; Director of Gastrointestinal
Pathology, Hospital Pathology Associates,
PA, Saint Paul; Clinical Assistant Professor,
Department of Laboratory Medicine and
Pathology, The University of Minnesota
Medical School, Minneapolis, Minnesota

NEAL S. GOLDSTEIN, MD
Advanced Diagnostics Laboratory, PLLC,
Redford, Michigan

ILYSSA O. GORDON, MD, PhD
Fellow in Gastrointestinal Pathology,
Department of Pathology, University
of Chicago Medical Center,
Chicago, Illinois

JOHN HART, MD
Professor of Pathology, Department of
Pathology, University of Chicago Medical
Center, Chicago, Illinois

†JOSEPH A. HOLDEN, MD, PhD
Department of Pathology, University of Utah
Health Sciences Center; Associated Regional
and University Pathologists (ARUP) Institute
for Clinical and Experimental Pathology,
Salt Lake City, Utah

VANI KONDA, MD
Instructor of Gastroenterology and Medicine,
Section of Gastroenterology, Department of
Medicine, University of Chicago Medical
Center, Chicago, Illinois

---

† Deceased.

LAURA W. LAMPS, MD
Professor and Vice-Chair; Director, Diagnostic
Laboratories, Department of Pathology,
University of Arkansas for Medical Sciences,
Little Rock, Arkansas

GREGORY Y. LAUWERS, MD
Gastrointestinal Pathology Service, James
Homer Wright Pathology Laboratories,
Massachusetts General Hospital; Department
of Pathology, Harvard Medical School, Boston,
Massachusetts

LESTER J. LAYFIELD, MD
Professor of Pathology, Head of Surgical
Pathology, University of Utah School of
Medicine; Department of Pathology, University
of Utah Health Sciences Center; Vice President
for Anatomic Pathology, Associated Regional
and University Pathologists (ARUP) Institute
for Clinical and Experimental Pathology,
Salt Lake City, Utah

ROGER K. MOREIRA, MD
Department of Pathology, Columbia University
Medical Center, New York, New York

AMY E. NOFFSINGER, MD
Professor, Department of Pathology,
University of Cincinnati College of Medicine,
Cincinnati, Ohio

REETESH K. PAI, MD
Assistant Professor of Pathology, Department
of Pathology, Stanford University Medical
Center, Stanford University School
of Medicine, Stanford, California

RISH K. PAI, MD, PhD
Assistant Professor, Division of Anatomic
and Molecular Pathology, Department of
Pathology and Immunology, Washington
University School of Medicine,
St Louis, Missouri

DALE C. SNOVER, MD
Staff Pathologist, Department of Pathology,
Fairview Southdale Hospital, Edina,
Minnesota; Clinical Professor, Department of
Laboratory Medicine and Pathology, The
University of Minnesota Medical School,
Minneapolis, Minnesota

KAY WASHINGTON, MD, PhD
Professor, Department of Pathology,
Vanderbilt University Medical Center,
Nashville, Tennessee

REBECCA WILCOX, MD
Department of Pathology, University of
Chicago Medical Center, Chicago, Illinois

**CARLYNN WILLMORE-PAYNE, BS,
MT(ASCP)**
Department of Pathology, University of Utah
Health Sciences Center; Associated Regional
and University Pathologists (ARUP) Institute for
Clinical and Experimental Pathology, Salt Lake
City, Utah

SHU-YUAN XIAO, MD
Professor of Pathology, Department of
Pathology, University of Chicago Medical
Center, Chicago, Illinois

Contents

Until very recently, there was general acceptance in the pathology community that all serrated lesions of the colon and rectum without overt cytologic dysplasia were hyperplastic polyps and had no malignant potential. Although there are still several unanswered questions in regard to the relationship between the various serrated lesions, there is a better understanding of the relationship of sessile serrated adenoma to carcinoma. This article discusses hyperplastic polyps, sessile serrated adenoma, traditional serrated adenoma, mixed polyps, and serrated lesions in such conditions as idiopathic inflammatory bowel disease and mechanical trauma. The major focus of the content is on diagnostic features of these lesions.

Gastrointestinal stromal tumors (GISTs) have emerged from being a poorly understood and therapeutically refractory sarcoma to a tumor whose biology has not only provided insight into a mechanism of oncogenesis but has also led to a rational basis for therapy. Most GISTs are characterized by KIT protein (CD117) expression and constitutive activating mutations in either the c-kit or platelet-derived growth factor receptor α genes. This information can now be obtained from routine formalin-fixed and paraffin-embedded tissue. Because the correct diagnosis is the key to successful treatment of this tumor, it is incumbent on the pathologist to be familiar with the various gross and histologic patterns shown by these tumors. GISTs range from small incidental stromal nodules to large cystic and solid tumor masses. GISTs show a variety of microscopic patterns and therefore several other tumors enter the differential diagnosis. Fortunately, with an understanding of GIST histology, and with the proper use of immunohistochemistry and molecular analysis, a correct diagnosis can usually be made. In addition to the correct diagnosis, several key attributes of the tumor need to be determined because they provide the basis for proper clinical management. This article summarizes the gross, microscopic, and molecular findings of GISTs, and discusses the differential diagnosis and key attributes of this interesting group of neoplasms.

The presence of esophageal eosinophilia encompasses a broad differential diagnosis, and at times a specific histologic diagnosis is not possible. This content provides a systematic approach to esophageal squamous eosinophilia with emphasis on specific, distinguishing features within this expansive differential.

Gastrointestinal (GI) infections are a major cause of morbidity and mortality worldwide. Although infectious organisms are often recovered by microbiological methods, surgical pathologists play an invaluable role in diagnosis. The lower GI tract, including the appendix, large bowel, and anus, harbors a wide variety of pathogens. Some infections are part of disseminated disease, whereas others produce clinicopathologic scenarios that are specific to the lower GI tract. This review focuses on selected infectious disorders of the lower GI tract that may be encountered by the general surgical pathologist, including viral, bacterial, fungal, and parasitic organisms, and including infections caused by food- and water-borne pathogens. Diagnostic gross and histologic features are discussed, as well as useful clinical features and ancillary diagnostic techniques. Pertinent differential diagnoses are also emphasized, including other inflammatory conditions of the gut (such as ischemia or idiopathic inflammatory bowel disease) that can be mimicked by lower GI infections.

Gastrointestinal (GI) neuroendocrine tumors (NETs) are a heterogeneous group of relatively slow-growing neoplasms with marked site-specific differences in hormonal secretion and clinical behavior. Most are sporadic neoplasms, with only 5% to 10% arising in patients with hereditary disorders, most commonly in multiple endocrine neoplasia type 1. Although a uniform terminology is not universally accepted, use of the 4-category WHO classification of these tumors is becoming more widespread, and recommendations for tumor grading and staging have been recently formulated. Most GI NETs are easily recognized on routine histologic examination; rarely, a limited panel of immunohistochemical markers may be useful in establishing the diagnosis. This article describes general and site-specific features of these tumors and outlines potential pitfalls in diagnosis.

Involvement of the upper gastrointestinal tract by inflammatory bowel disease was long held to be a feature of Crohn's disease, whereas ulcerative colitis was considered to be limited to the colon. It is now recognized that ulcerative colitis associated inflammation can involve the upper gastrointestinal tract, primarily the stomach. In addition to aphthoid esophageal ulcers in Crohn's disease, eosinophilic esophagitis and so-called lymphocytic esophagitis occur in association with ulcerative colitis and Crohn's disease. Possible immune mechanisms behind these conditions are presented. The differential diagnosis of inflammation in each site is discussed.

The effects of drugs on the gastrointestinal tract are diverse and depend on numerous factors. Diagnosis is centered on histologic findings, with mostly nonspecific patterns of injury that must be interpreted in the correct clinical context. Nonsteroidal antiinflammatory drugs are a common cause of drug-induced gastrointestinal injury, with effects primarily in the gastric mucosa but also throughout the gastrointestinal tract. Another common class of drugs causing a variety of pathologic findings in the gut is chemotherapeutic agents. This article discusses the differential diagnosis of the various patterns of injury, including ischemic damage, and the histologic findings specific for certain drugs.

Most epithelial neoplasms of the vermiform appendix are of mucinous type and can be stratified into 3 main diagnostic categories: (1) adenoma, (2) mucinous neoplasms of uncertain malignant potential or low-grade mucinous neoplasm, and (3) adenocarcinoma. Clinically, appendiceal mucinous adenomas and adenocarcinomas may present as right lower abdominal pain mimicking acute appendicitis, a mass, or pseudomyxoma peritonei. Nomenclature currently in use to describe and diagnose mucinous tumors of the appendix, particularly those of low morphologic grade, varies among surgical pathologists and centers, resulting in different histologic and clinical features being attributed to these entities in the literature. It may be of help, as already attempted by some investigators, to simply apply algorithmic parameters for such lesions (grade of the primary lesion, extensiveness and composite of extra-appendiceal involvement, and so forth), instead of adopting rigid classification categories. This approach allows for more objective data to be collected in hopes that it will provide a more nuanced understanding of the clinical behavior of the spectrum of mucinous appendiceal tumors. Remaining focused on histopathologic parameters of the primary and secondary sites of involvement may help in avoiding circular reasoning.

In recent years, significant clinical and technological advances have been made in endoscopic methods for diagnosis and treatment of early gastrointestinal neoplasms. However, essential information related to these novel techniques and their implications for practicing surgical pathologists have largely been missing in the general pathology literature. This article provides a general introduction to these novel therapeutic and diagnostic methods, and discusses their indications, contraindications, and potential limitations. The article aims to enable surgical pathologists to interact more efficiently with basic scientists and clinical colleagues to help implement and improve the existing clinical methods and to advance the new technologies.

An estimated 150,000 individuals are diagnosed with colorectal carcinoma (CRC) each year, and approximately 50,000 will die from this disease, making CRC the third leading cause of cancer deaths in the United States. For this reason, an enormous amount of effort has been spent to understand the molecular pathogenesis of this disease and to develop screening tests and prognostic markers. In the last 10 years, there has been a revolution in the understanding of CRC due to the identification of multiple distinct molecular pathways. With the introduction of biologic agents that target particular subtypes of CRC, molecular analysis of CRC is becoming standard of care in surgical pathology. In this context, the authors first describe the multiple molecular pathways leading to CRC and then discuss the role of molecular testing in the diagnosis of Lynch syndrome (formerly hereditary nonpolyposis colorectal carcinoma), prognosis, and therapy.

Surgical Pathology Clinics

THE CLINICS ARE NOW AVAILABLE ONLINE!

Access your subscription at:
www.theclinics.com

Daily Challenges in GI Pathology

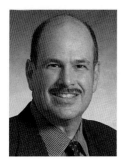
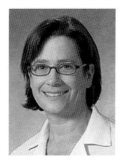

John Hart, MD   Amy E. Noffsinger, MD
Guest Editors

As a practicing gastrointestinal pathologist, I am faced with difficult-to-interpret biopsies and complex resection specimens every day. In speaking to many other gastrointestinal pathologists from around the country and around the world, I have come to the conclusion that the same difficult problems that plague me on a daily basis also plague my colleagues, which I suppose offers some measure of comfort. Nevertheless, when given the opportunity to serve as consulting editor for the *Surgical Pathology Clinics* series, I relished the chance to find guest editors and authors who could address at least some of these challenging topics. I was incredibly fortunate when Dr. John Hart from the University of Chicago and his former colleague, Dr. Amy Noffsinger, now at the University of Cincinnati, agreed to serve as guest editors for this edition.

They have chosen the exact topics and authors to address the aforementioned challenging topics that any reader could have hoped for. A comprehensive review of topics, including serrated colorectal neoplasia, the rapidly evolving field of gastrointestinal stromal tumors, eosinophilic conditions of the esophagus including eosinophilic esophagitis, infectious diseases of the gastrointestinal tract, neuroendocrine tumors, involvement of the upper gastrointestinal tract by inflammatory bowel disease, the all-too-omnipresent drug-induced injury of the gastrointestinal tract, mucinous tumors of the appendix (my personal favorite), the challenges (and opportunities) for surgical pathologists in the era of new endoscopic techniques, and an update of molecular pathology of colonic tumors, is all thoroughly covered by experts in these fields. I am completely confident

you will find these discussions relevant, practical, and up-to-date. The photomicrographs are of superb quality, and the references provide the reader with the seminal articles on each topic.

I am truly grateful to Drs. Hart and Noffsinger for their efforts and dedication to organizing and editing a superb edition to the *Surgical Pathology Clinics* series. Finally, I would also like to extend my gratitude to Joanne Husovski, the guiding spirit behind this entire series, and to the superb production team at Elsevier.

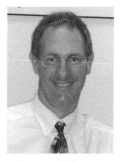

John R. Goldblum, MD
Consulting Editor

John R. Goldblum, MD
Department of Anatomic Pathology
Cleveland Clinic Lerner College of Medicine
Cleveland Clinic
9500 Euclid Avenue, L25
Cleveland, OH 44195, USA

E-mail address:
goldblj@ccf.org

Surgical Pathology 3 (2010) ix
doi:10.1016/j.path.2010.06.012
1875-9181/10/$ – see front matter © 2010 Elsevier Inc. All rights reserved.

SERRATED COLORECTAL NEOPLASIA

Dale C. Snover, MD[a,b], Kenneth P. Batts, MD[b,c,d],*

KEYWORDS

• Serrated • Sessile • Adenoma • Hyperplastic • Polyp • Colorectal

ABSTRACT

Until very recently, there was general acceptance in the pathology community that all serrated lesions of the colon and rectum without overt cytologic dysplasia were hyperplastic polyps and had no malignant potential. Although there are still several unanswered questions in regard to the relationship between the various serrated lesions, there is a better understanding of the relationship of sessile serrated adenoma to carcinoma. This article discusses hyperplastic polyps, sessile serrated adenoma, traditional serrated adenoma, mixed polyps, and serrated lesions in such conditions as idiopathic inflammatory bowel disease and mechanical trauma. The major focus of the content is on diagnostic features of these lesions.

OVERVIEW

Until approximately 2004, there was general acceptance in the pathology community that all serrated lesions of the colon and rectum without overt cytologic dysplasia were hyperplastic polyps (HPP) and had no malignant potential. This general belief was present even though as early as 1984 it was suggested by Urbanski and colleagues[1] that some serrated lesions had a propensity to develop into carcinoma, followed in 1990 by the seminal paper by Longacre and Fenoglio-Preiser[2] demonstrating that some serrated lesions were indeed neoplastic, and the term serrated adenoma was coined. In 1996 the term sessile serrated adenoma (SSA) was proposed by Torlakovic and Snover[3] for the lesions of the hyperplastic polyposis syndrome, suggesting that they were a subset of the lesions described by Longacre and Fenoglio-Preiser,[2] but without cytologic dysplasia as a prerequisite for diagnosis. The category of SSA was further expanded in 2003 by Torlakovic and colleagues[4] as a lesion occurring outside the context of the polyposis syndrome, and in that same year Goldstein and colleagues[5] demonstrated an association of SSA with microsatellite instable (MSI) colorectal carcinoma. The paper by Torlakovic and colleagues[4] found that the HPP category of serrated lesions could be subdivided into 3 types defined by their mucin character.

1. Microvesicular hyperplastic polyp (MVHP)
2. Goblet cell rich hyperplastic polyp (GCHP)
3. Mucin poor hyperplastic polyp (MPHP)

It was later discovered that these lesions had somewhat different molecular and genetic profiles, and it is now generally recognized that some of these lesions, particularly SSA, are an integral lesion in the serrated pathway to the development of sporadic CpG-island methylated phenotype (CIMP) carcinomas, a substantial proportion of

[a] Department of Pathology, Fairview Southdale Hospital, 6401 France Avenue South, Edina, MN 55435-2199, USA
[b] Department of Laboratory Medicine and Pathology, The University of Minnesota Medical School, Minneapolis, Mayo Mail Code 609, 420 Delaware Street SE, Minneapolis, MN 55455, USA
[c] Department of Pathology and Laboratory Medicine, and Virginia Piper Cancer Center, Abbott Northwestern Hospital, 800 East 28th Street, Minneapolis, MN 55407, USA
[d] Hospital Pathology Associates, PA, 2345 Rice Street, Suite 160, Saint Paul, MN 55113-3769, USA
* Corresponding author. Department of Laboratory Medicine and Pathology, Abbott Northwestern Hospital, 800 East 28th Street, Minneapolis, MN 55407.
E-mail address: Kenneth.Batts@allina.com

Surgical Pathology 3 (2010) 207–240
doi:10.1016/j.path.2010.05.001
1875-9181/10/$ – see front matter © 2010 Published by Elsevier Inc.

Key Features
SERRATED COLORECTAL NEOPLASIAS

1. HPPs tend to be small (<1 cm) and are more common in the left colon.

2. HPPs can be divided into microvesicular, goblet cell, and mucin depleted types, but to date the clinical relevance of these subtypes has not been demonstrated nor has a strong link to cancer been demonstrated.

3. SSAs were previously encompassed by the term hyperplastic polyp, but show architectural (basal dilatation and branching particularly) and proliferative abnormalities that distinguish them from HPPs; there is also molecular evidence that they are distinct from HPPs; several synonyms for SSAs exist.

4. SSAs have a propensity to be large (>2 cm), right sided, and multiple, and form a prominent component of most examples of hyperplastic polyposis.

5. SSAs have been linked to hypermethylated, BRAF-positive colorectal cancer (the serrated pathway), with development of cytologic dysplasia often being an intermediary step.

6. Traditional serrated adenomas have a propensity for the left colon, exophytic grown, and demonstrate surface cytologic dysplasia with a pencillate appearance and with ectopic crypts; they are generally morphologically, demographically and molecularly distinct from SSAs.

7. Serrated change can be seen in reactive processes (particularly mechanical injury) and serrated change in idiopathic inflammatory bowel disease is emerging as a potential preneoplastic change.

which are MSI but many of which are microsatellite stable (MSS).[6] Although there are still many unanswered questions in regard to the relationship between the various serrated lesions, a general schematic of the relationship of SSA to carcinoma is shown in **Fig. 1**.

The pathway from SSA to MSI carcinoma involves methylation of the promoter region of the mismatch repair gene hMLH1, followed by the development of microsatellite instability and a morphologic conversion from SSA to SSA with cytologic dysplasia (mixed SSA, tubular adenoma [TA], or advanced SSA), followed by the development of high-grade cytologic dysplasia and eventually carcinoma. Questions remain about the

speed with which this conversion occurs, although it would seem to be variable given that occasional carcinomas less than 1 cm in size are seen in association with SSA,[7,8] whereas most SSAs are larger lesions without cytologic dysplasia. There remains controversy about the relationship of the microvesicular HPP to SSA (with some investigators[9] suggesting that SSA derives from MVHP, a credible theory yet to be proved, and others suggesting that SSA and MVHP are separate lesions from inception), and about the role of traditional serrated adenoma (TSA) in the development of carcinoma. Details of this controversy are covered in the section on that lesion.

Details of the molecular aspects of these lesions and their role in carcinogenesis are beyond the scope of this article. The major focus of this article is on the diagnostic features of these lesions.

HPPS

OVERVIEW

The detailed morphologic study by Torlakovic and Snover[3] forms the basis for the current division of HPPs into 3 categories: goblet cell type (GCHP), microvesicular type (MVSP), and mucin-poor type (MPHP). As MPHP is rare, little is known about this polyp. Molecular data as well as differences in distribution and morphology provide evidence that MVHP and GCHPs are different lesions, although it remains unknown at this time what clinical differences derive from this. Thus, in daily practice in 2010 all of these polyps are generally reported as HPPs.

GROSS APPEARANCE

There are no known differences in the gross appearances of the 3 types of HPPs. HPPs tend to be small (generally <5 mm but occasionally larger), raised but not pedunculated (sessile or semisessile) (**Fig. 2**), and can be found throughout the colon but are more numerous distally, particularly for the goblet cell–rich type. The number of polyps in an individual patient varies considerably, from single to several to numerous, in which case the term hyperplastic polyposis has been applied.[10] Patients with serrated polyps (hyperplastic and serrated) have a greater tendency than patients with TAs to have additional serrated polyps,[11] and patients with colon cancers with microsatellite instability often have numerous serrated polyps in the background mucosa.[12] The clustering of serrated polyps (hyperplastic and SSAs predominantly), could be referred to the as the serrated milieu.

Fig. 1. The role of serrated lesions in the development of CIMP carcinoma. Solid arrows indicate steps that are well established in the literature. Dashed arrows indicate steps that are currently somewhat speculative and not directly supported by data.

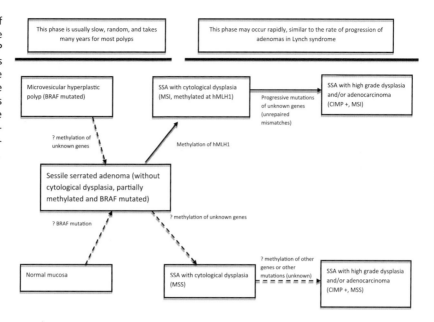

The far end of the serrated milieu is a condition termed hyperplastic polyposis (**Fig. 3**), defined somewhat arbitrarily as

1. At least 30 HPPs in a pancolonic distribution

   or

2. Five HPPs proximal to the sigmoid colon, at least 2 of which are greater than 1 cm in maximum dimension[10,13]

Hyperplastic polyposis is somewhat of a misnomer in that there is typically a mixture of HPPs and SSAs, with the latter sometimes predominating, leading to the term serrated adenomatous polyposis being proposed for this condition.[3] This is particularly true for the second of these definitions of hyperplastic polyposis, and these 2 definitions may define 2 different syndromes (ie, a true hyperplastic polyposis and serrated adenomatous polyposis).[13]

Fig. 2. HPPs: gross appearance. HPPs of the colorectum tend to be small (generally <5 mm but occasionally larger), are raised rather than flat, and generally sessile or semisessile rather than pedunculated. They lack the mucin or fecal cap seen in SSAs.

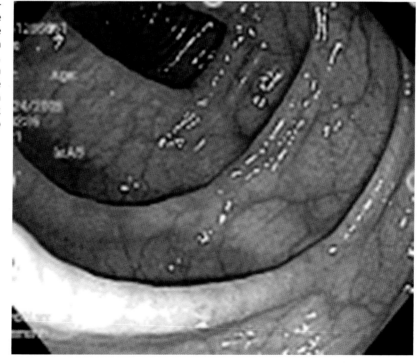

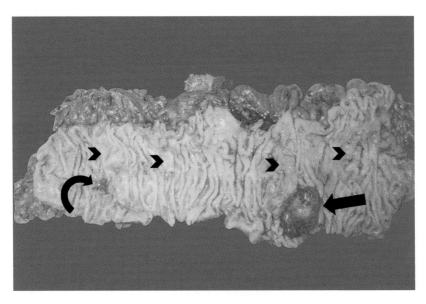

Fig. 3. Hyperplastic polyposis with adenocarcinoma: gross appearance. This image shows the typical features of hyperplastic polyposis. Most cases of hyperplastic polyposis have a significant number of SSAs and they may be the dominant polyp, be associated with cytologic dysplasia (mixed polyps) and even adenocarcinoma. In this example, the mass (*lower right, straight arrow*) was an adenocarcinoma that had been noted at previous endoscopy and the ulcerated lesion (*curved arrow*) was an unexpected small adenocarcinoma. Both of the adenocarcinomas arose in SSAs with cytologic dysplasia (mixed polyps)and all of the other flat polyps (*arrowheads* on some of these lesions) were SSAs, hence the diagnosis of hyperplastic polyposis; sessile serrated adenomatosis would also have been an appropriate moniker in this case.

MICROSCOPIC FEATURES

MVHPs are the prototype HPP. The major characteristic features are (see **Fig. 4**)

- Epithelial serrations predominantly toward the surface and to variable degrees deeper within crypts
- Elongation of the crypts resulting in a thickened mucosa in nearly all
- Decrease in goblet cells compared with normal mucosa
- Involved epithelial cells containing a delicate vesicular type of mucin instead of or intermixed with goblet cells
- Expanded proliferative zone that is orderly, does not spare the crypt base, and may occupy as much as the basal half of the mucosa
- Orderly crypt base architecture.

Specifically, there is a lack of the architectural distortion and abnormal proliferation seen in SSAs and absence of the cytologic and architectural features that define TSAs (see later discussion).

Additional features of MVHPs include nuclear atypia, which is variable but present in most cases and is always in the basal, proliferative zone. The muscularis mucosae is thickened in most, and about a third show tongues of the muscularis mucosae extending into the lamina propria. Nearly all show at least focal thickening of the subepithelial basement membrane. Kulchitsky cells are usually present in MVHP and often appear increased in number.

GCHPs are characterized by prominent, confluent goblet cells and often subtle serration that is limited to the upper third of the crypts (**Fig. 5**). The overall thickness of the mucosa is increased in only about 60% of cases. Nuclear atypia is not present and the crypt bases are essentially normal with no architectural or maturation abnormalities. Kulchitsky cells are increased in about 40% and a similar percentage show a small number of neuroendocrine cells with clear cytoplasm. The surface basement membrane is thickened in all cases and the muscularis mucosae is thickened in 75%.

Most MVHP contain some goblet cells interspersed with cells with microvesicular mucin and hence the diagnosis of GCHP is usually restricted to those lesions composed almost entirely of goblet cells, with minimal serration.

MPHPs are uncommon, thus little is known about them; they are clearly distinct morphologically from GCHPs but might be part of the spectrum of MVHPs. MPHPs share in common with

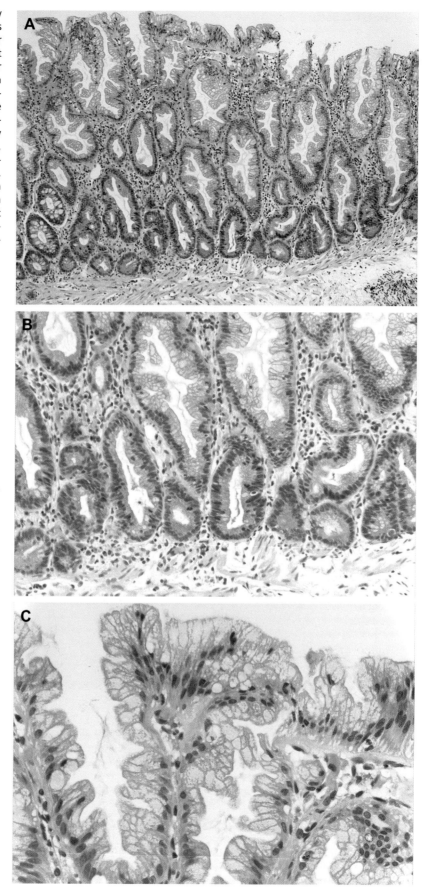

Fig. 4. MVHP. (*A*) Low magnification shows a serrated glandular architecture without crypt dilation, branching, or lateral spread as seen in SSAs. (*B*) High magnification of the basal zone shows some hyperchromasia and mitotic activity extending to the base, without abnormal proliferation as seen in SSAs. (*C*) High magnification of the surface epithelium highlights the somewhat fluffy-appearing name-giving feature of microvesicular mucin.

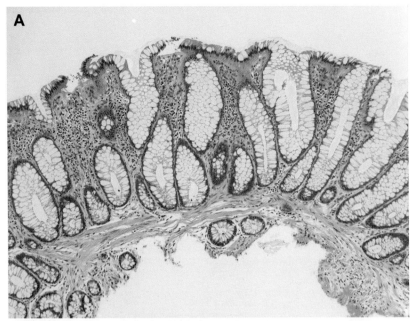

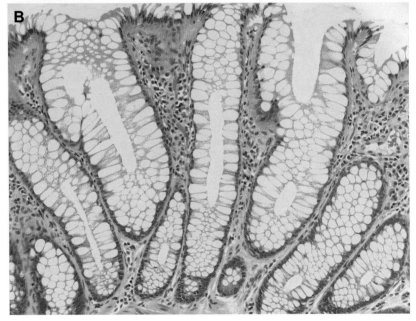

Fig. 5. GCHP. (*A*) Typically, GCHPs have little (and sometimes no) serrations and tend to the lack the darker basal zone seen in MVHPs (see **Fig. 4**A, B). (*B*) The surface epithelium consists of a uniform population of the name-giving goblet cells, lacking the fluffy microvesicular mucin of MVHPs (see **Fig. 4**C).

MVHP a micropapillary architecture, but are distinct from MVHP by virtue of a prominent lack of mucin/goblet cells, more hyperchromatic nuclei, and prominent hyperplasia of clear neuroendocrine cells (**Fig. 6**). These may represent MVHPs that have been damaged and are undergoing reactive change.

DIFFERENTIAL DIAGNOSIS

Currently it is not known whether distinguishing GCHP, MVSP, and MPHPs is clinically relevant, thus at the time of this publication there are no recommendations for subclassifying these HPPs in daily practice. If subtyping the 2 common

Fig. 6. MPHP. (*A*) At low magnification, the serrated architecture with deep crypt hyperchromasia resembles MVHP but not GCHPs, and lacks the glandular dilatation, branching, and lateral spread seen in SSAs. (*B*) The paucity of mucin and moderate hyperchromasia distinguish MPHPs from MVHPs; immunostains also show more prominent hyperplasia of clear neuroendocrine cells than seen in MVHPs. As these are uncommon, relatively little is known about MPHPs and they could represent variants of MVHPs.

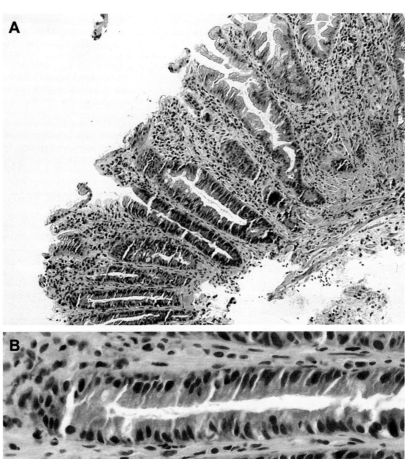

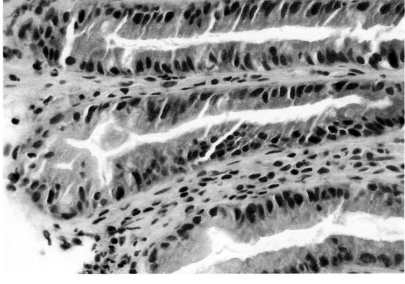

HPPs, MVHP and GCHP, is desired, key elements to consider are the obvious superficial serrations in all MVHPs as opposed to sometimes subtle serrations in GCHPs, the decrease in goblet cells in MVHPs as opposed to an increase in GCHPs, the presence of vesicular-type mucin in MVHPs in contrast to its absence in GCHPs, and deep-mid crypt atypia and hyperchromasia in MVHPs as opposed to absence of such in GCHPs. MPHPs tend to resemble MVSPs but have a greater degree of mucin depletion and neuroendocrine cell prominence.

The other main differential diagnoses are between HPPs and SSAs and between HPPs and flat serrated change in idiopathic inflammatory bowel disease (IIBD). These differentials are discussed later.

DIAGNOSIS

The diagnosis of HPPs is based on the identification of the histologic features described in the preceding sections. Currently, there is no defined role of special stains in daily practice, although MIB 1, MUC6, and CK20 stains could be useful if needed (see the section on SSA microscopy).

PROGNOSIS AND MANAGEMENT

When few in number, the presence of HPPs is a clinically innocuous condition. All forms of HPP are generally treated by endoscopic removal (or sampling of lesions if there are large numbers) and patients with only HPPs are considered at background population risk for the subsequent development of colon cancer. Currently, follow-up recommendations generally revert to population screening at 10-year intervals.

If HPPs are numerous in the form of hyperplastic polyposis, they are generally accompanied by SSAs. As this condition carries an increased risk of colorectal neoplasia, close surveillance with removal of all visible polyps is reasonable.

SSA

OVERVIEW

As discussed in the introduction to this article, most SSAs have traditionally been placed in the HPP category, with a movement to placing them into a separate category only occurring in the past decade. There is now considerable evidence that SSAs are an important component of the serrated neoplasia pathway to colorectal cancer. Nonuniform terminology for this polyp continues to make the literature difficult to decipher. Although the authors of this article prefer the term sessile serrated adenoma based on previous publications by one of us (DCS), other terms for this polyp in the literature include sessile serrated polyp[14] and serrated polyp with abnormal proliferation.[9] SSA is the second most common serrated lesion; from 7% to 25% of all serrated lesions were SSAs and they were present in approximately 9% of all patients undergoing screening colonoscopy in one large study.[15]

GROSS FEATURES

SSAs are nearly always sessile, have a tendency to be multiple, can be as small as 1 to 2 mm but are often 1.0 to 1.5 cm and can be as large as several centimeters. They are more numerous in the right colon and cecum but can be seen in the left colon and rectum. They can be subtle endoscopically, often being submitted as a possible enlarged fold or possible polyp or as an area of erythema. In situ, they have a tendency to have a small cap of adherent fecal material, even after otherwise adequate bowel preparation, or may have a prominent mucin cap (**Fig. 7**). More protuberant examples often have an underlying submucosal lipoma.

MICROSCOPIC FEATURES

The histologic features of SSAs can be roughly divided into architectural and cytologic categories, both of which are probably related to abnormal proliferation that is the basis for their abnormal growth. The architectural features are diagnostically more important, and include branching of crypts, dilatation of the base of the crypts, and a peculiar growth pattern in which the crypts seem to grow parallel to the muscularis mucosae, often creating an inverted T- or L-shaped crypt (**Fig. 8**).

Cytologically, the deep crypt epithelium is often fairly distinctive, with the presence of mature cells with a goblet cell or gastric foveolar cell phenotype at the base of the crypt, replacing the proliferative zone of normal mucosa (**Fig. 9**). This reflects a shift of the proliferative zone from the base to the mid crypt and results in immature-appearing cells with mitotic activity in the mid and sometimes upper crypts. Goblet cells may show considerable variation in appearance with a dystrophic appearance with somewhat hyperchromatic nuclei that may be present on lateral or apical aspects of the cells rather than abluminally toward the basement membrane as seen with normal goblet cells. Epithelial serrations always involve surface and crypts, and can extend to the crypt bases, in contrast to MVHPs. The surface epithelium can show foci of pseudostratification and occasionally eosinophilic or oncocytic-appearing cells, usually in association with elongation of the nuclei and displacement of the nucleus to the center of the cell. This change is reminiscent of the epithelium that is characteristic of TSAs.

Although special stains do not generally play a role in the daily diagnosis of SSAs, immunostains have provided some insight into them and their distinction from HPPs (**Fig. 10**).[16] In HPPs, marking with Ki-67 is limited to the basal third to half of the crypts and is regular throughout the polyp. Ki-67 emphasizes that the proliferative zone can occupy as much as 50% of the crypt length, somewhat greater than seen in normal

Fig. 7. Gross appearance of SSA. (*A*) Always sessile, endoscopically these polyps can subtly blend in to the background colonic folds and may be difficult to visualize at endoscopy. Often they will have adherent mucin (between *arrows*) that is difficult to rinse away during endoscopy, and at times a green-brown cap of fecal material may be seen. (*B*) Most SSAs are readily identifiable at endoscopy, however; the typical sessile appearance is shown here.

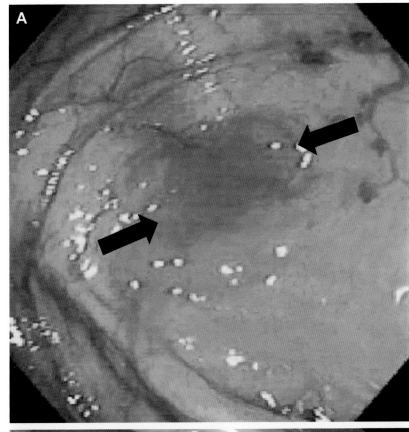

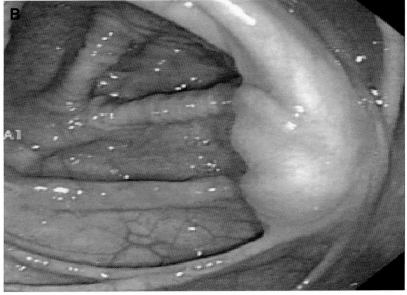

mucosa. In contrast, Ki-67 staining in SSAs is irregular, sometimes occupying entire crypts, but more often being located asymmetrically in crypts with no proliferation in the crypt bases but with proliferation seen more luminally, often only on one side of the crypt. This shifting of the proliferation zone (termed abnormal proliferation) is probably responsible for the architectural distortion

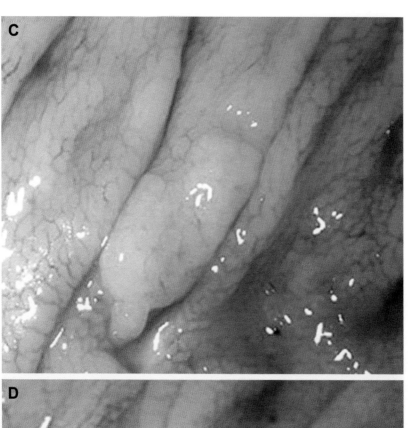

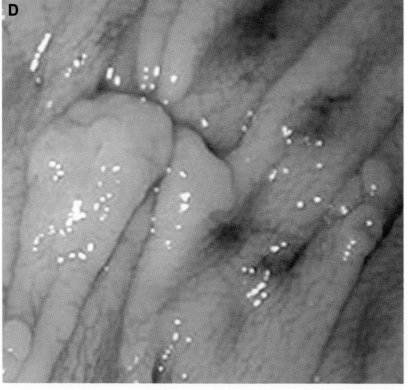

Fig. 7. (C, D). In resected specimens, the typical sessile, somewhat subtle fold-hugging appearance is exemplified in these polyps. A central depression may be seen in some cases.

Fig. 8. Low magnification microscopic appearance of SSA, highlighting architectural features. (*A*) It is not uncommon that these polyps seem to strip off the submucosa, resulting in a long strip of tissue at biopsy. This specimen affords a contrast between the optimally oriented mucosa at the bottom with the tangentially oriented tissue at the top. At this low magnification, the large sessile nature of the polyp can be appreciated along with the (in this case mild) crypt dilatation, deep branching, and lateral spread of crypts. (*B*) The typical features of excessive serrations and a laterally spread deep crypt are particularly well seen in this SSA.

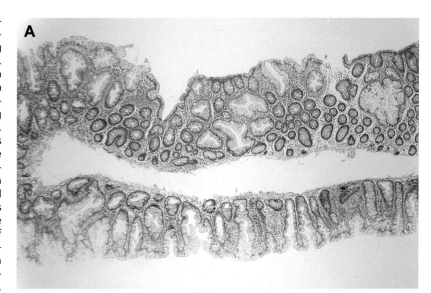

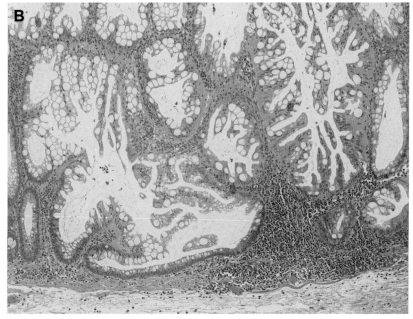

that occurs in these lesions. Cytokeratin 20 (CK20) staining also differs. In HPP, CK20 staining is confined to the surface epithelium and upper third of the crypts (differing from normal mucosa by extending somewhat down into the crypts, whereas in normal mucosa CK20 should be seen only in the surface epithelium). In SSA, CK20 staining is also irregular, often occupying the base of the crypts and sometimes marking entire crypts.[15] This corresponds morphologically to the histologic presence of mature cells at the crypt bases. Recently, MUC6 staining has also demonstrated significant differences, with MUC6 not staining HPPs but marking the bases of the crypts in SSAs,[17] although subsequent published study have not necessarily totally confirmed these findings.[18] Therefore, the significance of MUC6 staining and its possible role in diagnosis remains to be determined.

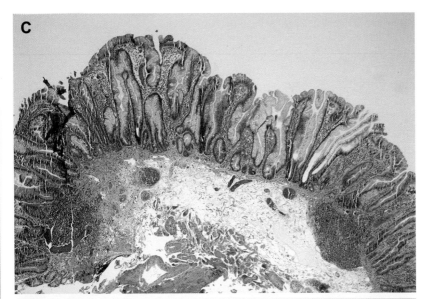

Fig. 8. (*C*) This SSA highlights the excessive deep crypt branching that can be seen in some examples, resulting in the glands having a forked appearance near the base. (*D*) This SSA showcases the glandular dilatation that can be prominent in some examples and the occasional paucity of crypt branching and excessive serrations.

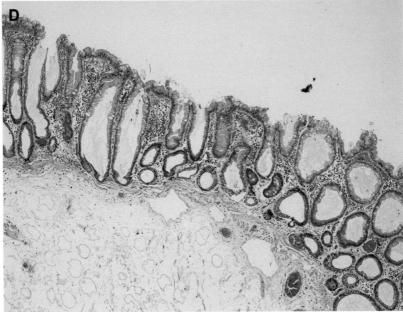

DIFFERENTIAL DIAGNOSIS

The distinction between MVHPs and SSAs is the most often encountered serrated polyp differential diagnosis of clinical relevance. The hyperchromasia in mid-deep crypts and surface maturation is similar between the 2 polyps, and it has not yet been proved that these are fundamentally unrelated polyps or whether SSAs arise from MVHPs.

The architectural caricature of SSAs (dilated, branching, L- or T-shaped crypts) in contrast to the absence of such in MVSPs is the most useful distinguishing feature in daily practice. The presence of the abnormal maturation of SSAs (shifting of the proliferative zone to the mid crypt with goblet cells or gastric foveolar-type epithelium at the crypt bases) can be helpful in difficult cases. One feature of some SSAs that is confusing is

Fig. 9. High magnification microscopic appearance of SSA, highlighting abnormal proliferation features. (*A*) The deep crypt here shows a boot-shaped crypt with prominent hyperchromasia in the deep crypt, similar to the deep hyperchromasia seen in MVHPs (see **Fig. 4**). In contrast to MVHPs, however, a zone of goblet cells at the far deep crypt is present in many SSAs, indicating abnormal proliferation. In this case the back-to-back mucin imparts a gastric foveolar-like appearance. (*B*) Even when the dominant architecture is nonserrated crypt dilatation, the goblet cells in the deep base can often be appreciated. (*C*) The other dominant feature of abnormal proliferation is dystrophic goblet cells. In the mid crypt seen at the upper field here, the goblet cells are haphazardly spaced, in contrast to the uniform appearance with basally located nuclei seen in normalcy.

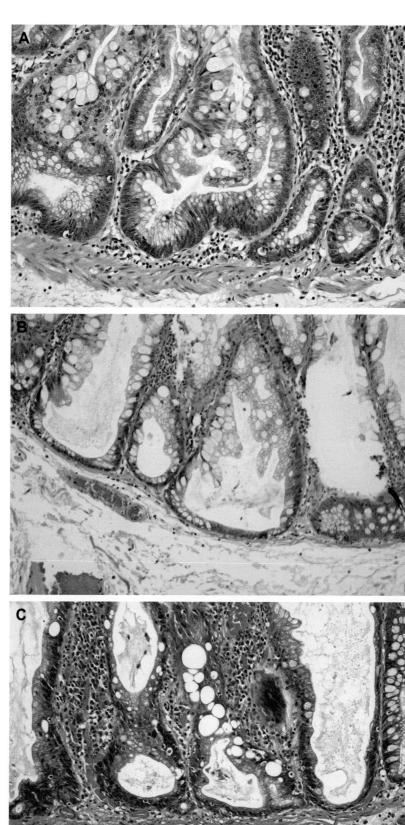
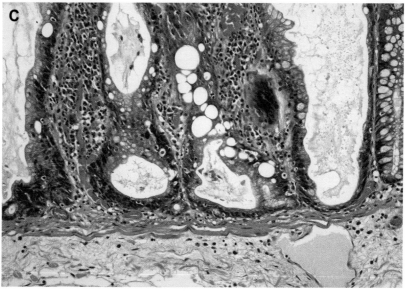

△△ **Differential Diagnosis**
SERRATED POLYPS

- Hyperplastic polyps

  Microvesicular

  Goblet cell

  Mucin poor

- SSA (sessile serrated polyp, serrated polyp with abnormal proliferation)

- SSA with cytologic dysplasia (mixed SSA-TA)

- TSA

- Flat serrated change in IIBD

- Fibroblastic polyp

- Mechanical injury (reactive serrated change)

---

that some areas of otherwise typical SSAs lack the crypt distortion and architectural abnormalities and taken out of context would appear similar to MVHPs. This feature has been used as an argument in favor of a transition from MVHPs to SSAs. Regardless of the association with MVHP, any lesion with more than an occasional distorted crypt should be diagnosed as SSA and not MVHP. The authors do not recommend using terms such as mixed MVHP-SSA for these lesions because this term has no clinical usefulness and because there is no proof that there is such a mixed lesion. One other consideration when there is crypt distortion in the form of branching, elongated, or irregular crypts is the location of the lesion. Because normal rectal mucosa is often somewhat distorted, some degree of distortion of the crypts is allowed in MVHP of the rectum, as long as that distortion does not include L- or T-shaped crypts or mature cells at the crypt bases.

Large size (>1 cm), particularly if the polyp is right-sided, should lead one to favor the polyp being an SSA if the polyp is histologically equivocal; conversely, small lesions on the left can safely be called HPP if the histologic features are not totally clear. Currently, the authors do not recommend using immunohistochemical staining to make this distinction in daily practice.

Sometimes, even after careful consideration, a serrated lesion cannot be classified absolutely on histologic criteria. This situation occurs most frequently with lesions from which only a biopsy is taken rather than being completely removed (which itself favors the lesion being an SSA),

resulting in only incomplete sampling and often resulting in a poorly oriented sample on the slide. If the polyp is tangentially sectioned and the crypt bases are not easily visible, then additional tissue levels should be cut in an attempt to see the bases. If the bases are not accurately seen and therefore an absolute diagnosis cannot be rendered, it is appropriate to make a diagnosis of serrated polyp (unclassified) or serrated polyp (HPP vs SSA, see microscopic description) with an explanation of the problem and perhaps a comment regarding the probability of the lesion being an HPP or SSA. Lesions that are unclassified but are large and in the right colon are most likely SSA and should be removed if possible, whereas small lesions in the rectum (which are usually completely removed initially) are probably HPP.

There has been considerable debate about the ability of most pathologists to distinguish SSA and MVHP on a daily basis. The earliest definition-generating studies examining this topic noted that SSAs comprised 18%[4] and 22.6%[5] of all serrated polyps. Subsequent studies have found frequencies ranging from 7%[19] to 34%[20]; this may reflect true variability in distinguishing SSAs and HPPs or potentially different populations of polyps being studied (SSAs are more heavily represented in the right colon). An Internet study looking specifically at interobserver variation using a broad, international pathologist population concluded that interobserver variation in identifying SSAs was significant but that education was useful in improving performance.[21] An interobserver study using 5 pathologists found moderate interobserver variation for distinguishing HPPs and SSAs, with an educational session not being of much benefit.[22]

See the section that follows on TSA for discussion of the differential diagnosis between SSA and TSA.

DIAGNOSIS

The diagnosis of SSA is based on the identification of the histologic features described earlier. Currently, there is no defined role of special stains in daily practice although conceivably MIB1, CK20, and MUC 6 could play a role in cases of particular interest (see discussion in the previous section on differential diagnosis for details).

PROGNOSIS AND MANAGEMENT

The serrated pathway of colorectal cancer is well established[23] and SSAs are likely the precursor for most cancers arising via this pathway, usually with the intermediate step of a mixed polyp

Fig. 10. Ki-67 staining of an MVHP (*A*) and SSA (*B*). (*A*) Note the relatively uniform staining of the basal half of the crypts. (*B*) The staining is more haphazard and some crypt bases do not show staining indicating lack of proliferation.

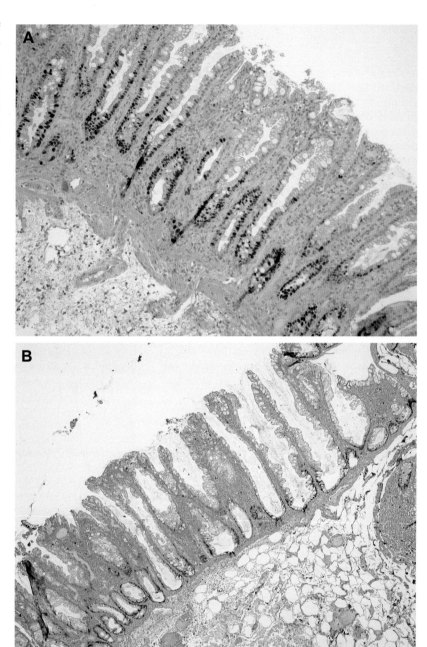

(**Fig. 11**; see also separate section on mixed polyps). Observational data would suggest that most SSAs progress at a slow rate. The rate of progression is probably driven by the rate of methylation and in particular methylation of the hMLH1 gene in the development of MSI carcinoma. The specific gene or genes related to development of MSS CIMP carcinomas are currently unknown. It would seem, however, that the rate of progression to carcinoma after development of MSI is relatively rapid. There are now several series of very small MSI carcinomas developing in SSAs that are less than 1 cm (**Fig. 12**).[7,8] These lesions demonstrate SSA with cytologic dysplasia and carcinoma, apparently in rapid sequence. Personal experience suggests that this process can even occur before the appearance of an endoscopically visible polyp, because we have seen cases of carcinoma arising in SSA that was interpreted as an area of erythema at endoscopy. These findings have led some to conclude that SSAs in general are rapidly progressive lesions, however as 15% to 20% of all serrated lesions are SSA without cytologic dysplasia and up to 9% of all patients undergoing screening have an SSA are indications that overall most lesions do not progress rapidly. The problem, of course, is finding those that do.

Adverse consequences from SSAs could conceivably arise in several forms: cancer risk for incompletely removed SSAs, cancer risk from SSAs missed at endoscopy, and the risk of synchronous or metachronous cancers in patients with SSAs.

Relatively little is known about the natural history of SSAs if incompletely removed, in part because it can be difficult to confirm complete removal endoscopically. In a retrospective review of a large number of patients with microsatellite colon cancers, Goldstein and colleagues[5] were able to find 91 cases in which earlier colonoscopy had noted HPPs (all on review being SSAs) at or near the site of the malignancy, raising the possibility that incompletely removed SSAs (initially regarded as HPPs as biopsies were taken before the SSA era) may have progressed to cancer. Recently, a case was reported in which a 1-cm right colon polyp was initially regarded as an HPP because of its endoscopic appearance and left intact. Eight months later the endoscopic appearance had changed and, at removal, an adenocarcinoma arising in a mixed SSA-TA (sessile serrated adenoma with cytological dysplasia) was identified.[24]

There are few data on endoscopically missed SSAs and cancer but some interesting circumstantial evidence exists. Sawhney and colleagues[25] noted that cancers occurring in patients having had recent colonoscopies (so-called interval cancers) showed a higher-than-expected number of microsatellite unstable cancers, which are known to be more common in serrated neoplasia, raising the possibility of serrated adenomas having been missed on earlier colonoscopy. Epidemiologically, although most colon cancer is decreasing in frequency there has been no change in the age-adjusted incidence of right colon adenocarcinoma for the last 2 decades.[26]

A retrospective review of the background mucosa in patients with MSI colon cancers noted an increase in serrated adenomas (and HPPs) in patients with MSI cancers compared with MSS controls.[12] If SSAs are numerous in the form of hyperplastic polyposis, there is an increased risk of colorectal neoplasia.

Management of SSAs depends on several factors including adequacy of excision in the original specimen and on the absence or presence of cytologic dysplasia (see the section on mixed polyp regarding the latter). Patients harboring lesions without cytologic dysplasia that are completely removed are at an unknown risk for the development of carcinoma, but anecdotal experience would suggest some increased risk of developing more SSAs. In addition, because these lesions are difficult to visualize endoscopically, removal may be inadequate even if the endoscopist believes that the lesion has been completely removed. Therefore, the authors have recommended returning these patients to repeat endoscopy at intervals used for patients with conventional adenomas.[27] This usually means a repeat endoscopy in 3 or 5 years.

Patients with SSAs without cytologic dysplasia in which the lesion is not completely removed by endoscopy face a more difficult decision. In general, it would be best to completely remove these lesions, because the absence of cytologic dysplasia in a biopsy does not rule out the possibility of cytologic dysplasia or even carcinoma elsewhere in the lesion. Alternatively, close surveillance may be adequate, if that surveillance is at close intervals (perhaps yearly) with adequate biopsy of the lesion at each visit to assure that cytologic dysplasia does not develop. For many patients, surgical excision of the lesion, if large, may be more tolerable than annual colonoscopy.

TSA

OVERVIEW

Of all the serrated lesions, perhaps at this point none is more controversial and misunderstood than the TSA. This is partly because the name is less than ideal. This name was proposed to distinguish what was the most characteristic of the lesions that were included in the rubric of serrated adenoma as first described by Longacre and Fenoglio-Preiser[2] from SSA.[4,15,27] The initial definition of serrated adenoma used by Longacre and Fenoglio-Preiser was one of any serrated lesion with dysplasia, although dysplasia was not clearly defined. Using their definition, serrated adenoma included not only the lesion referred to herein as the TSA but also SSA with cytologic dysplasia (see section on mixed polyps), some SSAs with focal eosinophilic change, which is often considered a form of cytologic dysplasia, and even some conventional adenomatous

Fig. 11. Adenocarcinoma arising in SSA. (*A*) In this low magnification, the background SSA is evident at the right edge of field, an area of cytologic dysplasia in the mid-left portion of the field, and an adeno-carcinoma in the left field – these areas are shown in **Fig. 11** (*B*, *C*), and D respectively. (*B*) The SSA demonstrates typical architectural features – irregular crypt branching and lateral spread.

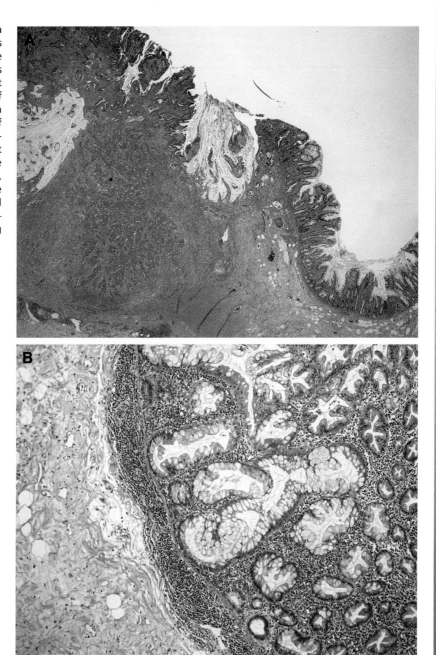

polyposis coli (APC)-related adenomas with serrated architecture. Much of the current litera-ture fails to recognize these distinctions, and hence one sees references to serrated adenoma without a modifier in many publications. Such ambiguous terminology is included in a popular schematic for the serrated pathway.[9] Herein the term TSA refers to that lesion described in several recent publications as the most unique lesion identified in the paper by Longacre and Fe-noglio-Preiser.[4,15,27] The lesion described by Yantiss and colleagues[28] as filiform serrated adenoma is in all likelihood the lesion referred to here as TSA.

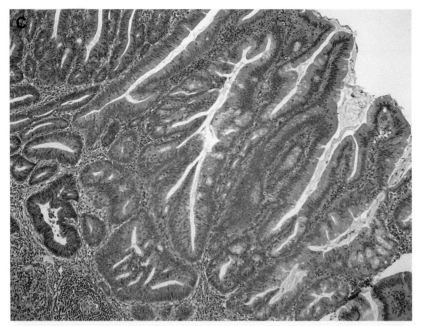

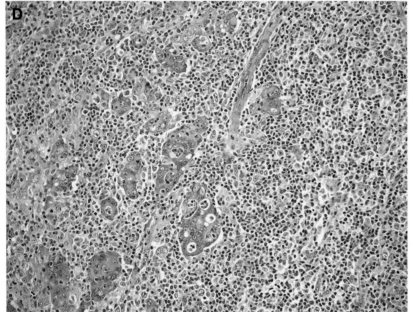

Fig. 11. (*C*) The dysplastic zone shows overt cytologic dysplasia ("SSA with cytologic dysplasia" or "mixed polyp"), which represents a usually-seen transition between SSA and adenocarcinoma when malignant transformation of SSAs occur. (*D*) The adenocarcinomas often show morphologic features that are associated with microsatellite instability – in this case the complex architecture indicative a higher-than-usual grade and the numerous tumor infiltrating lymphocytes are evident.

GROSS FEATURES

Grossly, TSA usually appears as a sessile but clearly demarcated lesion grossly similar to conventional villous adenoma (**Fig. 13**). These lesions are rarely pedunculated. They are most commonly seen in the left colon, especially the rectum, and are usually large when identified.

MICROSCOPIC FEATURES

As originally defined, the TSA is characterized by an exuberant, overall villiform growth pattern with extensive and sometimes complex serration (**Fig. 14A**).[4,27] In most lesions, the surface epithelium consists of oncocytic-appearing tall columnar cells with abundant eosinophilic cytoplasm,

Fig. 12. Early adenocarcinoma arising in small (4 mm) SSA. (*A*) The background polyp is a serrated polyp with only subtle crypt dilatation, a common problem encountered with small SSAs. (*B*) In this case, a small focus of irregular small glands was evident.

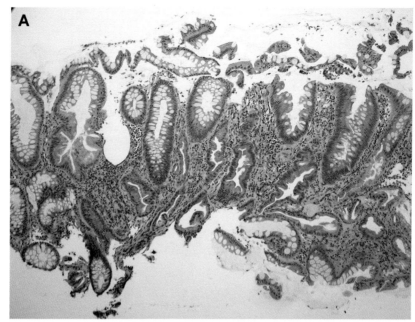

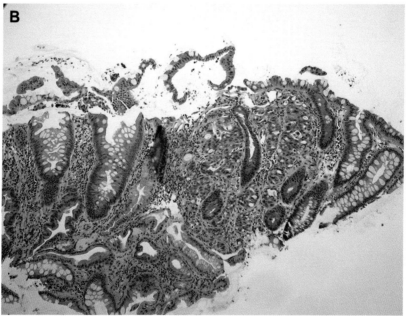

elongated but basally located nonpseudostratified nuclei, and little mitotic activity (**Fig. 14**B and C). Although these cells are often referred to as being dysplastic, they are not cytologically similar to dysplastic cells as seen in conventional adenomas, and immunostaining for Ki-67 reveals little proliferative activity in most of these abnormal cells (in distinction from conventional adenomas

which have widespread proliferative activity in the dysplastic cells) (**Fig. 15**A and B). A recent observation is that these lesions seem to be formed in part because of a loss of normal orientation of crypts to the muscularis mucosae, with the formation of so-called ectopic crypts (see **Fig. 14**D and E).[15] These short crypts, which run perpendicular to the surface of the individual villous

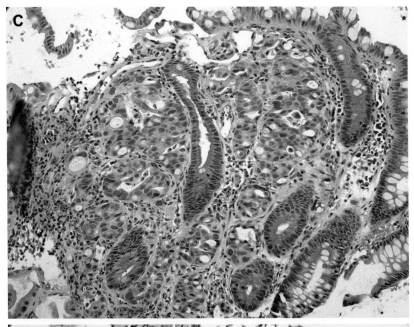

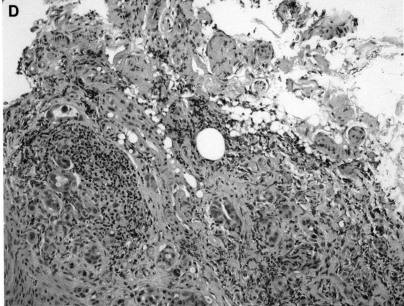

Fig. 12. (*C*) On higher magnification, it can be appreciated that this focus of atypical glands represented a focus of intramucosal adenocarcinoma, and that the adjacent glands showed dysplasia (a mixed polyp). (*D*) A small focus of irregular dysplastic glands with desmoplastic stroma was present, indicating a component of invasive adenocarcinoma in the small lesion.

structures, do not show normal anchoring to the underlying muscularis mucosae, which may be what allows the large villous structures to form. Immunostaining confirms that these structures seem to be crypts, with normal cytokeratin 20 staining on the surface and Ki-67 reactivity at the base of the ectopic crypts (**Fig. 15**C and D). If the presence of these ectopic crypts is used as the basis for the diagnosis of TSA, then lesions with the overall architecture of TSA but composed predominantly of goblet cells without the oncocytic-appearing cells that have been considered necessary for the diagnosis may be considered goblet cell–rich TSAs, a lesion that in the past has been difficult to classify.

Therefore, although the original definition of TSA required the presence of oncocytic pencillate cells, the authors currently believe that this is

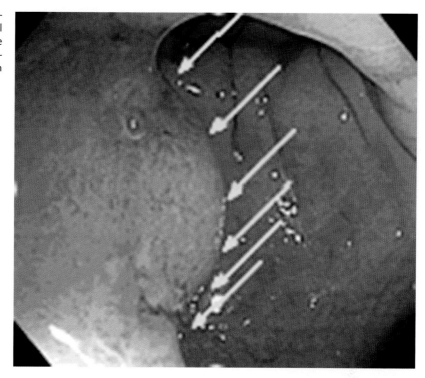

Fig. 13. Endoscopic appearance of traditional serrated adenoma. The lesion is sessile but protuberant and is located in the rectum.

a common and helpful diagnostic feature, but not one that is universally present. Our current definition requires the exuberant growth pattern, complex architecture, and most importantly the presence of easily identifiable ectopic crypts, usually in association with oncocytic epithelium. Conventional cytologic dysplasia histologically similar to that seen in conventional APC-related adenomas is not a required feature of TSA, but may develop in TSA.

DIFFERENTIAL DIAGNOSIS

Most TSAs are easily distinguished from MVSPs, GCHPs, and MPHPs by their uniform cytology, with pencil-like hyperchromatic nuclei with eosinophilic cytoplasm, and often large, protuberant growth endoscopically. TSAs are usually easily distinguished from SSAs, although SSAs may contain small foci that mimic TSAs cytologically.

The key distinguishing feature in most cases is the clone-like cytologic uniformity of the TSA as opposed to the hyperchromatic zone in the mid crypts seen in SSAs. TSAs also lack the deep crypt architectural abnormalities seen in SSAs but do have the propensity to create small ectopic crypts. Distinction of TSAs composed mainly of goblet cells from GCHP is based on the exhuberant

growth pattern of the TSA, with prominent ectopic crypt formation, compared with the subtle findings and normal overall architecture of GCHP.

Grossly, TSAs tend to be semisessile and prominently protuberant as opposed to the flat, nonprotuberant and often subtle endoscopic appearance of SSAs. TSAs often are left sided or rectal, less likely locations for SSAs. In our experience TSA is rarely if ever associated histologically with areas of SSA, but sometimes have adjacent areas difficult to distinguish from HPP. Therefore, the authors do not believe that TSA and SSA are related in the serrated pathway, but rather believe that TSA follows a somewhat different pathway to carcinoma.

From a conceptual perspective, there is now extensive molecular as well as histologic and demographic evidence that SSA and TSA are not closely related.[13,15] The major demographic difference is in the location of the lesions, with a preponderance of TSAs being located in the left colon, whereas most SSAs are located in the right colon. In addition to the differential staining patterns demonstrated with Ki-67 and CK20 as part of the new definition of TSA (ie, SSA demonstrates abnormalities in the location of the proliferation zone and marked abnormalities in maturation as demonstrated by CK20, whereas TSA

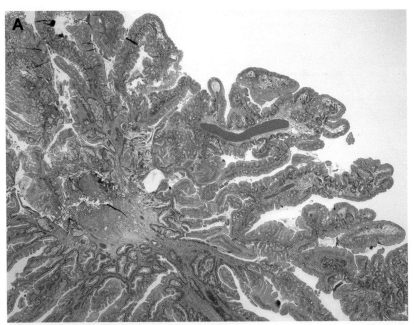

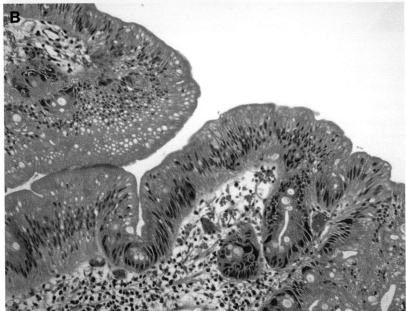

Fig. 14. Traditional serrated adenoma. (*A*) At low power these lesions often appear complex and may be mistaken for villous adenomas. (*B*) Surface area of TSA with eosinophilic pencillate cells but with few ectopic crypts. Ectopic crypts (see *D* and *E*), although usually present, are not totally uniform throughout the lesion.

demonstrates the ectopic crypt formation described earlier), there are differences in expression of MUC6 (present in SSA, absent in TSA),[16] and in survivin and Hedgehog protein that point to significant differences between these lesions.[29]

TSA, on occasion, may be difficult to distinguish from villous adenoma. In general, villous adenoma has uniform cytologically dysplastic epithelium with numerous mitoses lining the villi. Ectopic crypts should not be present in villous adenomas. Although the lining cells of typical TSA may be

Fig. 14. (*C*) High power illustrating the eosinophilic pencillate cells common to TSA, but not specific. Note the absence of mitoses. (*D*) The cells lining the villi are eosinophilic and numerous small ectopic crypts are present along the edge. (*E*) Ectopic crypts appear undifferentiated at the base with normal-appearing surface. In this particular area the cells do not have the eosinophilic pencillate appearance commonly seen in these lesions (see *C*).

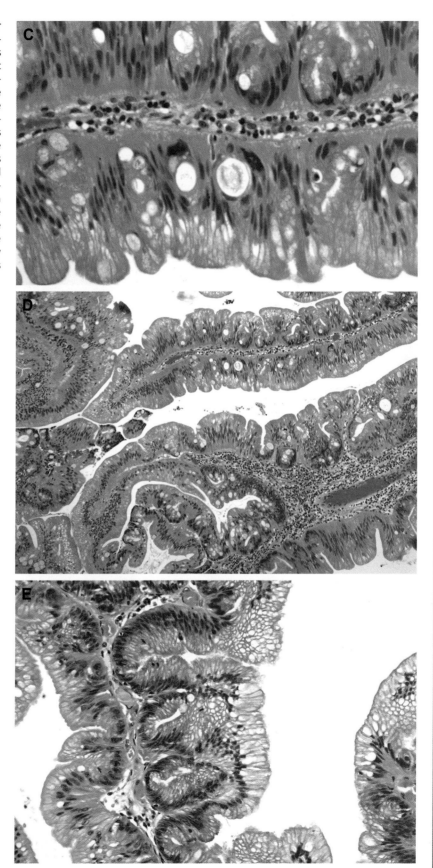

cytologically abnormal, they are not mitotically active unless the lesion has developed cytologic dysplasia similar to that of a villous adenoma as part of its progression toward carcinoma. If this cytologic dysplasia is extensive, it may be difficult to distinguish TSA from villous adenoma, although there may not be any practical significance to making this distinction.

PROGNOSIS AND MANAGEMENT

Relatively little is know about the natural history of TSAs, but it is presumed that they are premalignant. From a carcinogenic viewpoint, whereas SSA develops into carcinoma by methylation of hMLH1 and the development of microsatellite instability, methylation of hMLH1 and microsatellite instability are not part of the progression of TSA to carcinoma.[13] Therefore, although TSAs may develop more conventional cytologic dysplasia and carcinoma, they are not the lesions typically associated with MSI-high adenocarcinoma. They may, however, be associated with MSI-low adenocarcinoma because some of them demonstrate methylation of the MGMT gene.

Proper management of TSA is currently difficult to determine given our lack of knowledge of this lesion. Because most TSAs have cytologic dysplasia, albeit not typical dysplasia as seen in conventional adenomas, it is no doubt prudent to completely remove the lesions. Because most of these lesions are located in the left colon and/or rectum, this is usually not a problem. At this point the authors are recommending treating these lesions as conventional adenomas from the viewpoint of follow-up colonoscopy. Because TSAs do not generally become microsatellite unstable, the 1-year colonoscopy recommended for SSA with cytologic dysplasia may not be warranted for TSA unless there is a question regarding total removal of the lesion.

MIXED POLYPS

OVERVIEW

It is not rare to find serrated polyps demonstrating histologic features of more than 1 type of polyp. Terminology of these mixed lesions varies, and the term mixed polyp is an acceptable although perhaps not preferred term for serrated lesions as well as other forms of colonic polyps, assuming that the individual components of the mixture are defined in the diagnosis. Other preferred terms are discussed here.

Traditionally the term mixed polyp has most often been used for a mixture of HPP and conventional TA, a lesion referred to in the older literature as a mixed TA-HPP. Although the presumption initially was that these lesions likely represented an inadvertent collision of 2 different types of lesions, it is now apparent that most of these lesions are not mixed HPP with TA, but rather represent progression of SSA to a MSI state secondary to methylation of the hMLH1 gene, and hence are mixed SSA-TA. The authors prefer the term SSA with cytologic dysplasia, although mixed SSA-TA is acceptable. The term advanced SSA has also been proposed and has much in its favor, because this term more accurately portrays the significance of this finding. However, the term has not gained general acceptance. Although this type of mixed polyp may resemble a conventional TA arising in an SSA, from a molecular perspective the lesion is not related to conventional TA. Whereas most conventional TAs demonstrate mutation in the APC gene and are microsatellite stable, the cytologically dysplastic areas of mixed SSA-TA are often methylated at the hMLH1 gene with loss of mismatch repair and hence are MSI.[7] This difference is mechanistically important because with microsatellite instability comes the potential for rapid progression of these lesions to carcinoma. This fact explains the occasional very small cancers found in association with SSAs.[7,8] In some recent studies, serrated adenomas have been included as advanced adenomas along with conventional adenomas greater than 1 cm in size and those with villous architecture or high-grade dysplasia.[30] This may be appropriate, but only as long as serrated adenoma refers to SSA with cytologic dysplasia and not TSA or SSA without cytologic dysplasia.

Other mixed polyps that are occasionally seen include true HPP-TA, usually with the HPP being of the microvesicular type, TSA-TA or TSA-villous adenoma (VA), and occasionally hamartomatous polyps with areas of conventional TA.

GROSS FEATURES

As most mixed polyps represent SSAs with secondary development of TA-like dysplasia, the gross appearance of these polyps is generally identical to SSAs (flat or sessile). Other types of mixed polyps have the general appearance of the component parts.

MICROSCOPIC FEATURES

Most mixed polyps represent a background of SSA with the sharply demarcated, clonal-type growth of a population of uniform,

Fig. 15. (*A*) Ki-67 staining in TSA shows an absence of staining (and hence an absence of proliferation) in most of the lesion, including the eosinophilic pencillate cells often referred to as dysplastic. (*B*) For comparison with (*A*), a conventional TA stained with Ki-67 demonstrating uniform staining throughout the dysplastic cells.

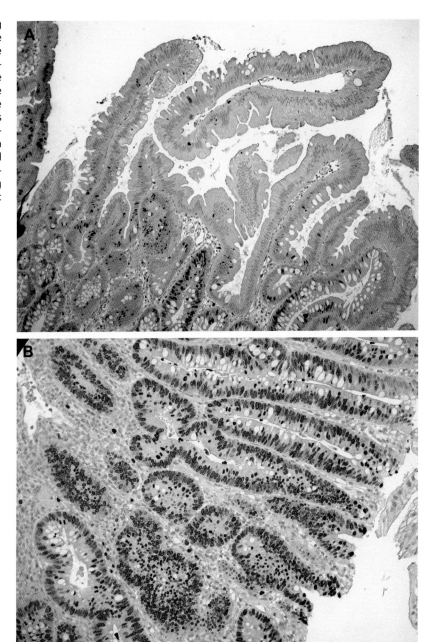

pseudostratified, hyperchromatic cells that are identical to those seen in TAs or with dysplastic mitotically active cells with more eosinophilic cytoplasm and round nuclei with prominent nucleoli, sometimes referred to as serrated dysplasia (**Fig. 16**). Other mixtures of polyp types are occasionally seen. Rarely, one finds a mixture of what seems to be a characteristic MVHP and TA. The significance of this lesion remains to be investigated. It could represent true conversion of an HPP to TA, it could represent a collision, or it could represent an SSA-TA in which the typical features of the SSA have been overtaken by the TA. Occasionally TSAs have adjacent areas of MVHP or, less commonly, GCHP or, rarely, SSA. Using the older definition of TSA as being characterized by

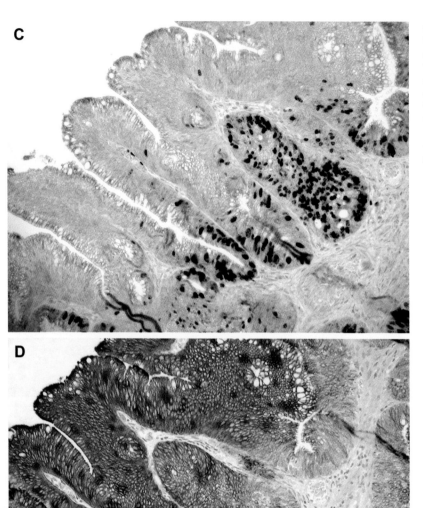

Fig. 15. (*C*) Ectopic crypts in TSA stained with Ki-67 and showing proliferation at the base of the ectopic crypts. (*D*) Ectopic crypts in TSA stained with cytokeratin 20 (same section as [*C*]). Note the normal pattern of CK20 staining on the surface.

the presence of oncocytic pencillate cells, lesions showing features of SSA plus TSA might have been considered common, but as explained in the section on TSA, these cells no longer are considered specific for TSA, and are quite common in otherwise typical SSAs, and hence do not constitute a mixed polyp. Similarly, in many typical SSAs there are areas that, taken out of context, might be considered as MVHP because they have straight crypts without distortion. Although these findings might indicate progression of MVHP to SSA, this has not been clearly demonstrated and recent findings using MUC6 as a marker of SSA would suggest that they do not represent

Fig. 16. SSA with cytologic dysplasia (mixed SSA-TA). (*A*) At low power, a clear demarcation can be seen between the SSA on the left and the cytologically dysplastic component on the right. (*B*) Junction of the cytologically dysplastic component on the right and the SSA on the left. In this case, the cytologically dysplastic cells are not as pseudostratified as those of a conventional TA. These types of cells have been referred to as serrated dysplasia. (*C*) In the area of the polyp with cytologic dysplasia, the crypt bases retain some architectural abnormalities including abnormal dilated and elongated crypt bases.

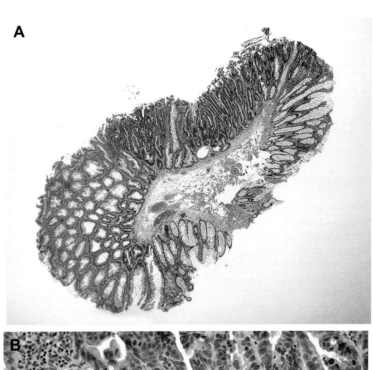

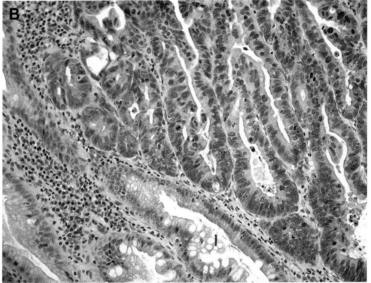

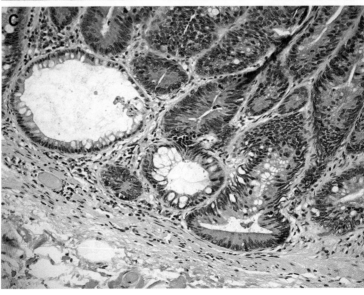

preexisting MVHP in the context of SSA but rather are part of the SSA, because the MVHP-like areas of SSAs express MUC6, whereas pure MVHPs do not.[16] Therefore, the authors do not currently recommend using the term mixed MVHP-SSA for lesions showing this mix of features, but rather would diagnosis only SSA in these cases.

DIFFERENTIAL DIAGNOSIS

Mixed SSA-TAs are distinguished from the others by the presence of clearly demarcated obvious cytologic dysplasia similar to that seen in adenomatous polyps of the colon, reflecting the arising of a clone of dysplastic cells in the background of a serrated polyp. The latter generally has histologic features of an SSA but rarely resembles an HPP. The authors do not recommend lumping these polyps together with TSAs, as has been done by some investigators,[9] as we believe there are straightforward morphologic differences in addition to the molecular differences discussed earlier.

PROGNOSIS

Relatively little is known about the natural history of SSAs with cytologic dysplasia (mixed SSA-TAs) because these are generally removed in their entirety when encountered by the clinician. There is circumstantial evidence that suggests that these may be on the fast track to malignancy, however. Although cancers arising from the serrated pathway nearly always have a component of cytologic dysplasia between the SSA and the cancer (ie, mixed polyps), the frequency with which mixed polyps are encountered without malignancy is low compared with the frequency of SSAs (about 20% of all serrated polyps). This implies that once an SSA develops overt dysplasia, it may progress to malignancy fairly quickly, which is in keeping with the molecular changes seen in these lesions.

SERRATED LESIONS IN OTHER CONDITIONS

FLAT SERRATED CHANGE IN IIBD

It is not uncommon to encounter serrated epithelium in random samples of the colorectum taken for dysplasia surveillance in patients with IIBD. Most commonly, the serrated changes seen in this context mimic small MVHPs in that the serrated change is usually not brisk, tends to be superficial, and is not associated with abnormal proliferation. Occasionally the serrated change mimics goblet cell HPPs, with a uniform, back-to-back population of goblet cells resulting in elongation of the crypts but often with little or no serration (hypermucinous change) (**Fig. 17**). Serrated changes reminiscent of SSAs are occasionally encountered in random samples as well.

The serrated change in random samples in IIBD raises several possibilities. They could be randomly sampled early (endoscopically invisible) sporadic serrated polyps, they could be a peculiar reactive change akin to serrated change seen in mechanical trauma, or they could be an early manifestation of the serrated pathway to colon cancer, analogous to flat dysplasia in random biopsies representing an early manifestation of the adenoma-carcinoma sequence.

There is some evidence supporting the contention that serrated change in IIBD may be premalignant. Kilgore and colleagues[31] histologically examined the background mucosa in 30 patients with Crohn disease with carcinomas. They noted that 33% of these patients had flat hyperplastic change in their flat noncancerous mucosa compared with 10% of the control cases, a statistically significant difference ($P = .03$). They concluded that "this mucosal alteration may, in some cases, represent an unusual form of dysplasia in this setting." Rubio and colleagues[32] examined the presumed precursor neoplasms adjacent to 50 colorectal cancers arising in ulcerative colitis, dividing them into adenomatous (TA, tubulovillous adenoma, or villous adenoma) and serrated (serrated polyp + serrated villous). They noted that 28% of the ulcerative colitis cancers had an adjacent serrated lesion compared with 4% of noncolitic cancer controls. It is unclear how these serrated lesions relate to the Torlakovic classification scheme used herein, however. Andersen and colleagues[33] studied the frequency of k-ras mutations in flat hypermucinous change in the mucosa of patients with resected colon cancer arising in ulcerative colitis, and concluded "The highest K-ras mutation frequency was found in villous, hypermucinous mucosa. We suggest that this entity should be investigated further as a potential risk lesion for cancer development. It may represent a pathway directly from non-classical dysplasia to cancer, not previously described." Serrated lesion adjacent to MSI cancer in inflammatory bowel disease has also been reported.[34] In our opinion, the clinical significance of flat serrated change in IIBD is currently unproved, but is most likely not a common problem because MSI cancers are likely no more common in the setting of IIBD than they are among the noncolitic population, and may be even less common.[35] However, in view of the theoretic role of these changes as precursor lesions of cancers arising via the serrated pathway, we are currently unwilling to dismiss them as clinically irrelevant

Fig. 17. Flat serrated and hypermucinous change in ulcerative colitis. (*A*) In this section, the randomly sampled colon shows a thickened epithelium composed of a uniform population of goblet cells with mild surface serration but no deep hyperchromasia or architectural abnormalities. (*B*) Elsewhere in this polyp is a transition to overt dysplasia, likely arising in the flat hypermucinous change. Although the background polyp did not strongly resemble an SSA overall, note the lateral branching present in deep crypts in (*A*) and (*B*).

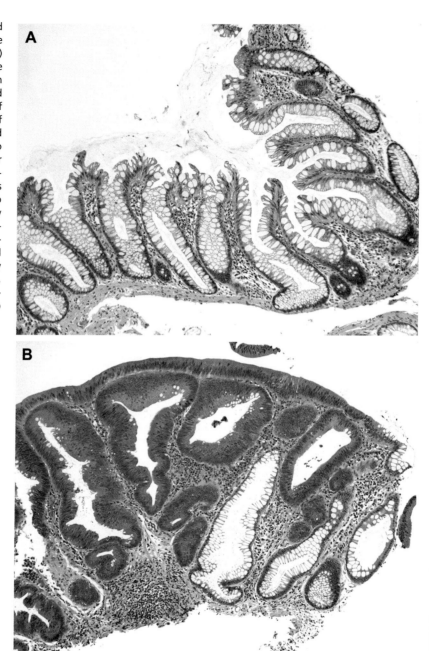

either. Currently, we report them as flat serrated change with a comment summarizing their uncertain status and allow the clinician to determine whether or not an alteration in surveillance strategy is reasonable. Follow-up similar to cases indefinite for dysplasia may not be unreasonable. Certainly, more data are needed on the prospective clinical significance of flat serrated change and the cost effectiveness of altering surveillance strategies because of it.

MECHANICAL TRAUMA

Polypoid lesions that arise secondary to mechanical trauma, such as solitary rectal ulcer syndrome, inflammatory cloacogenic polyps, or prolapsed diverticula, can sometimes show surface serrations that mimic true serrated polyps. The concurrent presence of fibromuscular hyperplasia of the lamina propria with often resultant architectural distortion in the form of diamond-shaped crypts are keys to identifying mechanical injury rather than a serrated neoplasm (**Fig. 18**).

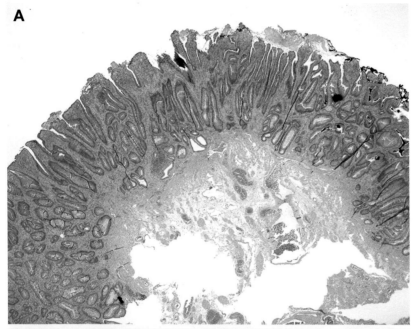

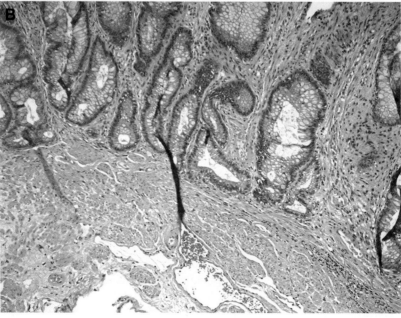

Fig. 18. Glandular distortion in mechanical injury mimicking SSA. (*A*) In this straightforward example of early solitary rectal ulcer syndrome clinically, there is glandular variability and dilatation with intervening fibrous stroma that is unlikely to be confused with an SSA. (*B*) Some examples of mechanical trauma can, however, mimic the architectural features of SSA, as seen here, and may also show some epithelial serration. The expanded fibrotic lamina propria and the clinical scenario are the most useful features in distinguishing mechanical injury from SSA.

FIBROBLASTIC POLYPS (PERINEURIOMAS)

Fibroblastic polyps of the colorectum are characterized primarily by an abnormal expansion of the lamina propria by a proliferation of bland spindled cells that histologically resemble fibroblasts (**Fig. 19**). There is evidence that these may actually represent perineuriomas.[36] Of relevance to this discussion, in more than 50% of fibroblastic polyps/perineuriomas, the associated epithelium is serrated, most commonly resembling MVHP or SSA. The relationship between the serrated epithelium and the fibroblastic/perineuriomal stroma is unclear at this point, but it should be noted that serrated epithelium/mesenchymal stromal interaction is not unique to these polyps, as submucosal lipomas not uncommonly underlie both HPPs and SSAs.

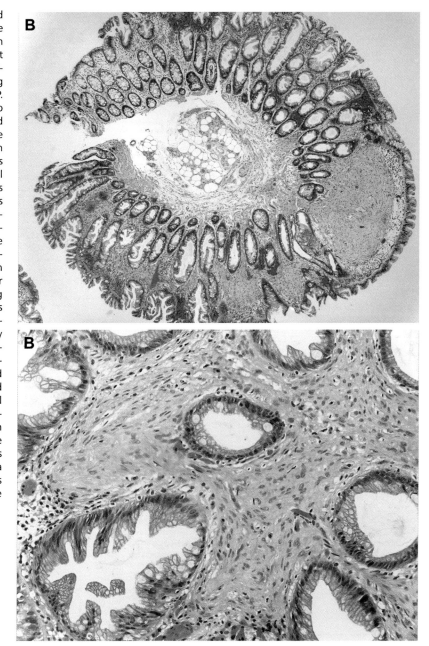

Fig. 19. Perineurioma and associated SSA. (*A*) The serrated polyp shown here shows some crypt dilatation and exaggerated serrations, favoring SSA more than MVHP. Focally within this polyp are areas of expanded stroma, the focal nature of this contrasting with the diffuse fibrous stroma in mechanical injury (see **Fig. 18**). This expanded stroma shows immunohistochemical features supporting the designation perineurioma. The focal nature of the perineurioma component in this case tends to favor this fundamentally being an SSA rather than this fundamentally being a perineurioma with secondary serrations, but the relationship and clinical significance of the combined serrated epithelial and spindled mesenchymal components remains unsettled at this time. (*B*) On high magnification, the bland histologic features of the perineurioma component, also known as fibroblastic polyp, are evident.

Pitfalls
DIAGNOSIS OF SERRATED POLYPS

Pitfall	Histologic Findings	Solution
Suboptimal specimen	Poor orientation (tangential sections without base of crypts)	Usually deeper levels to find the crypt bases are a better solution than reorientation. If the bases cannot be identified report the case as a sessile serrated polyp, unclassified. Recommend complete excision if there is residual lesion. You may favor SSA for larger and/or right-sided lesions and HPP for smaller and/or left-sided lesions
Suboptimal specimen	Biopsy only of a large lesion	If the biopsy shows SSA, make the diagnosis but indicate that the lesion should be removed if possible (cannot rule out cytologic dysplasia or worse elsewhere in the lesion). If the biopsy shows features of HPP, you can make the diagnosis but recommend excision because SSA cannot be ruled out
Suboptimal specimen	Cautery or crush artifact	Usually the best you can do is diagnose a sessile serrated polyp, unclassified and make recommendations as in first item, "Suboptimal specimen with poor orientation," regarding management and additional resection; rarely deeper levels will help
Calling a lesion with mixed features of HPP and SSA a mixed polyp	Some areas of the lesion have straight crypts with normal proliferation with other areas showing typical architectural features of SSA	Call these lesions SSA. Recent data using MUC6 would suggest that these mark as SSA even in the HPP-like areas, and when in doubt the diagnosis of SSA will be the more conservative call. In the rectum some degree of architectural distortion is allowed in HPP, so criteria are loose there (see no. 5)
Mistaking rectal HPP with crypt distortion as SSA	Elongated crypts with serrations and crypts that are distorted (curved, sometimes branching) but without excess basal serrations, or T-, L- or boot-shaped crypts and with normal proliferation	Normal rectal mucosa sometimes demonstrates crypt distortion in the normal mucosa that is carried over to the polyp. Generally the type of distortion is not that of SSA. For small rectal lesions completely removed, it is probably better to err on the side of HPP, when in doubt
Reactive conditions mimicking SSA	SSA-like lesions as part of mucosal prolapse, diverticulitis or other inflammatory/reparative processes (eg, cytomegalovirus colitis)	Recognition of the underlying condition usually allows the diagnosis to be made. If in doubt, evaluation of the lesion for the BRAF mutation helps because most SSAs have the mutation, whereas reactive conditions do not
Mistaking eosinophilic pencillate cells as significant cytologic dysplasia (implies development of satellite instability in SSA)	These cells are an integral part of TSA and should not cause a problem there. In SSA, areas of this eosinophilic change may occur but do not imply MSI	
TSA with a prominent villous pattern (filiform TSA) mimicking villous adenoma	Prominent exuberant villi with eosinophilic pencillate lining cells. Should have ectopic crypts foraccurate diagnosis. No pseudostratified dysplastic cells unless the lesion is a mixed TSA-TA	Attention to the type of lining cell and the presence of ectopic crypts should help in the diagnosis. If the TSA is overtaken by overtly pseudostratified dysplastic epithelium as part of neoplastic progression, distinction may be difficult but of little clinical consequence. Most of these lesions are rectal

REFERENCES

1. Urbanski SJ, Kossakowska AE, Marcon N, et al. Mixed hyperplastic adenomatous polyps: an under-diagnosed entity. Report of a case of adenocarcinoma arising within a mixed hyperplastic adenomatous polyp. Am J Surg Pathol 1984;8: 551–6.

2. Longacre TA, Fenoglio-Preiser CF. Mixed hyperplastic adenomatous polyps/serrated adenomas. A distinct form of colorectal neoplasia. Am J Surg Pathol 1990;14:524–37.

3. Torlakovic E, Snover DC. Serrated adenomatous polyposis in humans. Gastroenterology 1996;110: 748–55.

4. Torlakovic E, Skovland E, Snover DC, et al. Morphologic reappraisal of serrated colorectal polyps. Am J Surg Pathol 2003;27:65–81.

5. Goldstein NS, Bhanot P, Odish E, et al. Hyperplastic-like colon polyps that preceded microsatellite-unstable adenocarcinomas. Am J Clin Pathol 2003; 119:778–96.

6. Jass JR. Serrated adenoma of the colorectum and the DNA methylator phenotype. Nat Clin Pract Oncol 2005;2:398–405.

7. Goldstein NS. Small colonic microsatellite unstable carcinomas and high grade epithelial dysplasias in sessile serrated adenoma polypectomy specimens. A study of eight cases. Am J Clin Pathol 2006;125: 132–45.

8. Sheridan TB, Fenton H, Lewin MR, et al. Sessile serrated adenomas with low- and high-grade dysplasia and early carcinomas: an immunohistochemical study of serrated lesions "caught in the act". Am J Clin Pathol 2006;126:564–71.

9. O'Brien MJ, Yang S, Mack C, et al. Comparison of microsatellite instability, CpG island methylation phenotype, BRAF and KRAS status in serrated polyps and traditional adenomas indicates separate pathways to distinct colorectal carcinoma end points. Am J Surg Pathol 2006;30:1491–501.

10. Burt RW, Jass JR. Hyperplastic polyposis. In: Hamilton SR, Aaltonen LA, editors. WHO classification of tumours. Pathology and genetics. Tumours of the digestive system. Berlin: Springer-Verlag; 2000. p. 135–6.

11. Lazarus R, Junttila OE, Karttunen TJ, et al. The risk of metachronous neoplasia in patients with serrated adenoma. Am J Clin Pathol 2005;123:349–59.

12. Hawkins NJ, Ward RL. Sporadic colorectal cancers with microsatellite instability and their possible origin in hyperplastic polyps and serrated adenomas. J Natl Cancer Inst 2001;93:1307–13.

13. East JE, Saunders BP, Jass JR. Sporadic and syndromic hyperplastic polyps and serrated adenomas of the colon: classification, molecular genetics, natural history, and clinical management. Gastroenterol Clin North Am 2008;37:25–46.

14. Chung SM, Chen YT, Panczykowski A, et al. Serrated polyps with "intermediate features" of sessile serrated polyp and microvesicular hyperplastic polyp: a practical approach to the classification of nondysplastic serrated polyps. Am J Surg Pathol 2008;32:407–12.

15. Spring KJ, Zhao ZZ, Walsh MD, et al. High prevalence of sessile serrated adenomas with BRAF mutations: a prospective study of patients undergoing colonoscopy. Gastroenterology 2006;131:1400–7.

16. Torlakovic EE, Gomez JD, Driman DK, et al. Sessile serrated adenoma (SSA) vs. traditional serrated adenoma (TSA). Am J Surg Pathol 2008;32:21–9.

17. Owens SR, Chiosea SI, Kuan SF. Selective expression of gastric mucin MUC6 in colonic sessile serrated adenoma but not in hyperplastic polyp aids in morphological diagnosis of serrated polyps. Mod Pathol 2008;21:660–9.

18. Bartley AN, Thompson PA, Buckmeier JA, et al. Expression of gastric pyloric mucin, MUC6, in colorectal serrated polyps. Mod Pathol 2010;23:169–76.

19. Sandmeier D, Seelentag W, Bouzourene H. Serrated polyps of the colorectum: is sessile serrated adenoma distinguishable from hyperplastic polyp in a daily practice? Virchows Arch 2007;450:613–8.

20. Yang S, Farraye FA, Mack C, et al. BRAF and KRAS mutations in hyperplastic polyps and serrated adenomas of the colorectum: relationship to histology and CpG island methylation status. Am J Surg Pathol 2004;28:1452–9.

21. Glatz K, Pritt B, Glatz D, et al. A multinational, internet-based assessment of observer variability in the diagnosis of serrated colorectal polyps. Am J Clin Pathol 2007;127:938–45.

22. Farris AB, Misdraji J, Srivastava A, et al. Sessile serrated adenoma challenging discrimination from other serrated colonic polyps. Am J Surg Pathol 2008;32:30–5.

23. Jass JR. Classification of colorectal cancer based on correlation of clinical, morphological and molecular features. Histopathology 2007;50:113–30.

24. Oono Y, Fu K, Nakamura H, et al. Progression of a sessile serrated adenoma to an early invasive cancer within 8 months. Dig Dis Sci 2009;54(4): 906–9.

25. Sawhney MS, Farrar WD, Gudiseva S, et al. Microsatellite instability in interval colon cancers. Gastroenterology 2006;131:1700–5.

26. Gupta AK, Melton LJ 3rd, Petersen GM, et al. Changing trends in the incidence, stage, survival, and screen detection of colorectal cancer: a population-based study. Clin Gastroenterol Hepatol 2005;3: 150–8.

27. Snover DC, Jass JR, Fenoglio-Preiser C, et al. Serrated polyps of the large intestine: a morphologic and molecular review of an evolving concept. Am J Clin Pathol 2005;124:380–91.

28. Yantiss RK, Oh KY, Chen YT, et al. Filiform serrated adenomas: a clinicopathologic and immunophenotypic study of 18 cases. Am J Surg Pathol 2007; 31:1238–45.

29. Parfitt JR, Driman DK. Survivin and hedgehog protein expression in serrated colorectal polyps: an immunohistochemical study. Hum Pathol 2007; 38:710–7.

30. Lieberman D, Moravec M, Holub J, et al. Polyp size and advanced histology in patients undergoing colonoscopy screening: implications for CT colonography. Gastroenterology 2008;135: 1100–5.

31. Kilgore SP, Sigel JE, Goldblum JR. Hyperplastic-like mucosal change in Crohn's disease: an unusual form of dysplasia? Mod Pathol 2000;13:797–801.

32. Rubio CA, Befrits R, Jaramillo E, et al. Villous and serrated adenomatous growth bordering carcinomas in inflammatory bowel disease. Anticancer Res 2000;20:4761–4.

33. Andersen SN, Løvig T, Clausen OPF, et al. Villous, hypermucinous mucosa in long standing ulcerative colitis shows high frequency of K-ras mutations. Gut 1999;45:686–92.

34. Bossard C, Denis MG, Béziaeu S, et al. Involvement of the serrated neoplasia pathway in inflammatory bowel disease-related colorectal oncogenesis. Oncol Rep 2007;18:1093–7.

35. Mikami T, Yoshida T, Numata Y, et al. Low frequency of promoter methylation of O6-methylguanine DNA methyltransferase and hMLH1 in ulcerative colitis-associated tumors: comparison with sporadic colonic tumors. Am J Clin Pathol 2007;127:366–73.

36. Groisman GM, Polak-Charcon S. Fibroblastic polyp of the colon and colonic perineurioma: 2 names for a single entity? Am J Surg Pathol 2008;32:1088–94.

GASTROINTESTINAL STROMAL TUMORS: A GUIDE TO THE DIAGNOSIS

Joseph A. Holden, MD, PhD[a,b,†],
Carlynn Willmore-Payne, BS, MT(ASCP)[a,b],
Lester J. Layfield, MD[a,b,*]

KEYWORDS

• Gastrointestinal stromal tumor • c-kit • Platelet-derived growth factor gene • Imatinib

ABSTRACT

Gastrointestinal stromal tumors (GISTs) have emerged from being a poorly understood and therapeutically refractory sarcoma to a tumor whose biology has not only provided insight into a mechanism of oncogenesis but has also led to a rational basis for therapy. Most GISTs are characterized by KIT protein (CD117) expression and constitutive activating mutations in either the c-kit or platelet-derived growth factor receptor α genes. This information can now be obtained from routine formalin-fixed and paraffin-embedded tissue. Because the correct diagnosis is the key to successful treatment of this tumor, it is incumbent on the pathologist to be familiar with the various gross and histologic patterns shown by these tumors. GISTs range from small incidental stromal nodules to large cystic and solid tumor masses. GISTs show a variety of microscopic patterns and therefore several other tumors enter the differential diagnosis. Fortunately, with an understanding of GIST histology, and with the proper use of immunohistochemistry and molecular analysis, a correct diagnosis can usually be made. In addition to the correct diagnosis, several key attributes of the tumor need to be determined because they provide the basis for proper clinical management. This article summarizes the gross, microscopic, and molecular findings of GISTs, and discusses the differential diagnosis and key attributes of this interesting group of neoplasms.

OVERVIEW

In 2001, a remarkable case report appeared in the *New England Journal of Medicine*.[1] The report described a 50-year old woman who several years previously was found to have multiple nodules of gastrointestinal stromal tumor (GIST) in the stomach and in the omentum. The tumors were surgically excised. Unfortunately, a few years later the patient suffered from recurrent and metastatic disease. Various types of chemotherapeutic regimens were tried at this time but the tumors kept progressing. The patient then agreed to participate in an experimental trial of STI571 (imatinib mesylate, Gleevec). She was started on a daily dose of 100-mg capsules in March of 2000. The results were astounding. Within weeks, the tumors showed a decrease in metabolic activity and imaging studies showed a decrease in tumor size. Histologic examination of the treated GIST showed a myxoid fibrous stroma with only

[a] Department of Pathology, University of Utah Health Sciences Center, 15 North Medical Drive East, Salt Lake City, UT 84112, USA
[b] Associated Regional and University Pathologists (ARUP) Institute for Clinical and Experimental Pathology, 500 Chipeta Way, Salt Lake City, UT 84108, USA
[†] Deceased.
* Corresponding author. Department of Pathology, University of Utah Health Sciences Center, University of Utah School of Medicine, Salt Lake City, UT 84132.
E-mail address: layfiel@aruplab.com

Surgical Pathology 3 (2010) 241–276
doi:10.1016/j.path.2010.05.008
1875-9181/10/$ – see front matter

pyknotic tumor cells. This result seemed miraculous for a tumor that previously was known to be resistant to radiation and chemotherapy.

The successful treatment of this type of sarcoma was the result of many years of work leading to the discovery that GISTs are likely derived from cells that show lineage relationships with the interstitial cells of Cajal (ICC), the pacemaker cells of the gut, and not to smooth muscle as previously thought. This idea was first suggested in a report published in 1983 indicating that, unexpectedly, most gastric stromal tumors do not show smooth muscle differentiation.[2] The story culminated 15 years later with the landmark report clearly demonstrating that GISTs, like the ICC, are CD117 (KIT)-positive and contain c-kit activating mutations coding for a constitutively activated KIT tyrosine kinase.[3] The c-kit activating mutations were exclusively found in GISTs and not in true smooth muscle or neural tumors. The c-kit mutations were heterozygous and oncogenic when expressed in cell lines. These results indicate that c-kit activating mutations are probably the primary event that drives tumorigenesis. This demonstration that constitutive activating mutations in c-kit characterize many GISTs led to the realization that imatinib, a small-molecule tyrosine kinase inhibitor, already known to inhibit the BCR-ABL tyrosine kinase in chronic myelogenous leukemia (CML),[4,5] might be effective in inhibiting activated KIT in GISTs as well. After the initial report in the *New England Journal of Medicine* demonstrating the correctness of this hypothesis, many subsequent clinical trials have clearly confirmed the activity of imatinib in therapy for GISTs.[6–9]

The discovery of KIT-activating mutations in GIST revolutionized the therapy for this tumor and provided insight into the mechanism of oncogenesis in GISTs,[10] and perhaps other tumors as well. GIST is a solid tumor for which an understanding of the underlying molecular biology is crucial not only for developing a diagnostic algorithm but also to provide information needed for therapy.

KIT is a member of the type III membrane receptor tyrosine kinases, and consists of an extracellular ligand binding domain containing 5 immunoglobulin-like regions (D1, D2, D3, D4, D5), a transmembrane domain, an intracellular juxtamembrane domain, and a split tyrosine kinase active site composed of a tyrosine kinase (TK) 1 domain, a kinase insert domain (KID) followed by a TK2 domain.[11] Binding of the KIT ligand, stem cell factor (SCF), leads to KIT dimerization with activation of the KIT tyrosine kinase.[12,13] This activation results in a downstream signaling cascade that eventually leads to cell proliferation and the activation of antiapoptotic factors.[14–16]

The activating mutations in the c-kit gene that lead to a constitutively activated KIT tyrosine kinase in GISTs occur in exon 11 (68%), exon 9 (10%), exon 13 (1%), and exon 17 (1%).[17] The activating mutations are varied, but all are in frame and therefore code for a mutant protein. The mutations consist of small insertions, duplications, deletions, and substitutions.[18] As expected for a dominant gain of function mutation, most of the mutations in the tumors are heterozygous.

C-kit exon 11 codes for the intracellular juxtamembrane (JM) portion of the protein. This portion serves an autoinhibitory function. When KIT is in the inactive state, the JM domain of the molecule encoded by exon 11 inserts directly into the tyrosine kinase domain. In this conformation the activation loop (A loop) located in the TK2 domain is prevented from developing an extended conformation by steric hindrance from the JM domain.[19] The A-loop needs to be in an extended conformation in order for substrates to enter the active site and thus when prevented from extension, KIT is inactive. The activating c-kit mutations in exon 11 relieve this autoinhibition, and KIT becomes activated independent of ligand.

Exon 9 codes for part of the D5 Ig domain. Extracellular domains D1 to D3 bind SCF, leading to homodimerization; this brings domains D4 and D5 on opposite KIT monomers into close proximity.[12,13] The activating mutations in exon 9, most of which are an AY duplication at amino acid residues 502 to 503,[20] are located at the interface between the D5 domains in the homodimer. Although the specific mechanism of activation due to exon 9 mutation is not entirely clear, it is possible that this mutation results in an increase in the affinity of the D5 domains between the KIT monomers.[12] This situation might then in turn lead to a stabilization of the homodimer independent of ligand. Mutations in exon 13 and 17 are in the active site kinase domain and presumably stabilize the active conformation of the protein.

Most GISTs stain strongly positive for CD117, reflecting their lineage relationship with the ICC, and this staining characteristic is useful in the diagnosis; however, some tumors morphologically diagnosable as GISTs fail to show significant CD117 staining. Many of these tumors have been found to contain activating mutations in a related type III receptor kinase, platelet-derived growth factor receptor α (PDGFRA).[21,22] The gene for PDGFRA is adjacent to the c-kit gene on chromosome 4 (4q12) and most likely represents an ancestral gene duplication.[23] The protein probably functions in a similar manner as KIT, although structural biologic studies of PDGFRA have not yet been reported. Of note, the distribution of activating mutations in PDGFRA is opposite that observed for KIT. The most common PDGFRA exon affected is exon 18, homologous to c-kit exon 17 encoding the TK2 domain while PDGFRA exon 12 mutations, homologous to c-kit exon 11 encoding the JM domain, are much less frequent.[24] PDGFRA activating mutations are mutually exclusive with c-kit activating mutations. This reason for the difference in the distribution of mutations is not clear. PDGFRA mutation positive GISTs express PDGFRA in preference to KIT[21] suggesting that the development of new specific PDGFRA immunostains might find diagnostic use in evaluating CD117-negative GISTs.[25–28]

The distribution of the types of c-kit and PDGFRA activating mutations that occur in GISTs are summarized in **Fig. 1**. A small percentage of GISTs does not contain c-kit or PDGFRA mutations. Recent data suggest that some of the "wild-type" GISTs may use the BRAF pathway[29] or the amplification and overexpression of the insulin-like growth factor as alternative means for oncogenesis.[30]

GROSS FEATURES

GISTs can range from small tumors measuring only millimeters in diameter to large tumors

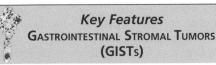

Key Features
GASTROINTESTINAL STROMAL TUMORS (GISTs)

1. GISTs range from small incidental stromal nodules to large cystic or solid tumor masses, usually occurring in the wall of the gastrointestinal tract.

2. GISTs are most commonly composed of spindled or epithelioid cells, or a mixture of both.

3. GISTs usually lack extensive necrosis and do not have high-grade, anaplastic, nuclei.

4. GISTs are CD117- and CD34-positive in the majority of cases.

5. Most CD117-positive GISTs contain c-kit activating mutations.

6. GISTs that are CD117-negative are usually gastric or omental and have an epithelioid histology with PDGFRA activating mutations.

7. Approximately 10% of GISTs are "wild type" without c-kit or PDGFRA activating mutations.

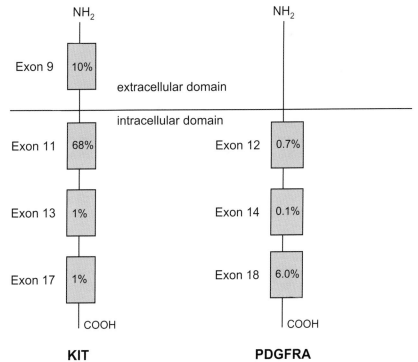

Fig. 1. Distribution of c-kit and PDGFRA activating mutations in gastrointestinal stromal tumors. The exons involved in the constitutive activation of c-kit and PDGFRA are shown. The percentage of mutations in each exon found in GISTs is indicated. (*Data from* Corless CL, Heinrich MC. Molecular pathobiology of gastrointestinal stromal sarcomas. Annu Rev Pathol 2008; 3:557–86.)

NH₂   NH₂

Exon 9   10%   extracellular domain

                    intracellular domain

Exon 11   68%   Exon 12   0.7%

Exon 13   1%   Exon 14   0.1%

Exon 17   1%   Exon 18   6.0%

COOH   COOH

KIT   **PDGFRA**

weighing many kilograms. Many of the smaller tumors are incidental findings during routine surgical procedures such as gastric bypass surgery. Their frequency in gastric resections, performed for reasons not related to a GIST, ranges from 10% to 35%.[31–33] Findings can also be incidental in resected specimens from the colon, appendix, and rectum, ranging in incidence from 0.2 %, 0.1%, and 0.01%, respectively.[34] Incidental GISTs generally appear as small, firm, well-demarcated, tan to white nodules, located in the muscular wall of the gastrointestinal (GI) tract. Some show calcifications and many of the incidental GISTs have KIT mutations.[35–37] Of note, surrounding ICC in patients with clinically significant GISTs also have c-kit mutations.[38] The common occurrence of small incidental GISTs, coupled with the rarity of clinically significant GISTs, about 7 to 15 cases per million individuals worldwide,[39] suggests that additional factors besides an underlying activating c-kit or PDGFRA mutation must play a role for an incidental GIST to become clinically significant.

For primary GIST resections, the tumors are much larger but also appear to arise from the muscular wall of the GI tract and do not appear widely invasive into surrounding tissues. The smaller ones tend to be fairly well demarcated. Their texture is somewhat soft and variable in color with shades of tan, gray, and white, as shown in **Fig. 2**A and B. Many of the larger ones appear multilobulated and multinodular. The larger ones may outgrow their blood supply with resulting cystic degeneration and hemorrhage (**Fig. 2**C and D).

GISTs can protrude into the bowel lumen, causing an intraluminal mass that can clinically present as bowel obstruction (**Fig. 3**A). When these tumors are resected, the overlying mucosa may show varying degrees of ulceration with hemorrhage. Gastrointestinal bleeding from mucosal ulceration is a common clinical presentation of GIST patients.[40] On the other hand, some GISTs grow as an exophytic mass and appear attached to the GI tract by only a small amount of normal tissue (**Fig. 3**B–D). It is thought that some extra gastrointestinal GISTs (eGISTs) that occur in the omentum or in the mesentery may have at one time been exophytic gastric or intestinal tumors that lost their attachment to the GI tract.[41] The frequency and types of activating mutations in eGISTs are similar to those found in GISTs associated with the GI tract.[42]

Two omental GISTs are shown in **Fig. 4**A and B. No gastric tissue was attached to either tumor. Perhaps these GISTs may at one time have been associated with the gastric wall, which would explain the finding that mutations in PDGFRA seem to predominate in both gastric and omental GISTs.[17] This mechanism might also explain the origin of GISTs in the omentum and mesentery, tissues not generally thought to contain ICC progenitor cells, although recent data suggest a population of ICC-like cells may be present outside the GI tract.[43,44] Nonetheless, it is easy to see from **Fig. 4**C how a small intestinal GIST, or from **Fig. 4**D how a gastric GIST, could have lost their attachments with the GI tract over time and then present as eGISTs.

Malignancy is difficult to predict in GISTs and is related to size, mitotic counts, location, and the specific type of activating mutation. Apart from the size, there are no gross characteristics that predict biologic behavior.

In the GI tract the most common origins are the stomach and small intestine. Esophageal and colorectal GISTs are rare; most stromal tumors in these locations are true leiomyomas.[45,46] However, because of the possible therapeutic options, it might be prudent to consider the possibility of a GIST for all intra-abdominal stromal tumors.

MICROSCOPIC FEATURES

ROUTINE HISTOLOGY

GISTs can show a remarkable variety of histologic patterns. Incidental GISTs are generally composed of bland spindle cells in a hyalinized and fibrotic stroma.[36] Mitotic activity is minimal and they are generally all of low risk. This finding suggests that many incidental GISTs involute and never progress to a clinically significant tumor. Secondary molecular changes superimposed on a c-kit or PDGFRA activating mutation are probably necessary for tumor progression. Clinical studies of patients with germline c-kit or PDGFRA activating mutations suggest the same conclusion. Many of the affected patients develop GISTs but the tumors are fairly indolent, have low mitotic counts, and cause morbidity because of their size rather than because of metastatic disease.[47–50] **Fig. 5** shows a section of the colon resected from a patient with a germline c-kit mutation (K642E). There is a remarkable hyperplasia of the ICC and numerous GIST tumor nodules are present in the muscularis (see **Fig. 5**A–C). However, the proliferative index of the GIST tumor nodules, measured by topo II staining, a marker of cell proliferation,[51] is low (see **Fig. 5**D). The histology of an incidental gastric GIST is shown in **Fig. 6**. The mitotic count for this tumor is negligible and the stroma shows calcification and fibrosis suggesting that with time, this tumor probably would have undergone fibrosis and involution.

Fig. 2. Common gross appearances of GISTs. The gross appearances of several GISTs are demonstrated. (*A*) GIST arising from the small intestine. The tumor is yellow and fairly well demarcated. Molecular analysis revealed an activating mutation in c-kit exon 9. (*B*) GIST arising from the stomach. The tumor is white with areas of hemorrhage, and was found to contain an activating mutation in c-kit exon 11.

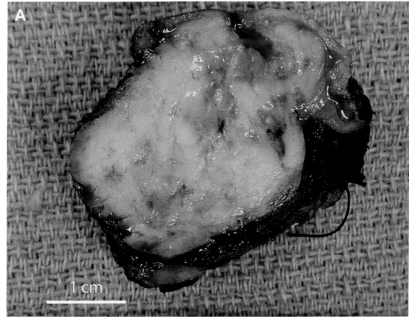

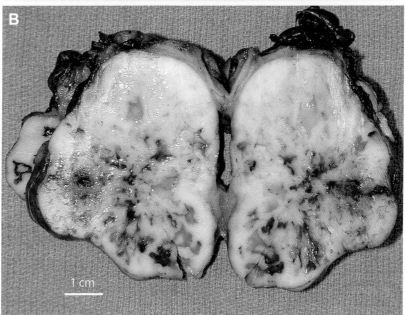

These observations with both familial and incidental GISTs suggest that secondary genetic events are necessary to trigger a more clinically aggressive tumor.

For clinically significant GISTs, the 2 most common histologic patterns are the spindle cell and epithelioid types. Some GISTs show a mixture of spindle and epithelioid cells. In some spindle cell GISTs the resemblance to a schwannoma is striking, and invariably resulted in this diagnosis before an understanding of GIST biology became common. It is now known that some GISTs, like schwannomas, will express S100.[52] In a similar fashion, many of the low-grade spindle cell GISTs resemble leiomyomas and were probably diagnosed as such before the advent of KIT staining and molecular analysis. Like true smooth muscle tumors, GISTs can also express muscle markers such as muscle-specific actin and smooth muscle actin.[52] Examples of these common histologic patterns are shown in **Fig. 7**.

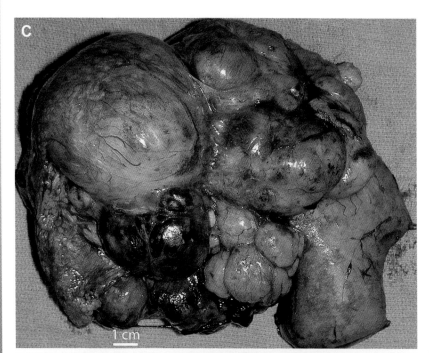

Fig. 2. (*C*) GIST arising from the small intestine. The tumor is multinodular, and by molecular analysis was found to contain an activating mutation in c-kit exon 9. (*D*) Small intestinal GIST as shown in *C*, but sectioned to reveal extensive cystic change and hemorrhage.

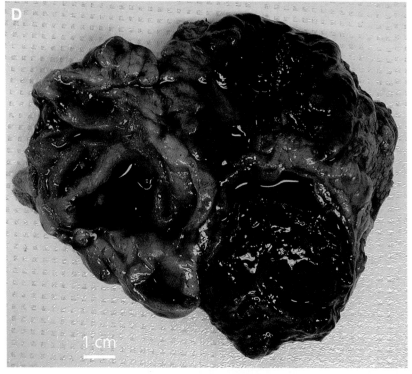

In addition, unusual histologic patterns occur so that some GISTs resemble chondrosarcomas, chordomas, hemangiomas, and even paragangliomas, as shown in **Fig. 8**. In some tumors, needle biopsy interpretation can be challenging. As shown in **Fig. 9**A, in some GISTs the stroma can be abundant and acellular, which could make interpretation of a small needle biopsy difficult if cellular areas are not sampled. Some GISTs also superficially

Fig. 3. Exophytic and intraluminal GISTs. GISTs can grow into the bowel lumen to cause obstructive symptoms or can grow as an exophytic mass attached to the GI tract. (*A*) GIST arising in the wall of the small intestine and protruding into the bowel lumen. The tumor was strongly CD117- and CD34-positive. Genotyping was not performed. (*B*) Gastric GIST attached to the wall of the stomach. The tumor contained an activating mutation in c-kit exon 11 and was attached to the gastric wall as an exophytic mass.

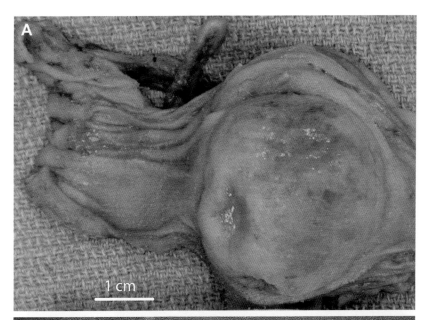

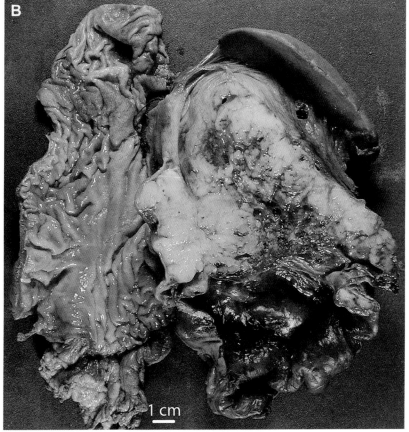

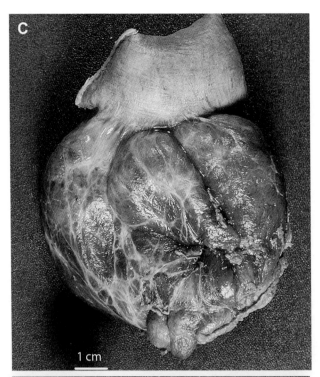

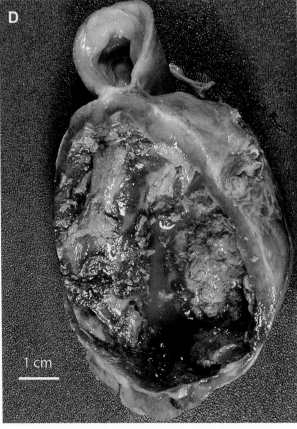

Fig. 3. (C) GIST arising from the small intestine. The tumor grew as an exophytic mass attached to the intestine by a small strand of tissue. The tumor contained an activating mutation in c-kit exon 11. (D) Same tumor as in C but sectioned to reveal cystic degeneration. The tumor has a prominent pseudocapsule.

Fig. 4. Possible origin of extragastrointestinal stromal tumors (eGISTs). (*A*) Omental GIST. The tumor was excised from the omentum and found to contain an activating mutation in PDGFRA (D842 V). There was no attachment to the stomach. (*B*) Omental GIST. The tumor has a prominent pseudocapsule, and was found to contain an activating mutation in c-kit exon 11. No attachment to the stomach was observed.

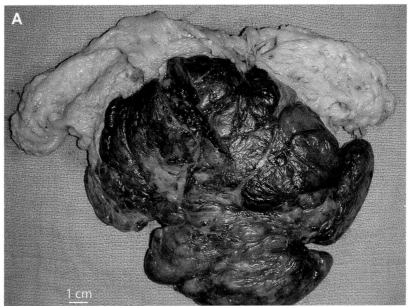

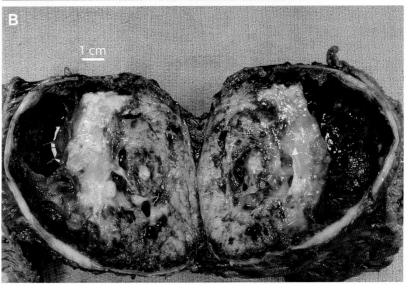

resemble a granulomatous process, which could also make interpretation of a small needle biopsy problematic (**Fig. 9**B). In general, pronounced nuclear atypia is not a feature of GISTs, although some degenerative changes and occasional atypical cells can be present (**Fig. 9**C and D). However, despite these varied histologic appearances, GISTs do not show high-grade, anaplastic nuclei. Although some GISTs do show necrosis, the presence of extensive necrosis is also unusual. As a general rule, a high-grade tumor with extensive necrosis is probably not a GIST. A recent review

summarizes the variety of histologic appearances that can be seen in GISTs.[53]

As more patients receive imatinib, it is important to become familiar with the effect of this drug on GIST histology. Resected specimens from imatinib treated patients can show complete or partial responses. Some treated tumors can show an altered immunophenotype.[54] In the initial GIST patient treated with imatinib,[1] needle biopsies of a liver metastasis obtained 1 and 2 months after therapy showed areas of scar with myxoid change and probably pyknotic tumor cells. No proliferative activity

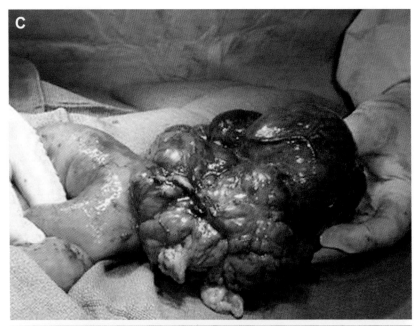

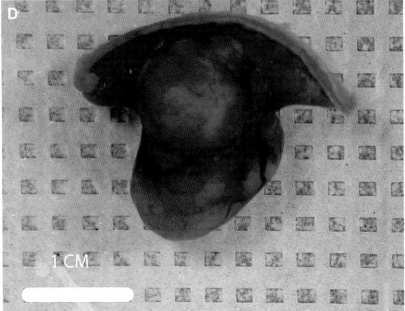

Fig. 4. (C) Intraoperative photo of the small intestinal GIST as shown in Fig. 2C and D. The tumor grows as an exophytic mass. It is easy to visualize how loss of attachment to the small intestine could result in this tumor becoming a mesenteric GIST with a similar gross appearance as shown for the omental GIST in A. The tumor had an activating mutation in c-kit exon 9. (D) Exophytic GIST arising in the wall of the stomach. The tumor was strongly CD117- and CD 34-positive, without significant mitotic activity. It is possible that with time, the tumor could lose its gastric attachment and become an omental GIST as in A and B.

was detected by MIB-1 staining. The authors have also studied a case of GIST metastatic to the liver. The patient was first treated with imatinib and then the liver mass was resected. As shown in Fig. 10A, the pretreatment biopsy showed a cellular spindle cell tumor. The tumor stained strongly positive for CD117, confirming the diagnosis of a GIST (not shown). Molecular analysis revealed a c-kit exon 11 mutation. After therapy, only bland spindle cells in a loose myxoid stroma are seen, as shown in Fig. 10B. The cells were negative for CD117 (not shown); however, the original c-kit activating mutation in exon 11 was still detected by molecular analysis.

Some patients show an initial response to imatinib but then become drug resistant. In many cases, the resistance is due to secondary mutations in the c-kit kinase domains.[55–58] In these cases, resection of the resistant tumor can show loose myxoid areas, probably representing treated tumor, but these

Fig. 5. Histology of the colon in a patient with a germline c-kit mutation (K642E). (*A*) hematoxylin and eosin–stained section of the colon showing diffuse ICC hyperplasia with a GIST tumor nodule (original magnification ×40). (*B*) CD117 stain highlighting the GIST tumor nodule (original magnification ×40).

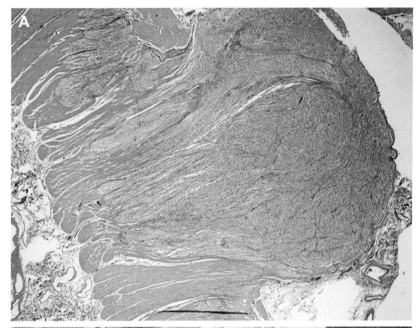

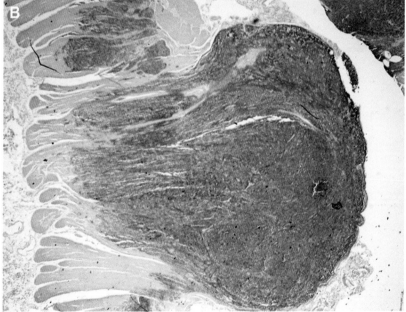

areas are overrun with viable, imatinib-resistant GIST tumor cells (**Fig. 10**C and D).

IMMUNOHISTOCHEMISTRY

Because of the variety of histologic patterns seen in GISTs, and of the number of tumors that mimic them, the use of immunohistochemistry is essential to arriving at a correct diagnosis. The majority of GISTs are strongly positive when stained with antibodies directed against the KIT protein (CD117). Although KIT is a membrane-bound signaling protein, the CD117 stain is interpreted as positive whether the staining is membranous, cytoplasmic, or both.[59–61] In some GISTs, the CD117 stain shows a "dot-like" pattern.[62] Assessment of this pattern is quite different to the interpretation of HER2 expression, another membrane signaling protein, whereby cytoplasmic staining is generally felt not to be biologically

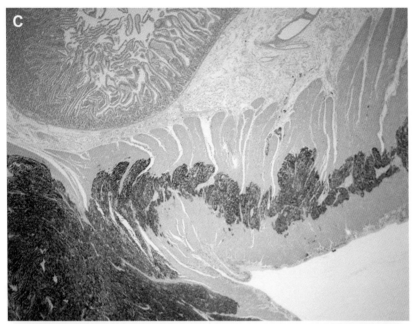

Fig. 5. (*C*) CD117 staining demonstrating the diffuse ICC hyperplasia (original magnification ×40). (*D*) Topo IIα stain. Staining for topo IIα, a cell proliferation marker, shows a lack of proliferating cells in the GIST tumor nodule. The surrounding colonic mucosa shows prominent topo IIα staining in the base of the crypts (original magnification ×20).

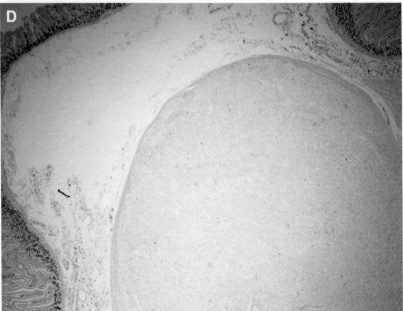

relevant.[63] The basis for the CD117 cytoplasmic staining in GISTs may reflect the cellular retention of the mutant proteins in the Golgi apparatus and endoplasmic reticulum.[64] It is interesting that the mutant KIT protein may be able to signal even when restrained in abnormal cellular locations.[65] It is important not to use antigen retrieval techniques for CD117 staining because retrieval techniques can result in false-positive CD117 staining.[66] An understanding of the problems associated with CD117 staining is important for accurate interpretation.[67] Examples of CD117 staining patterns commonly encountered in GISTs are shown in **Fig. 11**.

Not all GISTs are strongly CD117-positive. Some are completely negative, and these are usually those tumors that have activating mutations in PDGFRA rather than c-kit.[21,22] On the other hand, some GISTs show only weak and focal CD117 staining. Some of these cases represent

Fig. 6. Incidental gastric GIST. An incidental GIST was observed in the stomach excised from a re-do Nissen fundoplication. (*A*) A small stromal nodule is present in the wall of the stomach (original magnification ×20). (*B*) Stromal nodule showing areas of calcification (original magnification ×100).

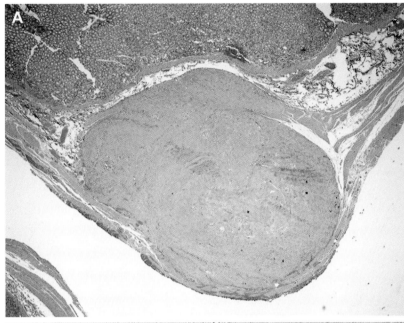

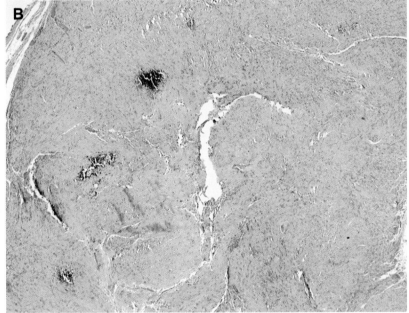

PDGFRA mutation positive tumors (**Fig. 11D**) but others represent c-kit mutation positive tumors. This result is not unexpected given recent reports indicating that there may be a continuum of CD117 expression in GISTs[68] and that a simple classification of a GIST as CD117-positive or CD117-negative may be too simplistic.

Most GISTs (70%) are positive when stained for CD34, and although not specific for GISTs, CD34 positivity can be helpful in evaluating those tumors

that are CD117-negative or focally CD117-positive. GISTs also can show expression of muscle markers as well as S100 protein, but these are not specific for GISTs and can be seen in true muscle and neural tumors as well. A useful stain to separate GISTs from true smooth muscle tumors is desmin, which is rare in GISTs but commonly expressed in smooth muscle tumors.[52] The possibility of using a specific stain against PDGFRA to detect KIT-negative GISTs that are PDGFRA

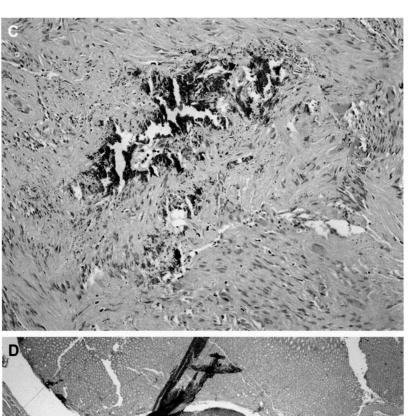

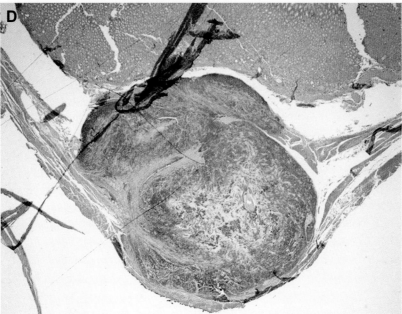

Fig. 6. (*C*) The stromal tumor is composed of bland tumor cells lacking mitotic activity (original magnification ×200). (*D*) The tumor stains strongly positive for CD117, confirming the diagnosis of a GIST (original magnification ×20).

mutation positive has been reported.[25–28] Two recent antibodies developed against protein kinase C (PKC)-θ and DOG1, proteins expressed in both KIT-positive and KIT-negative GISTs, may see widespread use in the future.[69–71]

PROLIFERATION INDICES

Although mitotic figure counting is clearly an important predictive marker of aggressive clinical behavior in GISTs, it is somewhat surprising that the routine use of other, more easily standardized proliferation markers has not yet been routinely adopted in GIST evaluation. Attempts to do so have been published, mostly with the MIB-1 proliferation marker.[72–74] The authors have been studying DNA topoisomerase IIα (topo IIα) in human neoplasms for several years. DNA topo IIα serves as a proliferation marker. Topo IIα correlates well with mitotic counts in GISTs and other

Fig. 7. Common histologic appearance of GISTs. GISTs can show several types of histologic patterns. Some of the more common types are shown. (A) Spindle cell type (original magnification ×200). (B) Epithelioid type (original magnification ×200).

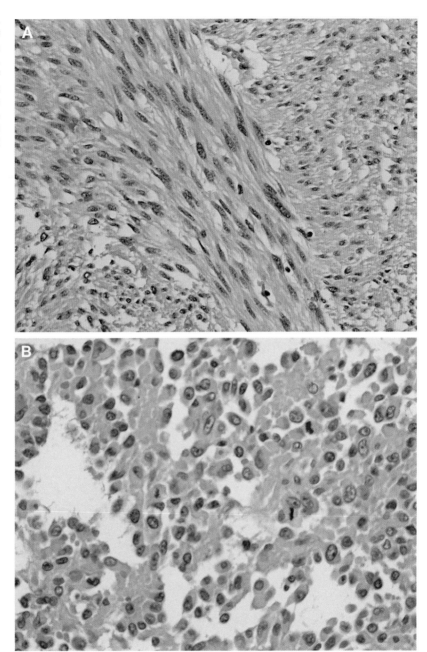

tumors.[75] The authors find it a useful adjunct stain in evaluating the clinical risk of GISTs and routinely use it in conjunction with mitotic counts. The protein is also the molecular target of several anticancer agents such as etoposide and doxorubicin,[51] and therefore provides additional information besides tumor proliferation. Topo IIα staining can be performed readily on paraffin-embedded tissues and is easily interpretable.

An example of the ease and usefulness of detecting topo II expression in GISTs is illustrated in **Fig. 12**. Two patients with small intestinal GISTs underwent surgical excision of the tumors. Pictures of the gross specimens are shown in **Fig. 2**. Both GISTs were strongly CD117-positive and molecular analysis indicated c-kit activating mutations in exon 9 for both. The smaller GIST was only 4 cm in greatest dimension and with a mitotic count of 0 per 50 high-power fields (hpf) was considered low risk (see **Fig. 2**A).The larger tumor measured 16 cm in greatest dimension and with a mitotic count of 17 mitotic figures per

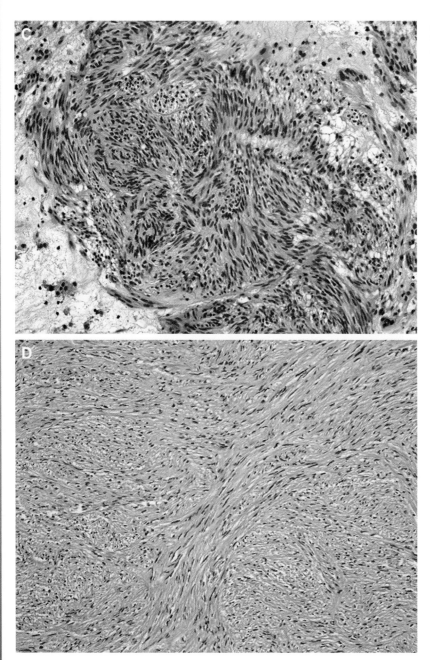

Fig. 7. (*C*) GIST resembling a schwannoma (original magnification ×100). (*D*) GIST resembling a leiomyoma (original magnification ×100).

50 hpf was considered a high-risk tumor (see **Fig. 2**C). The topo II indices of the tumors, as expected, were remarkably different. The low-risk tumor had a topo II index of 1.4 (see **Fig. 12**B) whereas the high-risk tumor had a topo II index of 30.8 (see **Fig. 12**D). Because of the inherent variability and subjectivity in counting mitotic figures,[76] the determination of a topo II index may eventually prove easier to standardize and be more reproducible than mitotic figure counting in stratifying GISTs.

MOLECULAR ANALYSIS

Although there is some debate as to whether molecular analysis is necessary for the evaluation of GISTs,[77] the authors have found it very useful for several reasons. First, the identification of the activated exon might help guide oncologists in choosing the proper dose of imatinib. Recent large clinical studies suggest 400 mg of imatinib is an appropriate starting dose for c-kit exon 11 mutation positive GISTs, but for c-kit exon 9 mutation

Fig. 8. GISTs resembling other soft tissue tumors. (*A*) Myxoid chondrosarcoma like (original magnification ×200). (*B*) Chordoma like (original magnification ×200).

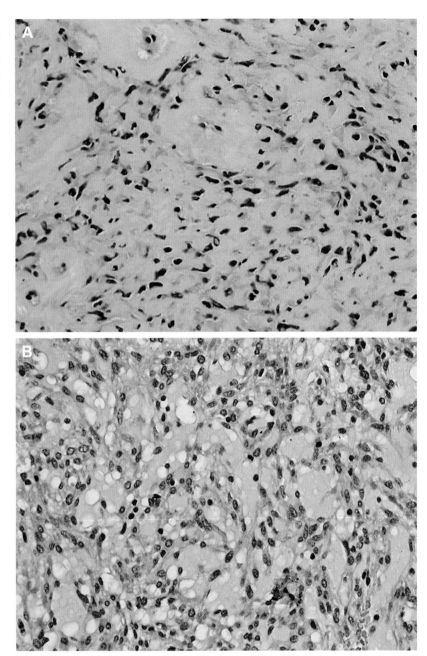

positive GISTs, the starting dose has been suggested to be 800 mg. This starting dose seemed to provide for a better progression-free survival for exon 9 mutation positive GISTs in some clinical trials,[78] although admittedly not in all.[79] Second, the identification of an activating mutation in either c-kit or PDGFRA confirms the diagnosis of GIST, irrespective of the immunohistochemical staining results. Because it now appears there is a spectrum of KIT expression in GISTs,[68] confusion might arise among pathologists as to whether the KIT stain is positive or negative. The presence of an activating mutation is an unequivocal result and does not suffer from the subjective interpretation so common to immunohistochemistry.[80] Third, molecular testing may be the only way at the present time to unequivocally diagnose KIT-negative GISTs[81] or GISTs with unusual immunohistochemical findings.[82,83]

There are a variety of ways to molecularly characterize GISTs, including denaturing high-performance liquid chromatography (dHPLC),[35]

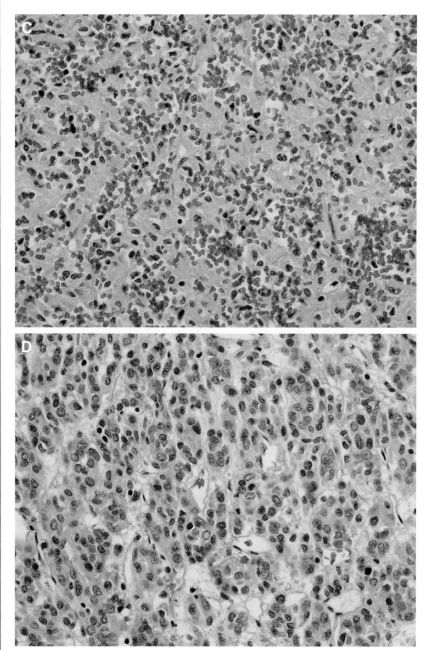

Fig. 8. (*C*) Hemangioma like (original magnification ×200). (*D*) Paraganglioma like (original magnification ×200).

direct DNA sequencing,[84] microfluidic deletion/insertion analysis,[85] and high-resolution DNA melting analysis.[75] The most widespread method of GIST mutation detection is dHPLC. However, DNA melting analysis with high-resolution technology was developed at the University of Utah as a mutation screening technology,[86] and for this reason the authors have applied this method as a way of screening for c-kit and PDGFRA mutations in GISTs. The principles and advantages of

mutation detection by melting analysis have been discussed previously.[87] In brief, genomic DNA isolated from a tumor of interest is subjected to polymerase chain reaction (PCR) with primers designed to amplify the exon of interest. The amplified products are heated and then allowed to re-anneal. If a mutation is present, a mixture of duplexes will form, consisting of the 2 homoduplexes (wild type-wild type, mutant-mutant) and 2 heteroduplexes (wild type-mutant, mutant-wild

Fig. 9. Additional histologic appearances of GISTs. (*A*) GIST with acellular stroma (original magnification ×100). (*B*) GIST with a granulomatous-like morphology (original magnification ×100).

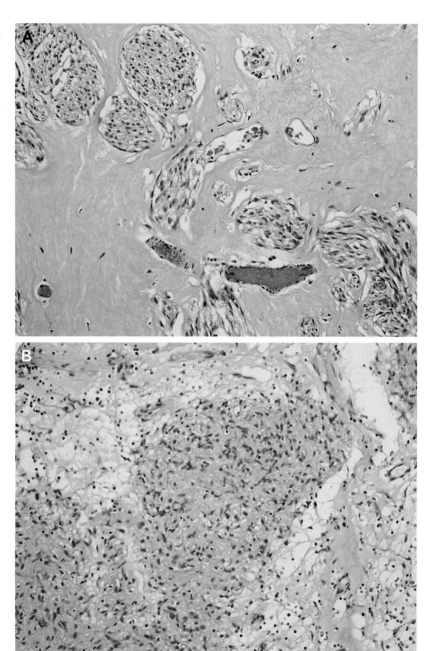

type). When subjected to DNA melting analysis, the presence of the heteroduplexes lowers the melting curve of the amplified products and indicates the presence of a mutation. PCR and melting analysis of the amplified products can be performed within 30 minutes after DNA isolation. An abnormal melting curve indicates a genetic alteration in the exon of interest. Subsequent direct DNA sequencing can be done if needed. Because many of the c-kit exon 11 mutations are insertions and deletions, they lead to such abnormal melting curves that an activating mutation can be correctly inferred simply by melting analysis, obviating the need for direct DNA sequencing.

DIFFERENTIAL DIAGNOSIS

GISTs can mimic several other neoplasms.[53,88] Some of the common examples of GIST mimics are discussed in this section.

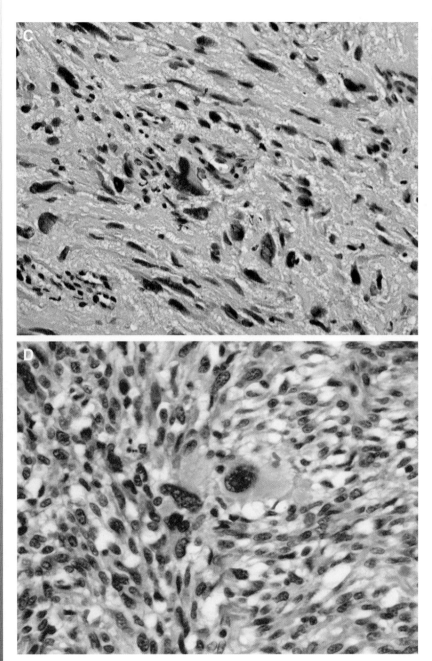

Fig. 9. (*C*) GIST with nuclear degenerative atypia (original magnification ×200). (*D*) GIST with scattered atypical cells (original magnification ×200).

GISTS VERSUS SMOOTH MUSCLE TUMORS

The most common tumor that resembles a GIST is a true smooth muscle tumor. Low-grade smooth muscle tumors, leiomyomas, can mimic a low-risk GIST. Leiomyomas can be distinguished from GISTs because leiomyomas are usually strongly desmin-positive and CD117-negative and do not contain c-kit or PDGFRA activating mutations. GISTs are only rarely desmin-positive.

On the other hand, high-grade leiomyosarcomas can resemble high-risk GISTs (**Fig. 13**). Again, it is useful to emphasize that any tumor with a high-grade histologic appearance is probably not going to be a GIST. However, as clearly shown in **Fig. 13**, the atypical areas in leiomyosarcoma may be focal and not sampled on a small needle biopsy. Leiomyosarcomas will also be CD117-negative, and c-kit and PDGFRA mutation negative, but may be desmin-positive.

Fig. 10. Histology of imatinib-treated GISTs. (*A*) Biopsy of a GIST metastatic to the liver. The tumor contained an activating mutation in c-kit exon 11. The tumor is cellular and shows a prominent spindle cell pattern (original magnification ×200). (*B*) Tumor as in *A* but resected after imatinib treatment. The tumor shows only loose myxoid areas and bland spindle cells. A c-kit exon 11 mutation was still detected in the tissue, suggesting that the GIST cells were present but quiescent (original magnification ×100).

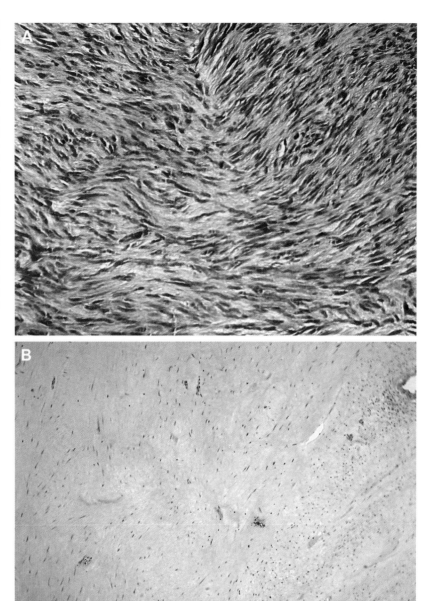

GISTS VERSUS CARCINOMAS

Spindle cell carcinomas may also resemble GISTs, and this possibility should always be considered, but carcinomas will usually be KIT-negative and cytokeratin-positive. Although in general GISTs are cytokeratin-negative, recent articles now clearly describe cytokeratin expression that can occur in GISTs.[82,83] The fact that some GISTs can have a signet-ring cell appearance adds to the dilemma, but carcinomas will generally not show strong KIT expression and of course,

molecular analysis for c-kit or PDGFRA mutations in such cases will be negative.

GISTS VERSUS SCHWANNOMAS

Some spindle cell GISTs can show a striking resemblance to a schwannoma (see **Fig. 7**C). However, careful histologic examination can help with the diagnosis. GISTs are usually more cellular than schwannomas and GIST nuclei are usually somewhat larger than those seen in a typical schwannoma. Mitotic activity is also more

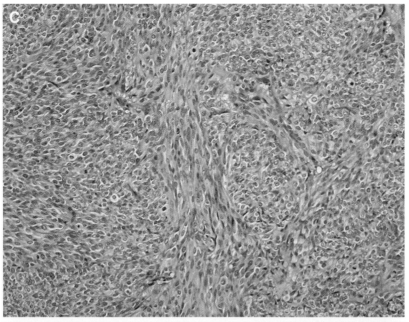

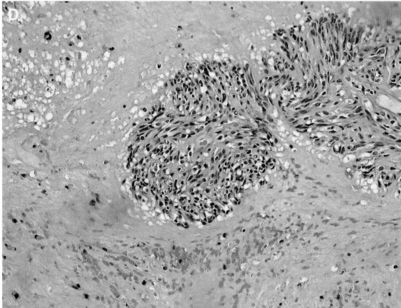

Fig. 10. (*C*) GIST with exon 11 mutation. The tumor is cellular and shows a spindle cell pattern (original magnification ×100). (*D*) The tumor in C was treated with imatinib. The tumor recurred 4 years after imatinib treatment. Molecular analysis of the recurrence revealed the presence of the original c-kit exon 11 mutation and a secondary mutation in c-kit exon 17 mutation (Y823D), a mutation known to be associated with imatinib resistance. The histology of the recurrent tumor is of a cellular spindle cell neoplasm infiltrating areas of loose myxoid tissue (original magnification ×200). (*Data from* Lim KH, Huang MJ, Chen LT, et al. Molecular analysis of secondary kinase mutations in imatinib-resistant gastrointestinal stromal tumors. Med Oncol 2008;25:207–13.)

characteristic of a GIST than of a schwannoma. Despite these differences, the histologic appearances overlap. In these cases, immunohistochemistry is helpful. Although some GISTs are S100 protein positive, a true schwannoma will be strongly S100 protein positive and CD117-negative. A true schwannoma will not contain c-kit activating mutations.

GISTS VERSUS OTHER SARCOMAS

Some GISTs resemble chondrosarcomas and chordomas (see **Fig. 8**A and B), but the fact that the occurrence of these tumors in the GI tract is exceedingly rare and the realization that GISTs can show this histology can prevent a misinterpretation. Of course GISTs can sometimes occur in

Fig. 11. Patterns of CD117 staining in GISTs. (*A*) Strong membrane and cytoplasmic CD117 staining in a GIST with a c-kit exon 11–activating mutation (original magnification ×200). (*B*) Predominantly cytoplasmic CD117 staining in a GIST with an exon 11–activating mutation (original magnification ×200).

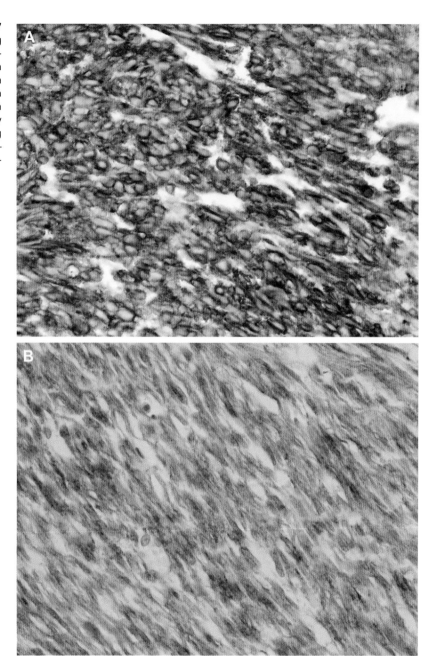

locations where these entities might be a diagnostic consideration, but a CD117 immunostain can help with the diagnosis.

GISTS VERSUS MELANOMA

Mucosal or metastatic melanoma should always be in the differential diagnosis of a GIST.[89] These tumors can occur anywhere in the GI tract. Many melanomas will be strongly CD117-positive,[90] and some also contain c-kit activating mutations.[90–93] The fact that Melan A positivity can be encountered in some epithelioid GISTs complicates the diagnosis.[94] The presence of melanin pigment in the tumor, a negative CD34 stain, and positive staining for S100 protein, HMB45, and Melan A will usually lead to the correct diagnosis of melanoma.

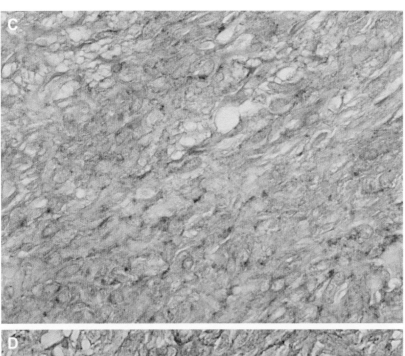

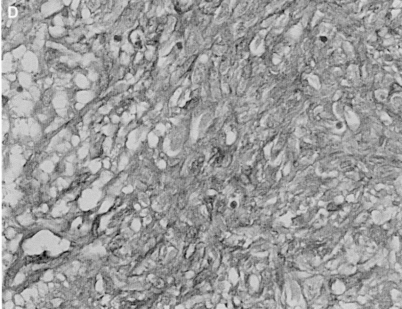

Fig. 11. (*C*) Dot-like CD117 staining in a GIST with an activating mutation in c-kit exon 9 (original magnification ×200). (*D*) GIST with a positive CD117 stain but which contained an activating mutation in PDGFRA exon 18 (original magnification ×200).

GISTS VERSUS OTHER CD117-POSITIVE TUMORS

When immunostaining for CD117 is performed correctly, the number of other tumors apart from GISTs that are positive becomes extremely small.[66] However, CD117-positive non-GIST tumors exist, and need to be considered in the differential diagnosis. Tumors that are CD117-positive, even without antigen retrieval technology, include adenoid cystic carcinoma,[95] Merkel cell carcinoma,[96] and some small cell lung carcinomas,[97] mast cell tumors,[98] and seminomas.[99] These tumors usually will not be considered in the diagnosis of a GIST and so should not cause diagnostic problems. However, a potential diagnostic problem can occur with disseminated endometrial stromal sarcoma (ESS) in the GI tract, as many of these tumors have been reported to be CD117-positive.[100] The pattern of growth of an

Fig. 12. Topoisomerase IIα as a proliferation marker in GISTs. (*A*) Hematoxylin and eosin–stained slide of a small intestinal GIST with an activating mutation in c-kit exon 9, gross photo in **Fig. 2A** (original magnification ×100). The mitotic count was 0 mitotic figures/50 high-power fields (hpf). (*B*) The topo IIα stain. Only scattered topo II–positive cells are present and the topo IIα proliferative index (percentage of topo II–positive tumor cells) is 1.4 (original magnification ×100).

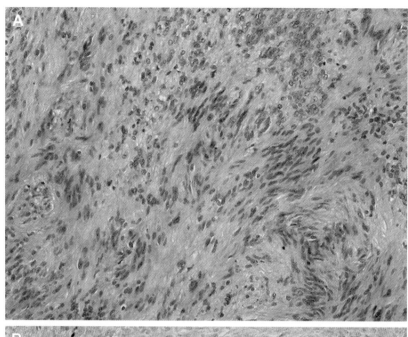

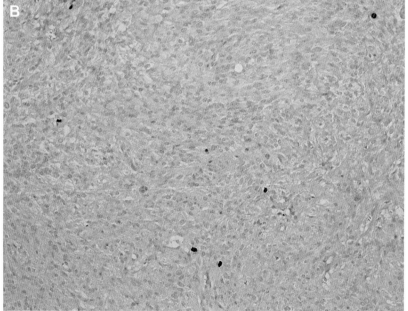

ESS usually is more infiltrative than a GIST, and the spindled cells are more compact and smaller. These tumors will be CD10-positive; remarkably, responses to imatinib have been reported in patients with ESS.[101,102]

GISTS VERSUS OTHER INFLAMMATORY, NEOPLASTIC, AND PROLIFERATIVE LESIONS

Other neoplasms in the GI tract can sometimes be confused with GISTs and include pecomas, a variety of spindle cell sarcomas and inflammatory polyps, and pseudotumors.[53,88,103] Pecomas usually can be distinguished from GISTs on a purely histologic basis and they will be CD117-negative on immunohistochemistry. However, some GISTs can also show a marked inflammatory infiltrate, and the diagnosis can be difficult without mutation analysis. **Fig. 14** shows the histology of a small intestinal tumor. The tumor is composed of loose spindle cells with a marked inflammatory infiltrate. Although the infiltrating mast cells are

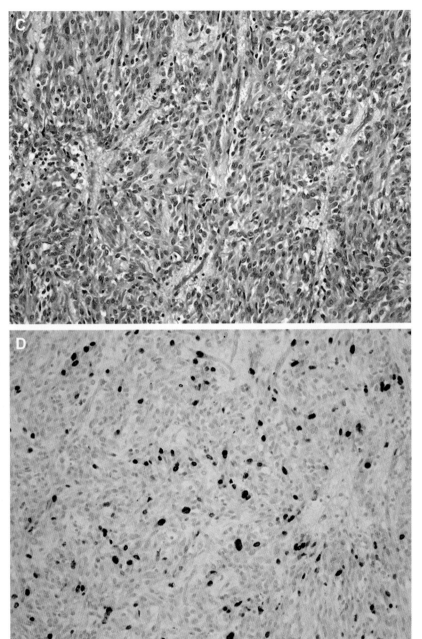

Fig. 12. (C) Hematoxylin and eosin–stained slide of a small intestinal GIST with an activating mutation in c-kit exon 9, gross photo in Fig. 2C and D. The mitotic count was 17 mitotic figures/50 hpf (original magnification ×100). (D) Topo IIα stain reveals many positive cells and the topo IIα index is 30.8 (original magnification ×100).

strongly KIT-positive (not shown), the spindle cells are negative, suggesting a possible inflammatory mass. Of note, mutation analysis revealed a PDGFRA activating mutation in exon 12 (S566R del 567–571). The diagnosis was a KIT-negative GIST with a marked inflammatory infiltrate.

Solitary fibrous tumors (SFT), which are CD117-negative, enter the differential diagnosis of KIT-negative GISTs, especially because they will be CD34-positive.[104] However, SFTs usually show

spindle cell morphology. Many KIT-negative GISTs show an epithelioid histology and are located in the stomach and omentum. SFTs are also BCL-2–positive on immunohistochemistry,[105] and of course will not contain c-kit or PDGFRA activating mutations. Desmoids, especially on biopsy, can be misinterpreted as a GIST on the basis of routine histology. In some immunohistochemical studies, desmoids may be interpreted as CD117-positive.[106] Desmoids usually show

Fig. 13. Comparison of cellular GIST with leiomyosarcoma. (*A*) Cellular GIST. The tumor was CD117-positive and contained an activating mutation in c-kit exon 11 (original magnification ×400). (*B*) Leiomyosarcoma. Some areas show a cellular pattern, similar to the GIST as in *A*, but the tumor was CD117-negative and contained no c-kit or PDGFRA activating mutations (original magnification ×400).

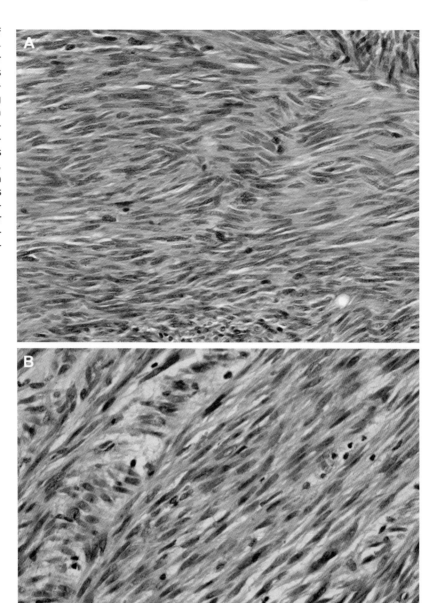

a more fibrous stroma, and the cells are more monotonous and blander appearing than GIST cells. Desmoids will be mutation-negative but β-catenin–positive,[107] and without antigen retrieval technology, desmoids lose their CD117 expression.

GISTS VERSUS IATROGENIC ARTIFACTS

Surgical sponges have also been reported to mimic GISTs in imaging studies.[108] A gross examination can lead to the correct diagnosis in such cases.

DIAGNOSIS

The diagnosis of a GIST is based on the location of the tumor, the histologic appearance, the immunophenotype, and the molecular alteration. Most GISTs arise from the muscular wall of the stomach and small intestine and are unusual, although not unheard of, in other sites.[109–117] eGISTs are

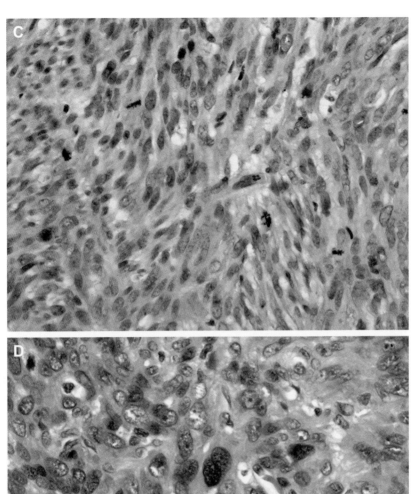

Fig. 13. (*C*) Leiomyosarcoma. Same tumor as in *B* but in a different area, demonstrating mitotic activity (original magnification ×400). (*D*) Leiomyosarcoma. Same tumor as in *B* but showing an area with marked nuclear atypia, beyond the spectrum usually observed in a GIST (original magnification ×600).

commonly found in the omentum and the mesentery, and may simply represent exophytic gastric or intestinal GISTs that over time have lost their connection with the GI tract.[41] The alternative explanation is that eGISTs may be derived from a small population of KIT-expressing cells in these sites.[42–44] In many cases, imaging studies can also help with the diagnosis.[118] The histology of most GISTs is usually that of a spindle cell or epithelioid tumor. Some GISTs show a mixed histologic pattern with both spindle cell and epithelioid areas. Because some GISTs show an unusual histologic appearance, immunohistochemical staining plays an important role in the diagnosis. Most GISTs will be strongly CD117- and CD34-positive. A spindle cell or epithelioid tumor arising in the wall of the GI tract, or in the mesentery or omentum, which is CD117- and CD34-positive, can be confidently diagnosed as a GIST without additional workup.

Fig. 14. KIT-negative GIST with inflammatory infiltrate. A 4-cm mass in the ileum was excised. The tumor was composed of a loose collection of spindle cells with a marked inflammatory infiltrate composed of mast cells, eosinophils, and lymphocytes as indicated in (*A*) (original magnification ×200) and (*B*) (original magnification ×600). Immunostaining for CD117 was positive only in mast cells and the initial diagnostic interpretation was of an inflammatory pseudotumor. Surprisingly, molecular analysis revealed an activating mutation in PDGFRA exon 12, indicating a GIST.

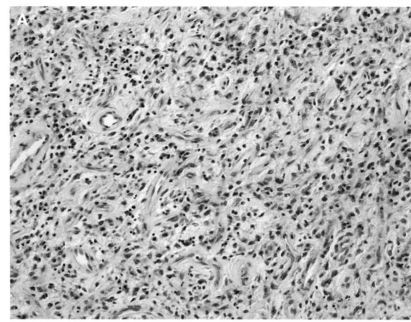

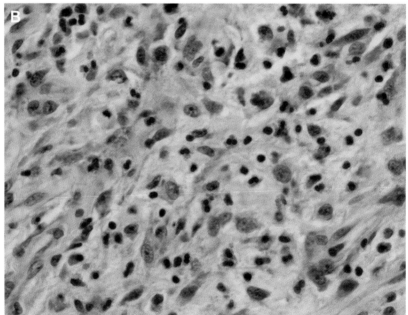

However, the diagnosis of a GIST is not always so straightforward. Some GISTs are CD117-negative,[22] and because it now seems that there is a variable degree of KIT expression in GISTs,[68] some tumors are only focally CD117-positive. This fact leads to disagreement among pathologists as to whether the CD117 stain is positive or negative. In addition, some tumors can be CD117-positive even though they are not GISTs; the most notable example is melanoma.[90] Although in the future additional immunohistochemical stains for PDGFRA,[25–28] PKC-θ,[69,70] and DOG1[71] may play an important role in GIST diagnosis, they are not yet widely available. On the contrary, molecular analysis for activating mutations in c-kit and PDGFRA is currently

Differential Diagnosis
GASTROINTESTINAL
STROMAL TUMORS (GISTs)

1. Leiomyosarcoma

2. Leiomyoma

3. Schwannoma

4. Melanoma

5. Desmoid tumor

6. KIT-positive carcinomas

7. Solitary fibrous tumor

8. Soft tissue sarcomas

9. Inflammatory polyps and pseudotumors

available and is used at several institutions, and is useful in characterizing any potential GIST. Detection of an activating mutation in either PDGFRA or c-kit, in the appropriate clinical and histologic background, provides in most cases for an unequivocal diagnosis.

In summary, the diagnosis of a GIST can usually be confidently made if attention is paid to the location of the tumor and its histologic appearance in conjunction with a judicious use of immunohistochemistry and molecular analysis.

PROGNOSIS

Unlike many types of sarcoma, prognosis in GISTs has been shown to be dependent on certain key tumor attributes,[119] and the pathologist has a central role in providing this important information. Most authorities in the field agree that the chance of metastatic disease for any GIST may never be absolutely zero, and for this reason the tumors are stratified according to clinical risk from very low to high.[17]

One important feature in stratifying GISTs according to clinical risk is the size of the tumor. As might be expected, the larger the tumor, the greater the chance of aggressive behavior. Another important feature is the mitotic count. The mitotic count for GISTs is defined as the number of mitotic figures per 50 hpf. As expected, the higher the mitotic count, the greater the chance of aggressive behavior. It should be emphasized that a mitotic count is merely an attempt to estimate the growth rate of a tumor. It does not truly measure tumor growth rate (the change in tumor growth over time) nor is it equivalent to a mitotic index, which is defined

as the percentage of tumor cells in mitosis.[120] The effects of fixation time on mitotic figure counting and misinterpretation of apoptotic cells as mitotic figures can be problematic.[76] As discussed earlier, because of these limitations it might be useful in the future to replace mitotic figure counting with a more standardized proliferation index, such as topo IIα or MIB-1.

Many studies have indicated that the risk of aggressive behavior also depends on the location of the tumor. Size and mitotic counts being equal, small intestinal GISTs seem to have a worse prognosis than gastric GISTs.[121]

Molecular analysis also helps to stratify these tumors even further. Recent data suggest that c-kit exon 11 mutation positive GISTs that contain small deletions of amino acid residues 557 to 558 define a population of tumors with a worse prognosis than those with c-kit exon 11 point mutations.[122] Also, not all PDGFRA activating mutations have the same clinical implications.[24,123]

Many low-risk GISTs are probably cured after surgical excision with clear margins, whereas macroscopically positive surgical margins for high-risk tumors is an adverse prognostic indicator.[124] For metastatic GISTs or high-risk GISTs after surgical excision, imatinib is

Pitfalls
GASTROINTESTINAL STROMAL
TUMORS (GISTs)

! GISTs can show focal CD117 staining so a small biopsy could be interpreted as negative due to sampling error. Molecular analysis can be used to help with the diagnosis.

! Some melanomas are not only CD117-positive but also contain c-kit activating mutations. Stains for melanoma markers are essential to separate melanoma from GIST.

! The use of antigen retrieval in CD117 staining can lead to false-positive results.

! The CD117 stain is negative or weakly positive in GISTs with PDGFRA activating mutations. These tumors generally are located in the stomach and omentum, they have an epithelioid histology, and molecular analysis can be used to demonstrate activating mutations in PDGFRA.

! GISTs can show a variety of morphologic patterns beyond the common spindle and epithelioid types.

recommended.[125] Of note, not all GISTs show the same response to imatinib. The objective response rates are best for exon 11 mutant GISTs (72%), followed by exon 9 (38%), then for wild type (28%).[17] The 3-dimensional structure of the KIT protein provides some insight into this therapeutic selectivity of the drug. Imatinib is a competitive inhibitor of adenosine triphosphate. However, the drug binds preferentially to the inactive conformation of KIT and therefore stabilizes KIT in the "off" mode.[19] KIT exon 11 activating mutations release the autoinhibitory portion from the active site, and this allows imatinib binding and stabilization of the inactive protein. Because KIT signaling is central to tumor proliferation, this essentially stops tumor progression. KIT exon 17 mutations (common in mastocytosis) or the common PDGFRA exon 18 mutation (D842 V) are in the TK2 domain and result in an activated protein, and probably affect the active site to make it less conducive to imatinib binding, hence a relative imatinib resistance. This domain of the protein is also the common location of secondary resistance mutations, which can occur after initially successful imatinib therapy.[55–58] New drugs targeting the resistant mutations have been described, and perhaps may eventually find use treating PDGFRA mutation positive GISTs and GISTs that contain secondary resistance mutations.[126]

SUMMARY

The identification of GISTs as tumors related to the ICC, and the demonstration of c-kit and PDGFRA activating mutations in them, has provided unity for a group of previously presumed heterogeneous GI stromal tumors. In addition, the demonstration that these tumors respond to the tyrosine kinase inhibitor imatinib has made GISTs one of the model tumors for targeted anticancer therapy. GISTs are rare tumors, and whether what has been learned about GIST biology and therapy applies to other, more common human malignancies remains to be determined. Nonetheless, pathologists play a key role in the treatment and management of GIST patients. Pathologists are responsible for providing not only an accurate diagnosis but also for providing the key attributes of the tumor, which allows oncologists to plan an appropriate treatment protocol.

ACKNOWLEDGMENTS

We thank the Associated and Regional University Pathologists (ARUP) Institute for Clinical and Experimental Pathology for their continued support. We thank Dr Carl Wittwer for his help with DNA melting analysis and Dr Timothy Gayowski for the intraoperative photographs.

In memory of Dr Holden

After submission of the manuscript for this article, Dr Joseph A. Holden, MD, PhD, died on March 28, 2009, of pancreatic cancer at age 60. Dr Holden was professor of pathology at the University of Utah School of Medicine, where he served as a highly regarded surgical pathologist and expert in the diagnosis of stromal tumors of the GI tract. His research focused on the role of DNA topoisomerase I and DNA topoisomerase II in cancer chemotherapy and evaluation of tyrosine kinase activating mutations in human malignancies. He graduated from Rutgers University and received his PhD in biochemistry from Duke University. Following a fellowship in biochemistry, he received his medical degree in 1982 from the University of Michigan and completed a residency in pathology at Washington University in St Louis. Dr Holden joined the University of Utah Department of Pathology faculty in 1987. He served 7 years as medical director of the Gene Rearrangement Section in the Hematopathology Laboratory. Dr Holden is survived by his wife of 30 years, Lisa, and daughter, Nella.

REFERENCES

1. Joensuu H, Roberts PJ, Sarlomo-Rikala M, et al. Effect of the tyrosine kinase inhibitor STI571 in a patient with a metastatic gastrointestinal stromal tumor. N Engl J Med 2001;344:1052–6.
2. Mazur MT, Clark HB. Gastric stromal tumors. Reappraisal of histogenesis. Am J Surg Pathol 1983;7: 507–19.
3. Hirota S, Isozaki K, Moriyama Y, et al. Gain-of-function mutations of c-kit in human gastrointestinal stromal tumors. Science 1998;279:577–80.
4. Druker BJ, Tamura S, Buchdunger E, et al. Effects of a selective inhibitor of the Abl tyrosine kinase on the growth of Bcr-Abl positive cells. Nat Med 1996;2:561–6.
5. Druker BJ, Talpaz M, Resta DJ, et al. Efficacy and safety of a specific inhibitor of the BCR-ABL tyrosine kinase in chronic myeloid leukemia. N Engl J Med 2001;344:1031–7.
6. Demetri GD, von Mehren M, Blanke CD, et al. Efficacy and safety of imatinib mesylate in advanced gastrointestinal stromal tumors. N Engl J Med 2002;347:472–80.
7. van Oosterom AT, Judson IR, Verweij J, et al. Update of phase I study of imatinib (STI571) in

advanced soft tissue sarcomas and gastrointestinal stromal tumors: a report of the EORTC Soft Tissue and Bone Sarcoma Group. Eur J Cancer 2002; 38(Suppl 5):S83–7.

8. Verweij J, Casali PG, Zalcberg J, et al. Progression-free survival in gastrointestinal stromal tumours with high-dose imatinib: randomised trial. Lancet 2004; 364:1127–34.

9. Heinrich MC, Corless CL, Demetri GD, et al. Kinase mutations and imatinib response in patients with metastatic gastrointestinal stromal tumor. J Clin Oncol 2003;21:4342–9.

10. Isozaki K, Hirota S. Gain-of-function mutations of receptor tyrosine kinases in gastrointestinal stromal tumors. Curr Genomics 2006;7:469–75.

11. Roskoski R Jr. Signaling by Kit protein-tyrosine kinase—the stem cell factor receptor. Biochem Biophys Res Commun 2005;337:1–13.

12. Yuzawa S, Opatowsky Y, Zhang Z, et al. Structural basis for activation of the receptor tyrosine kinase KIT by stem cell factor. Cell 2007;130:323–34.

13. Liu H, Chen X, Focia PJ, et al. Structural basis for stem cell factor-KIT signaling and activation of class III receptor tyrosine kinases. EMBO J 2007; 26:891–901.

14. Zhu MJ, Ou WB, Fletcher CD, et al. KIT oncoprotein interactions in gastrointestinal stromal tumors: therapeutic relevance. Oncogene 2007;26:6386–95.

15. Rossi F, Ehlers I, Agosti V, et al. Oncogenic Kit signaling and therapeutic intervention in a mouse model of gastrointestinal stromal tumor. Proc Natl Acad Sci U S A 2006;103:12843–8.

16. Kitamura Y, Hirotab S. Kit as a human oncogenic tyrosine kinase. Cell Mol Life Sci 2004;61:2924–31.

17. Corless CL, Heinrich MC. Molecular pathobiology of gastrointestinal stromal sarcomas. Annu Rev Pathol 2008;3:557–86.

18. Lasota J, Miettinen M. Clinical significance of oncogenic KIT and PDGFRA mutations in gastrointestinal stromal tumours. Histopathology 2008;53:245–66.

19. Mol CD, Dougan DR, Schneider TR, et al. Structural basis for the autoinhibition and STI-571 inhibition of c-Kit tyrosine kinase. J Biol Chem 2004;279: 31655–63.

20. Lasota J, Kopczynski J, Sarlomo-Rikala M, et al. KIT 1530ins6 mutation defines a subset of predominantly malignant gastrointestinal stromal tumors of intestinal origin. Hum Pathol 2003;34:1306–12.

21. Heinrich MC, Corless CL, Duensing A, et al. PDGFRA activating mutations in gastrointestinal stromal tumors. Science 2003;299:708–10.

22. Medeiros F, Corless CL, Duensing A, et al. KIT-negative gastrointestinal stromal tumors: proof of concept and therapeutic implications. Am J Surg Pathol 2004;28:889–94.

23. Giebel LB, Strunk KM, Holmes SA, et al. Organization and nucleotide sequence of the human KIT (mast/stem cell growth factor receptor) proto-oncogene. Oncogene 1992;7:2207–17.

24. Corless CL, Schroeder A, Griffith D, et al. PDGFRA mutations in gastrointestinal stromal tumors: frequency, spectrum and in vitro sensitivity to imatinib. J Clin Oncol 2005;23:5357–64.

25. Chang HM, Ryu MH, Lee H, et al. PDGFR alpha gene mutation and protein expression in gastrointestinal stromal tumors. Oncology 2008;74: 88–95.

26. Miselli F, Millefanti C, Conca E, et al. PDGFRA immunostaining can help in the diagnosis of gastrointestinal stromal tumors. Am J Surg Pathol 2008;32: 738–43.

27. Sevinc A, Camci C, Yilmaz M, et al. The diagnosis of C-kit negative GIST by PDGFRA staining: clinical, pathological, and nuclear medicine perspective. The diagnosis of C-kit negative GIST by PDGFRA staining: clinical, pathological, and nuclear medicine perspective. Onkologie 2007;30:645–8.

28. Peterson MR, Piao Z, Weidner N, et al. Strong PDGFRA positivity is seen in GISTs but not in other intra-abdominal mesenchymal tumors: immunohistochemical and mutational analyses. Appl Immunohistochem Mol Morphol 2006;14:390–6.

29. Agaram NP, Wong GC, Guo T, et al. Novel V600E BRAF mutations in imatinib-naive and imatinib-resistant gastrointestinal stromal tumors. Genes Chromosomes Cancer 2008;47:853–9.

30. Tarn C, Rink L, Merkel E, et al. Insulin-like growth factor 1 receptor is a potential therapeutic target for gastrointestinal stromal tumors. Proc Natl Acad Sci U S A 2008;105:8387–92.

31. Kawanowa K, Sakuma Y, Sakurai S, et al. High incidence of microscopic gastrointestinal stromal tumors in the stomach. Hum Pathol 2006;37:1527–35.

32. Abraham SC, Krasinskas AM, Hofstetter WL, et al. "Seedling" mesenchymal tumors (gastrointestinal stromal tumors and leiomyomas) are common incidental tumors of the esophagogastric junction. Am J Surg Pathol 2007;31:1629–35.

33. Agaimy A, Wünsch PH, Hofstaedter F, et al. Minute gastric sclerosing stromal tumors (GIST tumorlets) are common in adults and frequently show c-KIT mutations. Am J Surg Pathol 2007;31:113–20.

34. Agaimy A, Wünsch PH, Dirnhofer S, et al. Microscopic gastrointestinal stromal tumors in esophageal and intestinal surgical resection specimens: a clinicopathologic, immunohistochemical, and molecular study of 19 lesions. Am J Surg Pathol 2008;32:867–73.

35. Corless CL, McGreevey L, Haley A, et al. KIT mutations are common in incidental gastrointestinal stromal tumors one centimeter or less in size. Am J Pathol 2002;160:1567–72.

36. Chetty R. Small and microscopically detected gastrointestinal stromal tumours: an overview. Pathology 2008;40:9–12.

37. Agaimy A, Dirnhofer S, Wünsch PH, et al. Multiple sporadic gastrointestinal stromal tumors (GISTs) of the proximal stomach are caused by different somatic KIT mutations suggesting a field effect. Am J Surg Pathol 2008;32(10):1553–9.

38. Ogasawara N, Tsukamoto T, Inada K, et al. Frequent c-Kit gene mutations not only in gastrointestinal stromal tumors but also in interstitial cells of Cajal in surrounding normal mucosa. Cancer Lett 2005;230:199–210.

39. Reddy P, Boci K, Charbonneau C. The epidemiologic, health-related quality of life, and economic burden of gastrointestinal stromal tumours. J Clin Pharm Ther 2007;32:557–65.

40. Scarpa M, Bertin M, Ruffolo C, et al. A systematic review on the clinical diagnosis of gastrointestinal stromal tumors. J Surg Oncol 2008;98(5):384–92.

41. Agaimy A, Wünsch PH. Gastrointestinal stromal tumours: a regular origin in the muscularis propria, but an extremely diverse gross presentation. A review of 200 cases to critically re-evaluate the concept of so-called extra-gastrointestinal stromal tumours. Langenbecks Arch Surg 2006;391: 322–9.

42. Yamamoto H, Oda Y, Kawaguchi K, et al. c-kit and PDGFRA mutations in extragastrointestinal stromal tumor (gastrointestinal stromal tumor of the soft tissue). Am J Surg Pathol 2004;28:479–88.

43. Hinescu ME, Popescu LM, Gherghiceanu M, et al. Interstitial Cajal-like cells in rat mesentery: an ultrastructural and immunohistochemical approach. J Cell Mol Med 2008;12:260–70.

44. Sakurai S, Hishima T, Takazawa Y, et al. Gastrointestinal stromal tumors and KIT-positive mesenchymal cells in the omentum. Pathol Int 2001;51:524–31.

45. Miettinen M, Sarlomo-Rikala M, Sobin LH, et al. Esophageal stromal tumors: a clinicopathologic, immunohistochemical, and molecular genetic study of 17 cases and comparison with esophageal leiomyomas and leiomyosarcomas. Am J Surg Pathol 2000;24:211–22.

46. Miettinen M, Sarlomo-Rikala M, Sobin LH. Mesenchymal tumors of muscularis mucosae of colon and rectum are benign leiomyomas that should be separated from gastrointestinal stromal tumors—a clinicopathologic and immunohistochemical study of eighty-eight cases. Mod Pathol 2001;14:950–6.

47. Robson ME, Glogowski E, Sommer G, et al. Pleomorphic characteristics of a germ-line KIT mutation in a large kindred with gastrointestinal stromal tumors, hyperpigmentation, and dysphagia. Clin Cancer Res 2004;10:1250–4.

48. Li FP, Fletcher JA, Heinrich MC, et al. Familial gastrointestinal stromal tumor syndrome: phenotypic and molecular features in a kindred. J Clin Oncol 2005;23:2735–43.

49. Graham J, Debiec-Rychter M, Corless CL, et al. Imatinib in the management of multiple gastrointestinal stromal tumors associated with a germline KIT K642E mutation. Arch Pathol Lab Med 2007;131: 1393–6.

50. Kleinbaum EP, Lazar AJ, Tamborini E, et al. Clinical, histopathologic, molecular and therapeutic findings in a large kindred with gastrointestinal stromal tumor. Int J Cancer 2008;122:711–8.

51. Holden JA. DNA topoisomerases as anticancer drug targets: from the laboratory to the clinic. Curr Med Chem Anticancer Agents 2001;1:1–25.

52. Miettinen M, Lasota J. Gastrointestinal stromal tumors: review on morphology, molecular pathology, prognosis, and differential diagnosis. Arch Pathol Lab Med 2006;130:1466–78.

53. Kirsch R, Gao ZH, Riddell R. Gastrointestinal stromal tumors: diagnostic challenges and practical approach to differential diagnosis. Adv Anat Pathol 2007;14:261–85.

54. Pauwels P, Debiec-Rychter M, Stul M, et al. Changing phenotype of gastrointestinal stromal tumours under imatinib mesylate treatment: a potential diagnostic pitfall. Histopathology 2005;47:41–7.

55. Nishida T, Kanda T, Nishitani A, et al. Secondary mutations in the kinase domain of the KIT gene are predominant in imatinib-resistant gastrointestinal stromal tumor. Cancer Sci 2008;99:799–804.

56. Lim KH, Huang MJ, Chen LT, et al. Molecular analysis of secondary kinase mutations in imatinib-resistant gastrointestinal stromal tumors. Med Oncol 2008;25:207–13.

57. Liegl B, Kepten I, Le C, et al. Heterogeneity of kinase inhibitor resistance mechanisms in GIST. J Pathol 2008;216:64–74.

58. Antonescu CR, Besmer P, Guo T, et al. Acquired resistance to imatinib in gastrointestinal stromal tumor occurs through secondary gene mutation. Clin Cancer Res 2005;11:4182–90.

59. Fletcher CD, Berman JJ, Corless C, et al. Diagnosis of gastrointestinal stromal tumors: a consensus approach. Hum Pathol 2002;33:459–65.

60. de Silva CM, Reid R. Gastrointestinal stromal tumors (GIST): C-kit mutations, CD117 expression, differential diagnosis and targeted cancer therapy with Imatinib. Pathol Oncol Res 2003;9:13–9.

61. Badalamenti G, Rodolico V, Fulfaro F, et al. Gastrointestinal stromal tumors (GISTs): focus on histopathological diagnosis and biomolecular features. Ann Oncol 2007;18(Suppl 6). vi136–40.

62. Pauls K, Merkelbach-Bruse S, Thal D, et al. PDGFRalpha- and c-kit-mutated gastrointestinal stromal tumours (GISTs) are characterized by distinctive histological and immunohistochemical features. Histopathology 2005;46:166–75.

63. Taylor SL, Platt-Higgins A, Rudland PS, et al. Cytoplasmic staining of c-erbB-2 is not associated with

the presence of detectable c-erbB-2 mRNA in breast cancer specimens. Int J Cancer 1998;76:459–63.

64. Tabone-Eglinger S, Subra F, El Sayadi H, et al. KIT mutations induce intracellular retention and activation of an immature form of the KIT protein in gastrointestinal stromal tumors. Clin Cancer Res 2008;14:2285–94.

65. Xiang Z, Kreisel F, Cain J, et al. Neoplasia driven by mutant c-KIT is mediated by intracellular, not plasma membrane, receptor signaling. Mol Cell Biol 2007;27:267–82.

66. Hornick JL, Fletcher CD. Immunohistochemical staining for KIT (CD117) in soft tissue sarcomas is very limited in distribution. Am J Clin Pathol 2002; 117:188–93.

67. Sabah M, Leader M, Kay E. The problem with KIT: clinical implications and practical difficulties with CD117 immunostaining. Appl Immunohistochem Mol Morphol 2003;11:56–61.

68. Haller F, Happel N, Schulten HJ, et al. Site-dependent differential KIT and PDGFRA expression in gastric and intestinal gastrointestinal stromal tumors. Mod Pathol 2007;20:1103–11.

69. Motegi A, Sakurai S, Nakayama H, et al. PKC theta, a novel immunohistochemical marker for gastrointestinal stromal tumors (GIST), especially useful for identifying KIT-negative tumors. Pathol Int 2005;55:106–12.

70. Lee HE, Kim MA, Lee HS, et al. Characteristics of KIT-negative gastrointestinal stromal tumours and diagnostic utility of protein kinase C theta immunostaining. J Clin Pathol 2008;61:722–9.

71. Espinosa I, Lee CH, Kim MK, et al. A novel monoclonal antibody against DOG1 is a sensitive and specific marker for gastrointestinal stromal tumors. Am J Surg Pathol 2008;32:210–8.

72. Hasegawa T, Matsuno Y, Shimoda T, et al. Gastrointestinal stromal tumor: consistent CD117 immunostaining for diagnosis, and prognostic classification based on tumor size and MIB-1 grade. Hum Pathol 2002;33:669–76.

73. Nagasako Y, Misawa K, Kohashi S, et al. Evaluation of malignancy using Ki-67 labeling index for gastric stromal tumor. Gastric Cancer 2003;6: 168–72.

74. Filiz G, Yalçinkaya O, Gürel S, et al. The relationship between MIB-1 proliferative activity and mitotic index in gastrointestinal stromal tumors. Hepatogastroenterology 2007;54:438–41.

75. Willmore C, Holden JA, Zhou L, et al. Detection of c-kit-activating mutations in gastrointestinal stromal tumors by high-resolution amplicon melting analysis. Am J Clin Pathol 2004;122:206–16.

76. Thunnissen FB, Ambergen AW, Koss M, et al. Mitotic counting in surgical pathology: sampling bias, heterogeneity and statistical uncertainty. Histopathology 2001;39:1–8.

77. Hornick JL, Fletcher CD. The role of KIT in the management of patients with gastrointestinal stromal tumors. Hum Pathol 2007;38:679–87.

78. Debiec-Rychter M, Sciot R, Le Cesne A, et al. Kit mutations and dose selection for imatinib in patients with advanced gastrointestinal stromal tumours. Eur J Cancer 2006;42:1093–103.

79. Heinrich MC, Maki RG, Corless CL, et al. Primary and secondary kinase genotypes correlate with the biological and clinical activity of sunitinib in imatinib-resistant gastrointestinal stromal tumor. J Clin Oncol 2008;26(33):5352–9.

80. Kirkegaard T, Edwards J, Tovey S. Observer variation in immunohistochemical analysis of protein expression, time for a change? Histopathology 2006;48:787–94.

81. Liu T, Willmore-Payne C, Layfield LJ, et al. A gastrointestinal stromal tumor of the stomach morphologically resembling a neurofibroma: demonstration of a novel platelet-derived growth factor receptor alpha exon 18 mutation. Hum Pathol 2008;39(12):1849–53.

82. Lippai N, Füle T, Németh T, et al. Keratin-positive gastrointestinal stromal tumor of the stomach mimicking gastric carcinoma: diagnosis confirmed by c-kit mutation analysis. Diagn Mol Pathol 2008; 17(4):241–4.

83. Rossi G, Sartori G, Valli R, et al. The value of c-kit mutational analysis in a cytokeratin positive gastrointestinal stromal tumour. J Clin Pathol 2005;58:991–3.

84. Morey AL, Wanigesekera GD, Hawkins NJ, et al. C-kit mutations in gastrointestinal stromal tumours. Pathology 2002;34:315–9.

85. Zamò A, Bertolaso A, Franceschetti I, et al. Microfluidic deletion/insertion analysis for rapid screening of KIT and PDGFRA mutations in CD117-positive gastrointestinal stromal tumors: diagnostic applications and report of a new KIT mutation. J Mol Diagn 2007;9:151–7.

86. Erali M, Voelkerding KV, Wittwer CT. High resolution melting applications for clinical laboratory medicine. Exp Mol Pathol 2008;85:50–8.

87. Holden JA, Willmore-Payne C, Coppola D, et al. High-resolution melting amplicon analysis as a method to detect c-kit and platelet-derived growth factor receptor alpha activating mutations in gastrointestinal stromal tumors. Am J Clin Pathol 2007;128:230–8.

88. Abraham SC. Distinguishing gastrointestinal stromal tumors from their mimics: an update. Adv Anat Pathol 2007;14:178–88.

89. Gabali AM, Priebe P, Ganesan S. Primary melanoma of small intestine masquerading as gastrointestinal stromal tumor: a case report and literature review. Am Surg 2008;74(4):318–21.

90. Willmore-Payne C, Holden JA, Hirschowitz S, et al. BRAF and c-kit gene copy number in

mutation-positive malignant melanoma. Hum Pathol 2006;37:520–7.

91. Beadling C, Jacobson-Dunlop E, Hodi FS, et al. Kit gene mutations and copy number in melanoma subytpes. Clin Cancer Res 2008;14:6821–8.

92. Lutzky J, Bauer J, Bastian BC. Dose-dependent, complete response to imatinib of a metastatic mucosal melanoma with a K642E KIT mutation. Pigment Cell Melanoma Res 2008;21:492–3.

93. Hodi FS, Friedlander P, Corless CL, et al. Major response to imatinib mesylate in KIT-mutated melanoma. J Clin Oncol 2008;26:2046–51.

94. Guler ML, Daniels JA, Abraham SC, et al. Expression of melanoma antigens in epithelioid gastrointestinal stromal tumors: a potential diagnostic pitfall. Arch Pathol Lab Med 2008;132:1302–6.

95. Crisi GM, Marconi SA, Makari-Judson G, et al. Expression of c-kit in adenoid cystic carcinoma of the breast. Am J Clin Pathol 2005;124:733–9.

96. Swick BL, Ravdel L, Fitzpatrick JE, et al. Merkel cell carcinoma: evaluation of KIT (CD117) expression and failure to demonstrate activating mutations in the C-KIT proto-oncogene - implications for treatment with imatinib mesylate. J Cutan Pathol 2007; 34:324–9.

97. López-Martin A, Ballestín C, Garcia-Carbonero R, et al. Prognostic value of KIT expression in small cell lung cancer. Lung Cancer 2007;56:405–13.

98. Lim KH, Pardanani A, Tefferi A. KIT and mastocytosis. Acta Haematol 2008;119:194–8.

99. Kemmer K, Corless CL, Fletcher JA, et al. KIT mutations are common in testicular seminomas. Am J Pathol 2004;164:305–13.

100. Geller MA, Argenta P, Bradley W, et al. Treatment and recurrence patterns in endometrial stromal sarcomas and the relation to c-kit expression. Gynecol Oncol 2004;95:632–6.

101. Kalender ME, Sevinc A, Yilmaz M, et al. Detection of complete response to imatinib mesylate (Glivec((R))/Gleevec ((R))) with 18F-FDG PET/CT for low-grade endometrial stromal sarcoma. Cancer Chemother Pharmacol 2008;63(3):555–9.

102. Salvatierra A, Tarrats A, Gomez C, et al. A case of c-kit positive high-grade stromal endometrial sarcoma responding to imatinib mesylate. Gynecol Oncol 2006;101:545–7.

103. Greenson JK. Gastrointestinal stromal tumors and other mesenchymal lesions of the gut. Mod Pathol 2003;16:366–75.

104. Shidham VB, Chivukula M, Gupta D, et al. Immunohistochemical comparison of gastrointestinal stromal tumor and solitary fibrous tumor. Arch Pathol Lab Med 2002;126:1189–92.

105. Takizawa I, Saito T, Kitamura Y, et al. Primary solitary fibrous tumor (SFT) in the retroperitoneum. Urol Oncol 2008;26:254–9.

106. Yantiss RK, Spiro IJ, Compton CC, et al. Gastrointestinal stromal tumor versus intra-abdominal fibromatosis of the bowel wall: a clinically important differential diagnosis. Am J Surg Pathol 2000;24:947–57.

107. Carlson JW, Fletcher CD. Immunohistochemistry for beta-catenin in the differential diagnosis of spindle cell lesions: analysis of a series and review of the literature. Histopathology 2007;51:509–14.

108. Yamamura N, Nakajima K, Takahashi T, et al. Intra-abdominal textiloma. A retained surgical sponge mimicking a gastric gastrointestinal stromal tumor: report of a case. Surg Today 2008;38:552–4.

109. Papaspyros S, Papagiannopoulos K. Gastrointestinal stromal tumor masquerading as a lung neoplasm. A case presentation and literature review. J Cardiothorac Surg 2008;3:31.

110. Gupta N, Mittal S, Lal N, et al. A rare case of primary mesenteric gastrointestinal stromal tumor with metastasis to the cervix uteri. World J Surg Oncol 2007;5:137.

111. Showalter SL, Lloyd JM, Glassman DT, et al. Extragastrointestinal stromal tumor of the pancreas: case report and a review of the literature. Arch Surg 2008;143:305–8.

112. Perrone N, Serafini G, Vitali A, et al. Gastrointestinal stromal tumor metastatic to the scrotum. J Ultrasound Med 2008;27:961–4.

113. Irving JA, Lerwill MF, Young RH. Gastrointestinal stromal tumors metastatic to the ovary: a report of five cases. Am J Surg Pathol 2005;29:920–6.

114. Arce-Lara C, Shah MH, Jimenez RE, et al. Gastrointestinal stromal tumors involving the prostate: presentation, course, and therapeutic approach. Urology 2007;69:1209 e5–7.

115. Nasu K, Ueda T, Kai S, et al. Gastrointestinal stromal tumor arising in the rectovaginal septum. Int J Gynecol Cancer 2004;14:373–7.

116. Lasota J, Carlson JA, Miettinen M. Spindle cell tumor of urinary bladder serosa with phenotypic and genotypic features of gastrointestinal stromal tumor. Arch Pathol Lab Med 2000;124:894–7.

117. Foster R, Solano S, Mahoney J, et al. Reclassification of a tubal leiomyosarcoma as an eGIST by molecular evaluation of c-KIT. Gynecol Oncol 2006;101:363–6.

118. Gheorghe L, Gheorghe C, Cotruta B, et al. CT aspects of gastrointestinal stromal tumors: adding EUS and EUS elastography to the diagnostic tools. J Gastrointestin Liver Dis 2007;16:346–7.

119. Joensuu H. Risk stratification of patients diagnosed with gastrointestinal stromal tumor. Hum Pathol 2008;39:1411–9.

120. Alberts B, Bray LJ, Raff M, et al. Molecular biology of the cell. 3rd edition. New York (NY): Garland Publishing, Inc; 1994. p. 866.

121. Miettinen M, Lasota J. Gastrointestinal stromal tumors: pathology and prognosis at different sites. Semin Diagn Pathol 2006;23:70–83.

122. Kontogianni-Katsarou K, Dimitriadis E, Lariou C, et al. KIT exon 11 codon 557/558 deletion/insertion mutations define a subset of gastrointestinal stromal tumors with malignant potential. World J Gastroenterol 2008;14:1891–7.

123. Lasota J, Stachura J, Miettinen M. GISTs with PDGFRA exon 14 mutations represent subset of clinically favorable gastric tumors with epithelioid morphology. Lab Invest 2006;86:94–100.

124. Gouveia AM, Pimenta AP, Capelinha AF, et al. Surgical margin status and prognosis of gastrointestinal stromal tumor. World J Surg 2008;32(11): 2375–82.

125. von Mehren M. The role of adjuvant and neoadjuvant therapy in gastrointestinal stromal tumors. Curr Opin Oncol 2008;20:428–32.

126. Boyar MS, Taub RN. New strategies for treating GIST when imatinib fails. Cancer Invest 2007;25:328–35.

ESOPHAGEAL EOSINOPHILIA

Rebecca Wilcox, MD, John Hart, MD*

KEYWORDS

• Esophageal eosinophilia • Reflux esophagitis • Crohn's disease • Vasculitis

ABSTRACT

The primary nonepithelial components of normal esophageal mucosa are antigen presenting cells and occasional lymphocytes. The presence of eosinophils within the squamous epithelium usually indicates a pathologic process. The presence of esophageal eosinophilia encompasses a broad differential diagnosis, and at times a specific histologic diagnosis is not possible. Therefore, correlation of the microscopic features in the endoscopic esophageal biopsy specimens with the clinical history is critical to making the correct diagnosis. This content provides a systematic approach to esophageal squamous eosinophilia with emphasis on specific, distinguishing features within this expansive differential.

EOSINOPHILIC ESOPHAGITIS

OVERVIEW

Eosinophilic esophagitis (EE), a primary eosinophilic disorder of the esophagus, is a diagnosis that has increased in recognition and incidence in the last decade.[1–3] Although predominately a pediatric disease, EE is also well recognized in adults. Men comprise two-thirds of the patients with EE in the adult and pediatric age groups. Inhaled and swallowed environmental antigens, and more specifically food allergens, have been strongly implicated in the pathophysiology of EE and most patients who have EE will also have a clinical history of food allergy, asthma, or atopic disorders.[4–6] In children there is a significant overlap between the symptoms of EE and those of gastroesophageal reflux, including vomiting, epigastric/chest pain, food intolerance, and failure to thrive. In adults, a clinical history of food impaction is highly suspicious for EE; however, the prevailing symptom is dysphagia or gastroesophageal refluxlike symptoms.[7] Treatment with an elemental diet, steroids, or an elimination diet restricting the most common food allergens (peanuts, milk, soy, egg, and wheat) is usually effective.[8]

GROSS APPEARANCE

Endoscopic findings characteristic of EE include thickened mucosa producing longitudinal furrows

> ### Key Features
> #### ESOPHAGEAL EOSINOPHILIA
>
> • Esophageal eosinophilia may occur as an eosinophilic disorder primary to the esophagus, as in eosinophilic esophagitis, or as a component of a systemic disorder.
>
> • Adequate sampling of the mucosa of the esophagus and other gastrointestinal organs is imperative in making an accurate histologic assessment.
>
> • The presence of an eosinophil-predominant infiltrate versus a mixed inflammatory cell infiltrate with an eosinophilic component can be a helpful feature in the differential diagnosis.
>
> • The differential diagnosis of esophageal eosinophilia is extensive. Fundamental to making the appropriate diagnosis is the integration of histologic features with clinical findings.
>
> • At times, a definitive diagnosis cannot be made histologically.

Department of Pathology, University of Chicago Medical Center, 5841 South Maryland Avenue, Chicago, IL 60637, USA
* Corresponding author.
E-mail address: John.Hart@uchospitals.edu

Surgical Pathology 3 (2010) 277–295
doi:10.1016/j.path.2010.05.006

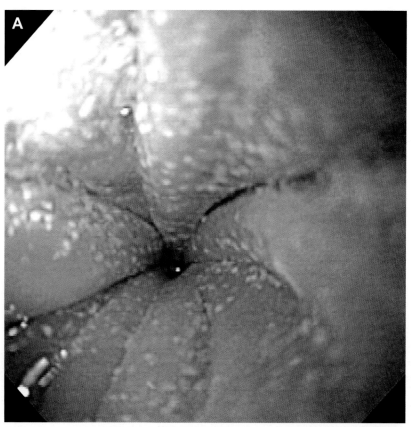

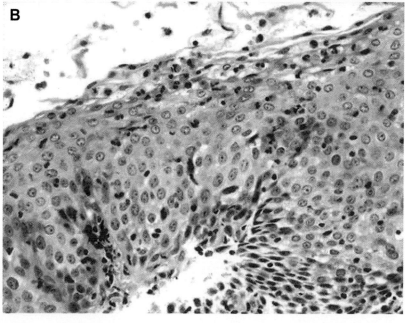

Fig. 1. Eosinophilic esophagitis. (*A*) Typical endoscopic appearance with numerous scattered white exudates. (*B*) A biopsy reveals a dense superficial infiltrate of eosinophils with microabscess formation.

or circumferential rings (so-called feline esophagus or trachealization) and patchy white exudates, reminiscent of esophageal candidiasis (**Fig. 1**A). The white exudates correspond histologically to dense clusters of intramucosal eosinophils and its presence has been found to be associated with an increased frequency of dysphasia.[9] Although the presence of any of these endoscopic features is suggestive of EE, none are pathognomonic. Furthermore, up to 30% of pediatric patients with active EE will have a normal endoscopic appearance.[2]

MICROSCOPIC FEATURES

Histologic features highly suggestive of EE include a dense intraepithelial eosinophil infiltrate often more prominent in the superficial portion of the epithelium, small clusters of eosinophils present at the epithelial surface (so-called eosinophilic microabscesses), and marked basal cell hyperplasia (**Fig. 1**B). According to the most recent consensus guidelines, 15 or more intraepithelial eosinophils in any one high power field is the threshold number of eosinophils required to make the diagnosis of EE.[10] The primary nonepithelial components of normal esophageal

mucosa are antigen presenting cells and occasional lymphocytes (**Fig. 2**).

DIFFERENTIAL DIAGNOSIS

Reflux esophagitis is the most common, and at times the most difficult condition to differentiate from EE. In general, reflux esophagitis has fewer, more diffusely scattered eosinophils than EE. Although basal cell hyperplasia is a well-described component of reflux esophagitis, it actually tends to be less pronounced than that seen in EE.[11] Degranulation of eosinophils has also been determined to be more common in EE than in reflux esophagitis, but this feature is difficult to quantitate.[12] Correlation with clinical history (eg, 24-hour pH monitoring or history of atopy) may help to establish the proper diagnosis; however, in some cases it is not possible to make a firm histologic distinction between the two. Secondary eosinophilic disorders, such as eosinophilic gastroenteritis or hypereosinophilic syndrome, must also be considered in the differential. Ruling out these entities requires examination of biopsies from additional sites from the patients' gastrointestinal tract. In addition, a clinical workup to exclude parasitic infections, allergic vasculitis/collagen vascular disease,

Fig. 2. Normal squamous mucosa. Note the absence of an inflammatory cell infiltrate.

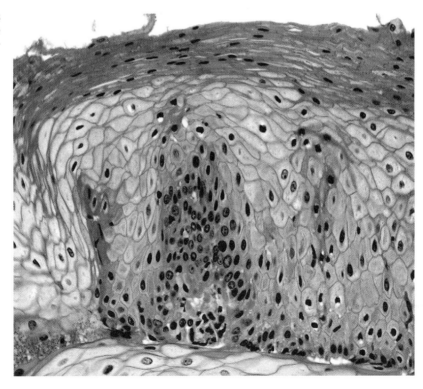

Differential Diagnosis
ESOPHAGEAL EOSINOPHILIA

- EE is a clinicopathologic diagnosis. Apply clinical context to the findings on histologic examination.
- Secondary eosinophilic disorders, such as eosinophilic gastroenteritis or hypereosinophilic syndrome, must also be considered in the differential.

Reflux esophagitis

- Reflux esophagitis has fewer, more diffusely scattered eosinophils than EE.
- Basal cell hyperplasia as a component of reflux esophagitis tends to be less pronounced than in EE.

Hypereosinophilic syndrome

Eosinophilic gastroenteritis

- Presence of sheets of eosinophils in the deep layers of the esophageal wall is the only histologic abnormality in eosinophilic gastroenteritis involving the esophagus.
- If the inflammatory cell infiltrate is mixed, or there is evidence of significant fibrosis or vasculitis, a systemic connective tissue or systemic vasculitis is favored.
- Absence of ganglion cells in the submucosal or myenteric plexus raises the possibility of Chagas disease.
- If only mucosal eosinophilic infiltrates are present, with no other portion of the gastrointestinal (GI) tract affected, eosinophilic esophagitis is more likely.

Drug-induced injury

- Presence of a discrete ulcer surrounded by endoscopically and histologically normal squamous mucosa is a clue to the diagnosis of pill esophagitis.

Infection

- When contemplating eosinophilia secondary to a parasitic infection all other causes of mucosal eosinophilia must be considered.
- Cytomegalovirus (CMV) and herpes simplex virus (HSV) infection may produce focal ulceration similar to that in drug-induced esophagitis.
- A clinical history of an immunosuppressed state is helpful to raise suspicion of a viral infection.

Crohn's disease

- Eosinophils may be prominent in Crohn esophagitis, however, more commonly the inflammatory cell infiltrates are mixed.

Collagen vascular disease/allergic vasculitis

- Patients with collagen vascular diseases may have a nonspecific esophagitis with a dense eosinophilic infiltrate.
- Drug-induced injury or opportunistic infections secondary to immunosuppression should be ruled out in patients with a history of a collagen vascular disease.

or myeloproliferative disorder should be considered in the proper clinical context.

DIAGNOSIS

Esophageal eosinophilia is a clinicopathologic diagnosis. To make a definitive diagnosis of EE, the patients' biopsy must meet the histologic criteria (at least ≥15 intraepithelial eosinophils/high-power field [HPF]) and the clinical history must meet diagnostic guidelines, including failure to respond to high-dose proton pump inhibitors (PPIs) or normal pH monitoring of the distal esophagus.[10] The eosinophilic infiltrates in EE can be exquisitely patchy, with some areas devoid of eosinophils and others exhibiting a dense infiltrate (Fig. 3). For this reason, multiple biopsies are necessary to exclude the diagnosis. Multiple biopsies separately submitted from the distal and mid-esophagus are most helpful in arriving at a firm histologic diagnosis of EE.[10] The presence of changes that are of equal severity in biopsies from the mid and distal esophagus is a useful finding when making a diagnosis of EE because reflux esophagitis is typically more severe at the distal end of the esophagus. If adequate biopsy sampling is not performed, then the pathologist may have to simply report a descriptive diagnosis of "squamous mucosa with a prominent intraepithelial infiltrate of eosinophils" and a comment describing the

Fig. 3. The patchiness of the eosinophilic infiltrates in eosinophilic esophagitis, even in the untreated state, is illustrated in these 2 biopsies, both taken from the distal esophagus. The biopsy in the top panel is completely normal, whereas the biopsy in the lower panel exhibits a dense infiltrate of eosinophils.

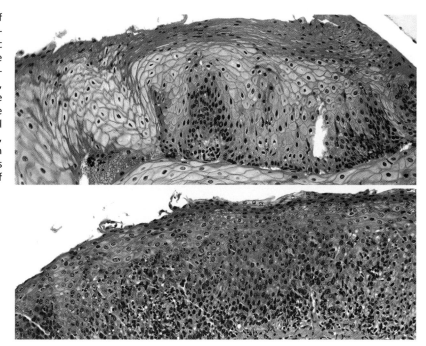

histologic features and the differential diagnostic considerations.

PROGNOSIS

The long-term natural history of EE is currently unknown. Correct diagnosis is important because it allows for appropriate therapy and prevention of the most devastating complications, including esophageal strictures in adults and growth restriction and failure to thrive in children.

REFLUX ESOPHAGITIS

OVERVIEW

Gastroesophageal reflux disease (GERD), caused by the reflux of gastric and duodenal contents into the distal esophagus, is a highly prevalent disease with a wide range of clinical symptoms. Approximately 40% of the adult population in the United States is affected by GERD symptoms, including epigastric pain, nausea/vomiting, regurgitation, and dysphagia.[13,14] The primary predisposing factors of GERD result from either increased intra-abdominal or intragastric pressure as in pregnancy or obesity; structural abnormalities, such as a hiatal hernia; or delayed gastric emptying as seen in diabetes. Although the true incidence is not well defined, GERD symptoms are commonly encountered in infants and the

pediatric population.[15] As in EE, one of the most devastating complications in this population is failure to thrive. When GERD causes endoscopic or histologic evidence of esophageal inflammation it is referred to as reflux esophagitis. This condition is the most common type of esophagitis, eosinophilic or otherwise, encountered in general practice.

GROSS APPEARANCE

The endoscopic findings of reflux esophagitis tend to correspond to the degree of esophageal injury, ranging from erythema and superficial erosions to ulcerations and strictures or scarring with Barrett's metaplasia. The absence of endoscopic findings does not exclude the diagnosis of reflux esophagitis, and therefore endoscopic biopsy is an important diagnostic modality.[16,17]

MICROSCOPIC FEATURES

Numerous histologic abnormalities are present in reflux esophagitis, but none are specific for the diagnosis.[16,17] Basal cell hyperplasia and increased length of the lamina propria papillae are probably the most sensitive features of reflux, but unfortunately these changes cannot be assessed accurately in poorly oriented esophageal biopsies. Basal cell hyperplasia is defined as a basal cell layer that is more than 15% of the total thickness of the

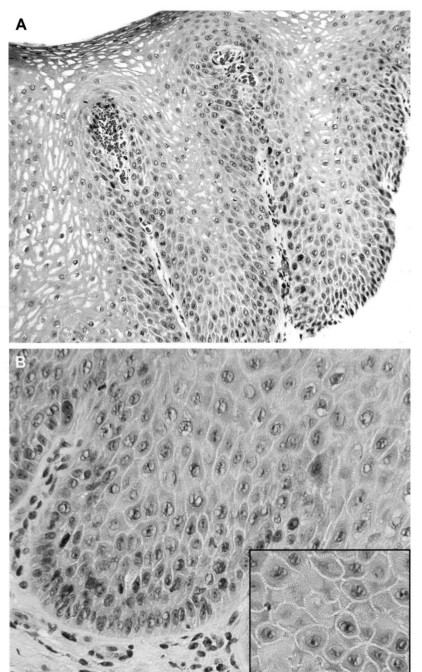

Fig. 4. Reflux esophagitis. (*A*) Increased length of papillae and rare scattered intraepithelial lymphocytes are evident in this field. (*B*) Prominence of dilated intracellular spaces (spongiosis) is a sensitive feature of reflux.

epithelium. The basal cells can be recognized as smaller squamous cells at the base of the epithelium with darker staining cytoplasm and a higher nucleus-to-cytoplasm ratio than the more superficial cells. The precise border of the basal cell layer can be difficult to determine in some cases, and therefore the reproducibility of this criterion is probably lower than some other features. The lamina propria papillae normally extend upward about one-half of the total thickness of the epithelium. Papillae that

Table 1
Eosinophilic infiltrate differences

Diagnosis	Histologic Features
Eosinophilic esophagitis	15 or more eosinophils/HPF; eosinophilic infiltrate more prominent in the superficial epithelium; eosinophilic microabscesses; marked basal cell hyperplasia; equal severity of histologic features in midesophagus and distal esophagus
Eosinophilic gastroenteritis	In addition to eosinophilic esophagitis, must have pathologic accumulation of eosinophils within the stomach, small bowel, or colon with all other possible causes of mucosal eosinophilia ruled out clinically
Reflux esophagitis	Diffusely scattered eosinophils (no microabscesses); basal cell hyperplasia present but generally less prominent than in EE; histologic changes more severe in the distal esophagus compared with midesophagus; presence of active carditis
Drug-induced injury	Eosinophils are one component of a mixed inflammatory infiltrate; tends to be focal and affect midesophagus; NSAIDs cause nonspecific esophagitis or features of reflux without basal cell hyperplasia
Infectious esophagitis	With the exception of parasites, eosinophils are generally part of a mixed inflammatory cell infiltrate; histologic changes are often focal; identification of organisms is key to the diagnosis
Crohn's disease	Eosinophils are a component of a nonspecific mixed inflammatory cell infiltrate; lamina propria granulomas are necessary for a specific diagnosis in the proper clinical context (correlate with findings of GI biopsies from other sites)
Collagen vascular disease/allergic/vasculitis	Intense inflammatory cell infiltrates, sometimes with eosinophil predominance; vasculitis not usually identified in biopsy specimens (clinical correlation required for diagnosis)

are more than two-thirds of the thickness are usually regarded as abnormal and as a feature of reflux. Basal cell hyperplasia and increased papillae length generally occur together because both represent a response to mucosal injury (**Fig. 4**A).

Because a certain degree of reflux of gastroduodenal contents occurs in normal individuals, mild basal cell hyperplasia and lengthening of the papillae are not uncommon in the distal esophagus. In one study of histologic features of reflux esophagitis,[18] which included a control group of normal individuals (with documented negative 24-hour pH monitoring), basal cell hyperplasia was present at the gastroesophageal junction in 50% (10 of 20) of the control biopsies and papillary elongation was present in 24% (4 of 17). Papillary elongation was also present in biopsies obtained from 2 cm above the gastroesophageal junction in 16% (3 of 19) of the normal control subjects. Thus, the location of the biopsy is an important piece of information in evaluating for histologic features of reflux esophagitis.[18]

Because basal cell hyperplasia and papillary elongation can only be recognized in well-oriented esophageal biopsies other features of reflux are usually more useful in making the histologic diagnosis. Recently, dilatation of intracellular spaces between the squamous cells (spongiosis) was emphasized as an important histologic marker of reflux disease.[19,20] Damage to tight junction by the refluxate causes increased paracellular permeability. By light microscopy the squamous cells appear to be slightly separated from one another and desmosomes can be seen at high power (**Fig. 4**B). This change, although often patchy, does not require optimal biopsy orientation and appears to be a quite sensitive marker. However, it can also be seen in normal individuals in biopsies from the distal esophagus and gastroesophageal junction, again emphasizing that knowledge of the biopsy site is necessary for proper interpretation by the surgical pathologist.

Another histologic feature of reflux that can be assessed in poorly oriented esophageal biopsies is the presence of an intraepithelial inflammatory cell infiltrate. Lymphocytes and Langerhans cells occur normally within the squamous mucosa and can be seen in increased number in many conditions, including reflux, Crohn's disease, celiac disease, drug-induced mucosal injury, and without an identified cause. Because of the nonspecific nature of lymphocytic infiltrates their presence alone is not regarded as diagnostic of reflux or any other condition.[21]

Eosinophils and neutrophils are commonly seen in severe reflux, but are not sensitive markers because they are usually absent in mild cases.[16,17] Neutrophils, which are never normally present in the esophageal squamous mucosa, are usually only seen in the vicinity of erosions or ulcers, and often biopsies are not obtained in such cases as a presumptive endoscopic diagnosis of erosive esophagitis is possible. Whether eosinophils can be found normally in the squamous mucosa has been the topic of much debate. Some authors have stated that even a single intraepithelial eosinophil is abnormal,[22] whereas others allow for rare scattered eosinophils as a normal finding. In the study mentioned previously, rare eosinophils were seen in 2 of the 20 normal adults with negative 24-hour pH monitoring.[18] Again, eosinophils are not a sensitive marker of GERD, being found in only 20% to 40% of patients.

DIFFERENTIAL DIAGNOSIS

In general, biopsies from patients with reflux esophagitis exhibit less than 10 eosinophils per high power field. However, occasionally biopsies with reflux esophagitis will exhibit intramucosal eosinophil densities that reach or exceed the numeric criterion for EE.[23] Subtle differences of the eosinophilic infiltrate may be helpful in delineating this differential and are summarized in **Table 1**. Another histologic feature useful in distinguishing the two is the presence of active or inactive carditis (**Fig. 5**). Gastric carditis is a well-described histologic marker of gastroesophageal reflux disease.[24–27] In contrast, the cardia mucosa

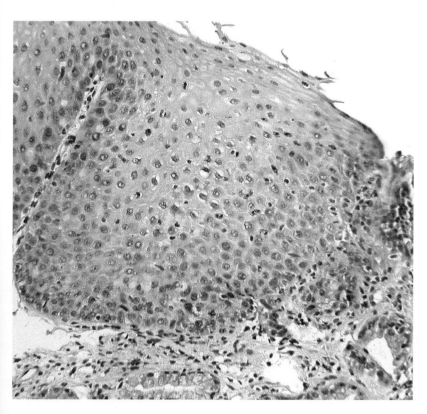

Fig. 5. Reflux esophagitis with a documented abnormal 24-hour pH probe study. The number of intraepithelial eosinophils exceeds 15/HPF in this field.

in patients with EE is not significantly inflamed. In severe cases of reflux with erosion or ulceration, the possibility of drug injury or infection must be ruled out.

DIAGNOSIS

No single histologic feature is specific for reflux esophagitis and biopsies must be evaluated in conjunction with the patients' clinical and medication history. Positive esophageal pH monitoring, measured as a percentage of time with an intraesophageal pH below 4, is a specific method of diagnosing GERD, although it is not always practical, particularly in the pediatric population. Decreased symptoms in response to antisecretory therapy (PPIs or H_2 antagonists) allow for a presumptive diagnosis of GERD; however, reflux esophagitis can only be diagnosed by endoscopy or biopsy.

PROGNOSIS

The diagnosis and assessment of severity in reflux esophagitis is important because it allows for the appropriate management of individual patients. The heterogeneity of symptom response to dietary and medical management is vast. Long-standing reflux has the potential to become a chronic relapsing process. Chronicity risks the development of complications, such as peptic strictures or Barrett's metaplasia, which carries the potential to become dysplastic or frankly malignant. Approximately 11% of patients with reflux esophagitis will also have Barrett's metaplasia.[28–30]

EOSINOPHILIC GASTROENTERITIS INVOLVING THE ESOPHAGUS

OVERVIEW

Although one might assume that eosinophilic esophagitis represents the esophageal form of eosinophilic esophagitis, most authorities actually regard eosinophilic esophagitis as a disorder distinct from eosinophilic gastroenteritis. Because dense mucosal eosinophilic mucosal infiltrates are characteristic of both conditions, other clinical and histologic features are used to separate these two diseases. To make a diagnosis of esophageal involvement by eosinophilic gastroenteritis tissue, eosinophilia must be documented in another portion of the GI tract, or eosinophilic infiltrates must be evident in the deeper layers of the esophageal wall.[31,32]

GROSS APPEARANCE

Eosinophilic gastroenteritis can involve any layer of the wall of the GI tract. In the few described cases of esophageal involvement, eosinophilic infiltration of the muscularis propria resulted in thickening and luminal stenosis.[33,34] Mucosal involvement would presumably lead to an endoscopic appearance similar to that seen in eosinophilic esophagitis.

MICROSCOPIC FEATURES

Dense sheetlike infiltrates of eosinophils are the histologic hallmark of idiopathic eosinophilic gastroenteritis wherever in the gastrointestinal tract it is found. Any bowel layer may be affected. In the esophagus most reported cases have involved the muscularis propria.[31,32] Cases limited to the esophageal squamous mucosa would be labeled as eosinophilic esophagitis unless involvement of other parts of the gastrointestinal tract was also documented to be involved by biopsy.

DIFFERENTIAL DIAGNOSIS

The differential diagnosis includes all of the other diseases that can cause eosinophilic infiltration of the esophageal wall discussed in this content. If only mucosal eosinophilic infiltrates are present, and no other portion of the gastrointestinal tract is affected, then a diagnosis of eosinophilic esophagitis is more appropriate. In eosinophilic gastroenteritis involving the esophagus, the only histologic abnormality is the presence of sheets of eosinophils in the deep layers of the esophageal wall. If the inflammatory cell infiltrate is mixed, or if there is evidence of significant fibrosis or vasculitis, then a systemic connective tissue or systemic vasculitis would be favored. The absence of ganglion cells in the submucosal or myenteric plexus would raise the possibility of Chagas disease. Hypereosinophilic syndrome with gastrointestinal-tract involvement must also be considered.

DIAGNOSIS

Many cases of esophageal involvement by idiopathic eosinophilic gastroenteritis are diagnosed first by biopsy documentation of involvement of another portion of the gastrointestinal tract. Radiographic evidence of thickening of the esophageal wall is then taken as prima facie evidence of esophageal involvement (**Fig. 6**).[31,32] In some cases, endoscopic examination confirms narrowing of the esophageal lumen, whereas biopsies

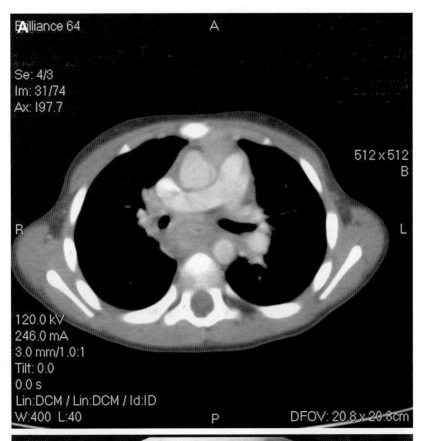

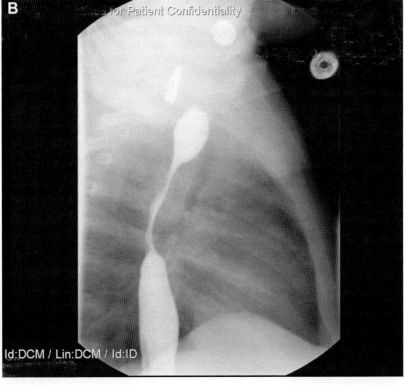

Fig. 6. Eosinophilic gastroenteritis involving the esophagus in a child. (*A*) A CT scan of the thorax demonstrates marked thickening of the esophageal wall. (*B*) Coronal view of the CT scan reveals a segmental stricture of the esophagus.

Fig. 6. (*C*) Endoscopic biopsies of the esophagus reveal dense infiltrates of eosinophils in the lamina propria and infiltration of the overlying epithelium. (*D*) Higher-power view of the esophageal biopsy highlighting the presence of numerous lamina propria eosinophils. (*E*) A gastric biopsy from the same child also reveals dense infiltrates of eosinophils. The duodenal biopsies likewise exhibited dense infiltrates of eosinophils in the submucosa and deep lamina propria (not shown).

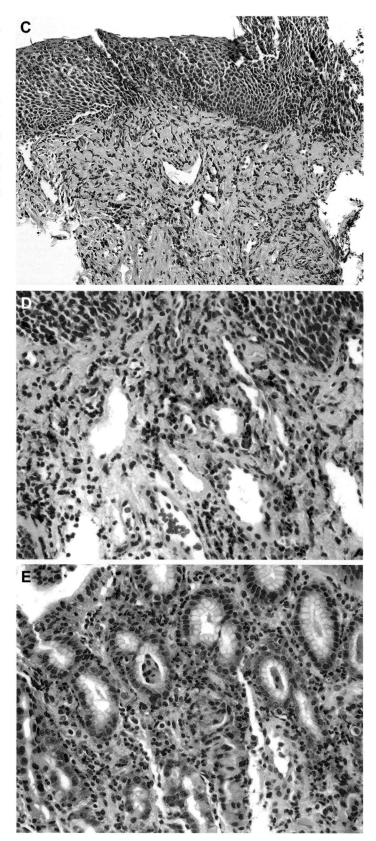

may reveal eosinophilic infiltrates only if submucosal tissue happens to be obtained. A full-thickness biopsy of the esophageal wall is not often performed in these patients.

PROGNOSIS

Most patients with eosinophilic gastroenteritis experience symptomatic improvement following high-dose steroid treatment. Surgery may be necessary for patients with perforation or high-grade obstruction. The long-term prognosis is not well described.[30,31]

DRUG-INDUCED INJURY

OVERVIEW

More than 50 drugs have been reported in the literature to cause esophagitis, but only a few widely used medications are responsible for most of the cases.[34,35] Nonsteroidal antiinflammatory drugs (NSAIDs) and the tetracycline antibiotics (especially doxycycline) together account for approximately two-thirds of the cases of pill-induced esophagitis documented in the literature.[36,37] Another class of drugs that have recently gained attention as a cause of esophagitis is the bisphosphonates, used in the treatment of osteoarthritis. Potassium cholate, ferrous sulfate, and emepronium bromide are other well-known causes of drug-induced esophagitis.[34,35]

Elderly patients are particularly at risk for drug-induced esophagitis, primarily because older individuals consume more medications, but also because decreased esophageal motility is more common in this population. Most injury to the esophagus is direct (pill esophagitis), secondary to surface contact with acidic pill fragments. Gastroesophageal reflux can also contribute to the development of drug-induced esophagitis because many medications cause relaxation of the lower esophageal sphincter.[38] Presenting symptoms include dysphagia, odynophagia, retrosternal pain, or food refusal. There is often an accompanying history of swallowing pill capsules with little or no water and taking medications while bed ridden.

GROSS APPEARANCE

In drug-induced injury, discrete areas of erosion, ulceration, and in severe cases, esophageal strictures may be apparent by endoscopy. Ulceration occurs most often at the narrowing of the midesophagus caused by external compression by the aortic arch. An endoscopically normal esophagus is also capable of harboring pill-induced esophagitis evident only by histologic examination of biopsy specimens.[34]

MICROSCOPIC FEATURES

Although usually well tolerated, drugs can cause severe esophagitis with deep ulceration. The histologic features of drug-induced esophagitis are generally nonspecific. Clear refractile crystalline material from the pill tablets can sometimes be seen in biopsy material, sometimes surrounded by multinucleated foreign body giant cells.[39] There may be a mucosal mixed inflammatory cell infiltrate at times accompanied by erosion or ulceration.[34,35] The inflammatory infiltrate in some NSAID-induced esophagitis cases may have a conspicuous eosinophil component; however, it is always mixed with neutrophils. Basal cell hyperplasia may be absent in patients on NSAIDS who develop reflux as the prostaglandin-inhibitors hinder cell proliferation.[40,41]

DIFFERENTIAL DIAGNOSIS/DIAGNOSIS

Although common, drug-induced injury of the esophagus is under recognized. Barring the rare instance in which portions of the culprit drug are actually present within the histologic section,[39] the nonspecific nature of the histology of drug-induced injury typically precludes a definitive diagnosis. The presence of a discrete ulcer surrounded by endoscopically and histologically normal squamous mucosa is a clue to the diagnosis of pill esophagitis.

PROGNOSIS

Discontinuation or a reduction in dose of the culprit drug normally leads to resolution of the esophageal injury.

ESOPHAGEAL INFECTIONS

OVERVIEW

Within any organ system, the classic infection to cause a truly eosinophil-dominant infiltrate is the parasite. With the exception of *Trypanosoma cruzi*, the parasite that causes Chagas disease that is endemic to South and Central America, parasitic infections of the esophagus are extremely rare and are likely to occur only in the severely immunocompromised.[42,43] In fungal and viral esophageal infections, eosinophils, although at times prominent, will be one component of a mixed inflammatory cell infiltrate. Better antiretroviral therapy for patients infected with HIV has led to a decrease in opportunistic gastrointestinal infections in this population; however, it is important to remember that those patients who are HIV positive without access to health care and patients using steroids or cytotoxic drugs are at risk for opportunistic infections of the esophagus. Candida esophagitis also occurs in patients with diabetes, organ transplant recipients, patients taking oral or inhaled steroids, and patients with altered esophageal motility (eg, scleroderma, achalasia).

GROSS APPEARANCE

In Chagas disease, the parasite infection damages the myenteric plexuses resulting in loss of intramural ganglia and interstitial cells of Cajal in the esophagus and the lower esophageal sphincter.[44,45] Therefore, the classic gross appearance of Chagas disease affecting the esophagus closely resembles achalasia and ultimately megaesophagus. Eosinophilic infiltrates are not evident in the squamous mucosa unless superimposed reflux esophagitis develops.

In the more commonly encountered esophageal infections, endoscopy findings are nonspecific and can range from erythema to ulcerations. Candida esophagitis, the most common esophageal infection, has a considerable range of endoscopic findings, including erythema that mimics severe reflux; white nodules or plaques reminiscent of EE; or in advanced cases narrowed, friable mucosa that may be grossly worrisome for a neoplastic process.[46] Candida albicans is by far the most common species to cause fungal

esophagitis, but other Candida species and other fungi may be responsible in rare cases.[47]

MICROSCOPIC FEATURES

In Chagas disease, the amastigotes of *T cruzi* are found primarily in neurons and muscle fibers of the esophageal wall and are therefore not visible in endoscopic mucosal biopsies. A dense eosinophilic infiltrate may be the only indication of the underlying disease.[44,45]

Candida esophagitis, which at times has a prominent eosinophilic infiltrate within the surface epithelium, is generally accompanied by superficial neutrophilic microabscesses. Identification of the fungal pseudohyphae is important because the budding yeast form of Candida is part of the normal oral gastrointestinal flora and does not necessarily indicate esophagitis. The fungal forms are usually admixed with surface inflammatory debris and desquamated squamous cells (**Fig. 7**).

In HSV esophagitis, the squamous epithelium infected by the virus is typically found at the edge of an ulcer (**Fig. 8**). Infected squamous cells are sometimes multinucleated, and the intranuclear inclusions may be in the form of a central eosinophilic body or produce a diffuse sanded appearance to the nucleus.[48] In contrast, CMV cannot infect squamous cells but instead is found within endothelial cells and fibroblasts present in the granulation tissue of ulcer beds. The typical

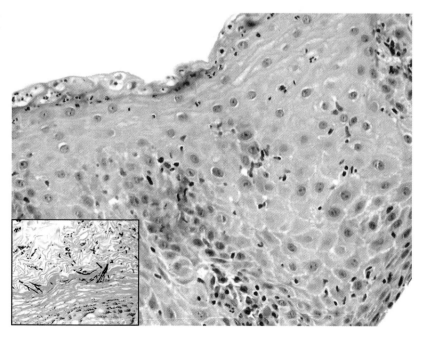

Fig. 7. Candida esophagitis. Note the presence of a focal and mixed inflammatory cell infiltrate. The inset demonstrates fungal elements in a Gomori methenamine silver stain, which were not obvious in the H&E stained section.

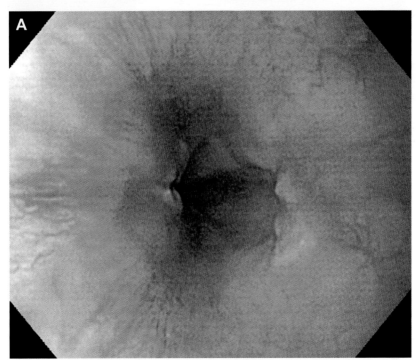

A

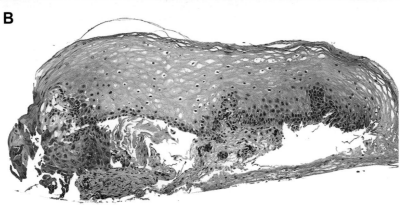

B

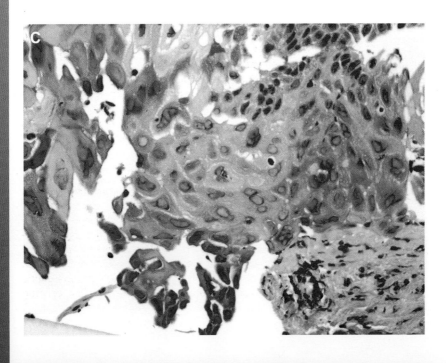

C

Fig. 8. Herpes simplex virus esophagitis. (*A*) This endoscopic photograph reveals a focal esophageal ulceration. (*B*) This low-power view reveals HSV-infected squamous cells at the edge of the ulcer. (*C*) This high-power view reveals typical multinucleated virally infected squamous cells and characteristic intranuclear viral inclusions.

owl's eye intranuclear inclusion may not be evident in patients who are already receiving antiviral therapy.[49] In doubtful cases, immunohistologic stains can be performed to confirm the diagnosis of HSV or CMV esophagitis. Finally, in patients who are severely immunocompromised multiple infections can coexist.

DIFFERENTIAL DIAGNOSIS

When contemplating the diagnosis of eosinophilia secondary to a parasitic infection all other causes of mucosal eosinophilia must be considered (see differential diagnosis box). As in any ulcerated lesion, injury secondary to a drug reaction or a neoplastic process must also be ruled out. CMV and HSV infection may produce focal ulceration similar to that seen in some cases of drug-induced esophagitis. A clinical history of an immunosuppressed state is helpful to raise suspicion of a viral infection.

DIAGNOSIS

Organisms may not always be identified on H&E sections. Special stains for fungus may increase sensitivity. If ulcers are present, biopsies should be targeted to include areas from the ulcer base, ulcer edge, and adjacent intact mucosa. For patients on antiviral therapy, viral culture may be a more sensitive test than examination of biopsy specimens; therefore, when infection is suspected specimens should be sent to surgical pathology for histologic review and microbiology. Because the surface plaque containing fungal organisms is easily dislodged and lost during the processing of esophageal biopsy specimens, cytologic examination of esophageal

---

⚠️⚠️ *Differential Diagnosis*
GRANULOMATOUS ESOPHAGITIS

- Crohn's disease
- Sarcoidosis
- Tuberculosis
- Fungal infection
- Behçet's Disease
- Chronic granulomatous disease
- Foreign body
- Neoplasia

---

brush preparations is a key method to increase diagnostic yield.[50]

PROGNOSIS

Most patients diagnosed with infectious esophagitis are immunocompromised. Identifying an infectious process in a timely manner is critical because infectious esophagitis is a major cause of complications and morbidity in these patients. Prognosis improves greatly with restoration of normal immune status either through effective management of antiretroviral therapy or decreasing immunosuppression in patients not infected with HIV.

CROHN'S DISEASE

OVERVIEW

Crohn's disease affecting the esophagus is rare but its complications can be severe, so early diagnosis is warranted. The true incidence is unknown; however, prospective studies indicate that at least 5% of the adult and pediatric population with Crohn's disease can be expected to have esophageal involvement. Symptoms can be nonspecific or nonexistent and commonly do not correlate well with endoscopy findings.[51–53]

GROSS APPEARANCE

Endoscopy findings can range from erythema, erosions, and aphthous ulcers to late-stage findings, such as stricture; cobblestoning; and fistula formation, which have the potential to mimic a neoplastic process.[51–53]

MICROSCOPIC FEATURES

In general, the histopathologic features of Crohn esophagitis are that of a nonspecific esophagitis or erosive esophagitis. When present, the granulomas of esophageal Crohn's disease are dense, sarcoidlike, with no central necrosis (**Fig. 9**). These features should always be reviewed concurrently with other specimens of the upper GI tract and ideally also with lower GI biopsies.[51–53]

DIFFERENTIAL DIAGNOSIS

Although eosinophils may be prominent in Crohn esophagitis, more commonly the inflammatory cell infiltrates will be mixed. If granulomas are identified in the lamina propria special stains for organisms may be warranted (see Differential diagnosis list previously mentioned). If erosion or ulceration is endoscopically evident, biopsies should exclude neoplasia, infection, reflux esophagitis, or drug injury.

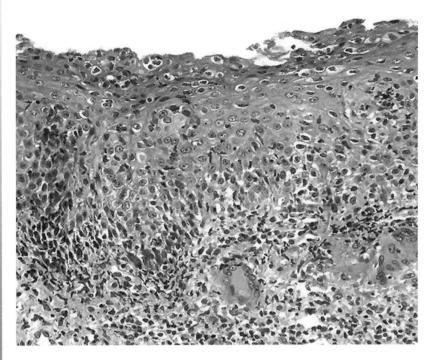

Fig. 9. Crohn esophagitis. A small granuloma is evident in the lamina propria. The overlying epithelium exhibits nonspecific esophagitis with a mixed inflammatory cell infiltrate.

DIAGNOSIS

The presence of granulomas in the correct clinical context is diagnostic of Crohn esophagitis. However, most biopsies will show a nonspecific esophagitis with or without giant cells. Therefore, the evaluation of extraesophageal involvement is critical for diagnosis.

PROGNOSIS

Severe Crohn esophagitis has long-term complications that may require surgical intervention. Early detection allows for appropriate medical management and improved prognosis.[54–57] Currently there is no evidence to suggest that patients with Crohn's disease with esophageal involvement differ from those that do not in terms of overall prognosis.

COLLAGEN VASCULAR DISEASE/ALLERGIC VASCULITIS

OVERVIEW

Collagen vascular and rheumatoid diseases, such as scleroderma, systemic lupus erythematous, mixed connective tissue disorders, and poly/dermatomyositis, can affect the esophagus. As elsewhere in the body, the inflammation associated with vascular disorders are often nonspecific with a dense eosinophilic component. Of the true vasculitides, Churg-Straus syndrome is the one

classically to be accompanied by a significant eosinophilia. Churg-Straus is a systemic disease characterized by asthma, blood and tissue eosinophilia, and a systemic-wide small vessel vasculitis. The vasculitis generally appears later in the disease; early in its course Churg-Straus syndrome can be difficult to distinguish from eosinophilic gastroenteritis or hypereosinophilic syndrome.[58,59] Although extremely rare, there are cases of esophageal involvement presenting as the initial manifestation of Churg-Straus syndrome.[60,61]

GROSS APPEARANCE

There is no distinct gross or endoscopic appearance in the collagen vascular diseases.

MICROSCOPIC FEATURES/DIFFERENTIAL DIAGNOSIS/DIAGNOSIS

In the biopsy specimens of everyday practice, patients with collagen vascular diseases will have, at best, a nonspecific esophagitis with a dense eosinophilic infiltrate. In 2 published cases of Churg-Strauss syndrome presenting in the esophagus, biopsies showed only intense inflammatory cell infiltrates composed mainly of eosinophils. Vasculitis was never identified and the diagnosis was made by applying the American College of Rheumatology classification criteria.[60] As in all of the diseases within the differential

Pitfalls
ESOPHAGEAL EOSINOPHILIA

! Esophageal biopsies should not be performed and read in isolation. Inadequate sampling of the esophagus (eg, distal only) may impede the diagnosis of eosinophilic esophagitis. Furthermore, limiting biopsies to the esophagus (ie, not submitting additional upper GI specimens, such as stomach and duodenum) prohibits the exclusion of systemic diseases, such as Crohn's disease or eosinophilic gastroenteritis.

! The clinical context must fit the diagnosis. An esophageal biopsy that shows 15 eosinophils per high power field meets the current histologic criteria for a diagnosis of eosinophilic esophagitis; however, if that patient has not been on a proton pump inhibitor and a 24-hour pH probe test demonstrates gastroesophageal reflux, the biopsy findings are more likely a result of severe reflux esophagitis.

diagnosis of esophageal eosinophilia, this emphasizes the need to apply clinical context to the findings on histologic examination.

Finally, patients with these disorders are at increased risk for drug-induced injury or opportunistic infections secondary to immunosuppression. These conditions should be ruled out in patients with a known history of a collagen vascular disease.

PROGNOSIS

Treatment and prognosis of these disorders are highly variable.

REFERENCES

1. Kapel RC, Miller JK, Torres C, et al. Eosinophilic esophagitis: a prevalent disease in the United States that affects all age groups. Gastroenterology 2008; 134:1316–21.
2. Spergel JM, Brown-Whitehorn TF, Beausoleil JL, et al. 14 years of eosinophilic esophagitis: clinical features and prognosis. J Pediatr Gastroenterol Nutr 2008;48:30–6.
3. Liacouras CA, Spergel JM, Ruchelli E, et al. Eosinophilic esophagitis: a 10-year experience in 381 children. Clin Gastroenterol Hepatol 2005;3: 1198–206.
4. Yamazaki K, Murray JA, Arora AS, et al. Allergen-specific in vitro cytokine production in adult patients with eosinophilic esophagitis. Dig Dis Sci 2006;51: 1934–41.
5. Mishra A, Hogan SP, Brandt EB, et al. An etiological role for aeroallergens and eosinophils in experimental esophagitis. J Clin Invest 2001;107:83–90.
6. Fogg MI, Ruchelli E, Spergel JM. Pollen and eosinophilic esophagitis. J Allergy Clin Immunol 2003; 112:796–7.
7. Desai TK, Stecevic V, Chang C, et al. Association of eosinophilic inflammation with esophageal food impaction in adults. Gastrointest Endosc 2005;61: 795–801.
8. De Angelis P, Markowitz JE, Torroni F, et al. Paediatric eosinophilic oesophagitis: towards early diagnosis and best treatment. Dig Liver Dis 2006;38:245–51.
9. Straumann A, Spichtin H, Bucher KA, et al. Eosinophilic esophagitis: red on microscopy, white on endoscopy. Digestion 2004;70:109–16.
10. Furuta GT, Liacouras CA, Collins MH, et al. Eosinophilic esophagitis in children and adults: a systematic review and consensus recommendations for diagnosis and treatment. Gastroenterology 2007;133:1342–63.
11. Steiner SJ, Kernek KM, Fitzgerald JF. Severity of basal cell hyperplasia differs in reflux versus eosinophilic esophagitis. J Pediatr Gastroenterol Nutr 2006;42:506–9.
12. Mueller S, Neureiter D, Aigner T, et al. Comparison of histologic parameters for the diagnosis of eosinophilic oesophagitis versus gastro-oesophageal reflux disease on oesophageal biopsy material. Histopathology 2008;53:676–84.
13. Camilleri M, Dubois D, Coulie B, et al. Prevalence and socioeconomic impact of upper gastrointestinal disorders in the United States: results of the US Upper Gastrointestinal Study. Clin Gastroenterol Hepatol 2005;3:543–52.
14. Locke GR, Talley NJ, Fett SL, et al. Prevalence and clinical spectrum of gastroesophageal reflux: a population-based study in Olmsted County, Minnesota. Gastroenterology 1997;112:1448–56.
15. Nelson SP, Chen EH, Syniar GM, et al. Prevalence of symptoms of gastroesophageal reflux during childhood: a pediatric practice-based survey. Pediatric Practice Research Group. Arch Pediatr Adolesc Med 2000;154:150–4.
16. Allende DS, Yerian LM. Diagnosing gastroesophageal reflux disease: the pathologist's perspective. Adv Anat Pathol 2009;16:161–5.
17. Fiocca R, Mastracci L, Riddell R, et al. Development of consensus guidelines for the histologic recognition of microscopic esophagitis in patients with gastroesophageal reflux disease: the Esohisto project. Hum Pathol 2010;41:223–31.
18. Mastracci L, Spaggiari P, Grillo F, et al. Microscopic esophagitis in gastro-esophageal reflux disease: individual lesions, biopsy sampling, and clinical correlation. Virchows Arch 2009;454:31–9.

19. Ravelli AM, Villanacci V, Ruzzenenti N, et al. Dilated intercellular spaces: a major morphological feature of esophagitis. J Pediatr Gastroenterol Nutr 2006; 42:510–5.

20. Orlando LA, Orlando RC. Dilated intercellular spaces as a marker of GERD. Curr Gastroenterol Rep 2009;11:190–4.

21. Purdy JK, Appelamn HD, Golembeski CP, et al. Lymphocytic esophagitis: a chronic or recurring pattern of esophagitis resembling allergic contact dermatitis. Am J Clin Pathol 2008;130:508–13.

22. DeBrosse CW, Case JW, Putnam PE, et al. Quantity and distribution of eosinophils in the gastrointestinal tract of children. Pediatr Dev Pathol 2006;9:210–8.

23. Rodrigo S, Abboud G, Oh D, et al. High intraepithelial eosinophil counts in esophageal squamous epithelium are not specific for eosinophilic esophagitis in adults. Am J Gastroenterol 2008;103: 435–42.

24. Csendes A, Smok G, Burdiles P, et al. 'Carditis': an objective histological marker for pathologic gastroesophageal reflux disease. Dis Esophagus 1998; 11:101–5.

25. Der R, Tsao-Wei DD, Demeester T, et al. Carditis: a manifestation of gastroesophageal reflux disease. Am J Surg Pathol 2001;25:245–52.

26. Glickman JN, Fox V, Antonioli DA, et al. Morphology of the cardia and significance of carditis in pediatric patients. Am J Surg Pathol 2002;26:1032–9.

27. Borrelli O, Hassall E, D'Armiento F, et al. Inflammation of the gastric cardia in children with symptoms of acid peptic disease. J Pediatr 2003;143:520–4.

28. Winters C, Spurling TJ, Chobanian SJ, et al. Barrett's esophagus. A prevalent, occult complication of gastroesophageal reflux disease. Gastroenterology 1987;92:118–24.

29. Mann NS, Tsai MF, Nair PK. Barrett's esophagus in patients with symptomatic reflux esophagitis. Am J Gastroenterol 1989;84:1494–6.

30. Csendes A, Smok G, Burdiles P, et al. Prevalence of Barrett's esophagus by endoscopy and histologic studies: a prospective evaluation of 306 control subjects and 376 patients with symptoms of gastroesophageal reflux. Dis Esophagus 2000;13:5–11.

31. Khan S, Orenstein SR. Eosinophilic gastroenteritis. Gastroenterol Clin North Am 2008;37:333–48.

32. Straumann A. Idiopathic eosinophilic gastrointestinal diseases in adults. Best Pract Res Clin Gastroenterol 2008;22:481–6.

33. Yan BM, Shaffer EA. Primary eosinophilic disorders of the gastrointestinal tract. Gut 2009;58:721–32.

34. Oh HE, Chetty R. Eosinophilic gastroenteritis: a review. J Gastroenterol 2008;43:741–50.

35. Zografos GN, Georgiadou D, Thomas D, et al. Drug-induced esophagitis. Dis Esophagus 2009;22:633–7.

36. Noffsinger AE. Update on esophagitis: controversial and underdiagnosed causes. Arch Pathol Lab Med 2009;133:1087–95.

37. Kadayifci A, Gulsen MT, Koruk M, et al. Doxycycline-induced pill esophagitis. Dis Esophagus 2004;17: 168–71.

38. Parfitt JR, Driman DK. Pathological effects of drugs on the gastrointestinal tract: a review. Hum Pathol 2007;38:527–36.

39. Abraham SC, Bhagavan BS, Lee LA, et al. Upper gastrointestinal tract injury in patients receiving Kayexalate (sodium polystyrene sulfonate) in sorbitol. Am J Surg Pathol 2001;25:637–44.

40. Sopeña F, Lanas A, Sáinz R. Esophageal motility and intraesophageal pH patterns in patients with esophagitis and chronic nonsteroidal anti-inflammatory drug use. J Clin Gastroenterol 1998; 27:316–20.

41. Mason JC. NSAIDs and the oesophagus. Eur J Gastroenterol Hepatol 1999;11:369–73.

42. Bittencourt AL, Vieira GO, Tavares HC, et al. Esophageal involvement in congenital Chagas' disease. Report of a case with megaesophagus. Am J Trop Med Hyg 1984;33:30–3.

43. Ferreira MS, Nishioka SDA, Silvestre MT, et al. Reactivation of Chagas' disease in patients with AIDS: report of three new cases and review of the literature. Clin Infect Dis 1997;25:1397–400.

44. Meneghelli UG. Chagas' disease: a model of denervation in the study of digestive tract motility. Braz J Med Biol Res 1985;18:255–64.

45. de Lima MA, Cabrine-Santos M, Tavares MG, et al. Interstitial cells of Cajal in chagasic megaesophagus. Ann Diagn Pathol 2008;12:271–4.

46. Underwood JA, Williams JW, Keate RF. Clinical findings and risk factors for Candida esophagitis in outpatients. Dis Esophagus 2003;16:66–9.

47. Kliemann DA, Pasqualotto AC, Falavigna M, et al. Candida esophagitis: species distribution and risk factors for infection. Rev Inst Med Trop Sao Paulo 2008;50:261–3.

48. McBane RD, Gross JB. Herpes esophagitis: clinical syndrome, endoscopic appearance, and diagnosis in 23 patients. Gastrointest Endosc 1991;37:600–3.

49. Forrest G. Gastrointestinal infections in immunocompromised hosts. Curr Opin Gastroenterol 2004;20:16–21.

50. Geisinger KR. Endoscopic biopsies and cytologic brushings of the esophagus are diagnostically complementary. Am J Clin Pathol 1995;103:295–9.

51. Ruuska T, Vaajalahti P, Arajärvi P, et al. Prospective evaluation of upper gastrointestinal mucosal lesions in children with ulcerative colitis and Crohn's disease. J Pediatr Gastroenterol Nutr 1994;19:181–6.

52. Alcántara M, Rodriguez R, Potenciano JL, et al. Endoscopic and bioptic findings in the upper gastrointestinal tract in patients with Crohn's disease. Endoscopy 1993;25:282–6.

53. Isaacs KL. Upper gastrointestinal tract endoscopy in inflammatory bowel disease. Gastrointest Endosc Clin N Am 2002;12:451–62.

54. Feagans J, Victor D, Joshi V. Crohn disease of the esophagus: a review of the literature. South Med J 2008;101:927–30.

55. Ramaswamy K, Jacobson K, Jevon G, et al. Esophageal Crohn disease in children: a clinical spectrum. J Pediatr Gastroenterol Nutr 2003;36:454–8.

56. Decker GA, Loftus EV, Pasha TM, et al. Crohn's disease of the esophagus: clinical features and outcomes. Inflamm Bowel Dis 2001;7:113–9.

57. D'Haens G, Rutgeerts P, Geboes K, et al. The natural history of esophageal Crohn's disease: three patterns of evolution. Gastrointest Endosc 1994;40:296–300.

58. Hellmich B, Holl-Ulrich K, Merz H, et al. [Hypereosinophilic syndrome and Churg-Strauss syndrome: is it clinically relevant to differentiate these syndromes?]. Internist (Berl) 2008;49:286–96 [in German].

59. Bailey M, Chapin W, Licht H, et al. The effects of vasculitis on the gastrointestinal tract and liver. Gastroenterol Clin North Am 1998;2:747–82.

60. Mir O, Nazal E, Cohen P, et al. Esophageal involvement as an initial manifestation of Churg-Strauss syndrome. Presse Med 2007;36(1 Pt 1): 57–60.

61. Pagnoux C, Mahr A, Cohen P, et al. Presentation and outcome of gastrointestinal involvement in systemic necrotizing vasculitides: analysis of 62 patients with polyarteritis nodosa, microscopic polyangiitis, Wegener granulomatosis, Churg-Strauss syndrome, or rheumatoid arthritis-associated vasculitis. Medicine (Baltimore) 2005; 84:115–28.

INFECTIOUS DISEASES OF THE LOWER GASTROINTESTINAL TRACT

Laura W. Lamps, MD

KEYWORDS

• Infection • Colitis • Ischemia • Inflammatory bowel disease • Granuloma

ABSTRACT

Gastrointestinal (GI) infections are a major cause of morbidity and mortality worldwide. Although infectious organisms are often recovered by microbiological methods, surgical pathologists play an invaluable role in diagnosis. The lower GI tract, including the appendix, large bowel, and anus, harbors a wide variety of pathogens. Some infections are part of disseminated disease, whereas others produce clinicopathologic scenarios that are specific to the lower GI tract. This review focuses on selected infectious disorders of the lower GI tract that may be encountered by the general surgical pathologist, including viral, bacterial, fungal, and parasitic organisms, and including infections caused by food- and water-borne pathogens. Diagnostic gross and histologic features are discussed, as well as useful clinical features and ancillary diagnostic techniques. Pertinent differential diagnoses are also emphasized, including other inflammatory conditions of the gut (such as ischemia or idiopathic inflammatory bowel disease) that can be mimicked by lower GI infections.

OVERVIEW

Gastrointestinal infections are one of the most important causes of morbidity and mortality worldwide. Enteric pathogens are the leading childhood cause of death in the world, and are the second leading cause of death among all ages. The number of bone marrow and solid organ transplant patients is also increasing, as well as the population of patients with other immunocompromising conditions. In addition, as global urbanization, immigration, and transcontinental travel become more frequent, infectious diseases that were once limited to certain regions of the world could be encountered by any practicing anatomic pathologist.

The goals of the surgical pathologist in evaluating lower gastrointestinal specimens for infection are essentially twofold:

First, acute self-limited and/or infectious processes should be distinguished from chronic idiopathic inflammatory bowel disease (ulcerative colitis and Crohn disease), ischemia, and other chronic colitides such as lymphocytic colitis.

Second, dedicated attempts must be made to identify the specific infectious organism(s). A discussion with the gastroenterologist regarding symptoms and macroscopic findings, as well as knowledge of travel history, food intake (such as sushi or poorly cooked meat), sexual practices, and immune status, can be valuable in the evaluation of specimens for infectious diseases.

Surgical pathologists should also be aware of the infections that are most likely to mimic other inflammatory bowel diseases, particularly Crohn disease, ulcerative colitis, and ischemic colitis (Table 1). This article focuses on selected infections of the lower gastrointestinal tract that are likely to be encountered by surgical pathologists, with an emphasis on those that mimic chronic idiopathic inflammatory bowel disease and/or ischemic colitis.

Department of Pathology, University of Arkansas for Medical Sciences, 4301 West Markham Street, Shorey 4S/09, Little Rock, AR 72205, USA
E-mail address: lampslauraw@uams.edu

Surgical Pathology 3 (2010) 297–326
doi:10.1016/j.path.2010.05.009
1875-9181/10/$ – see front matter © 2010 Elsevier Inc. All rights reserved.

Key Features
INFECTIOUS DISEASES OF THE LOWER GASTROINTESTINAL TRACT

Cytomegalovirus

1. Ulcers are most common gross and microscopic finding

2. Infected cells are enlarged, with "owl's eye" nuclear and basophilic cytoplasmic inclusions

Vasotropic fungi

1. Characteristic nodular infarction

2. Fungi radiate outward from vessel

Salmonella

1. Typhoid species: Ulcerated Peyer patch; mononuclear cells predominate

2. Nontyphoid species: Neutrophilic cryptitis, crypt abscesses

3. Can cause marked architectural distortion

Yersinia

1. One of the most common causes of isolated granulomatous appendicitis

2. Gross and histologic features may be histologically indistinguishable from Crohn disease

Enterohemorrhagic *Escherichia coli*

1. Most often affects right colon

2. Histologic features indistinguishable from ischemia of other causes

Amoebiasis

1. May closely mimic chronic idiopathic inflammatory bowel disease

2. Ingested red blood cells characteristic of *Entamoeba histolytica*

3. Organisms may be scarce, and difficult to distinguish from macrophages

CYTOMEGALOVIRUS

CYTOMEGALOVIRUS: OVERVIEW

Cytomegalovirus (CMV) infection can develop anywhere in the lower gastrointestinal tract.[1-3] CMV is best known as an opportunistic pathogen in the context of a suppressed immune system, and is the most common gastrointestinal pathogen overall in patients with AIDS.[1-3] The most common clinical symptoms of gastrointestinal infection are diarrhea (either bloody or watery), abdominal pain, fever, and weight loss.[1-3] Primary CMV infections in immunocompetent persons are generally self-limited; they are usually asymptomatic, but may be associated with a mononucleosis-like syndrome.[4]

CYTOMEGALOVIRUS: GROSS FEATURES

CMV causes a variety of gross lesions.[1-3] Ulceration is the most common, regardless of site; ulcers may be single or multiple, and either superficial or deep. Ulcers are often very large (>10.0 cm), with a well-circumscribed, "punched-out" appearance and intervening normal mucosa. Segmental ulcerative lesions and linear ulcers may mimic Crohn disease grossly (**Fig. 1**). Other macroscopic lesions include mucosal erosions, erythema, hemorrhage, pseudomembranes, and inflammatory polyps or masses.[5,6]

CYTOMEGALOVIRUS: MICROSCOPIC FEATURES

Similar to the spectrum of gross pathology, the histologic spectrum of CMV infection is also extremely variable, ranging from minimal inflammatory reaction to deep ulcers with prominent granulation tissue and necrosis.[1-3] Frequent histologic features include mucosal ulceration (**Fig. 2**), a mixed inflammatory infiltrate often including numerous neutrophils, and cryptitis (**Fig. 3**). Crypt abscesses, crypt atrophy and loss, and numerous apoptotic enterocytes may be seen as well. Prominent aggregates of macrophages may be seen surrounding viral inclusions, sometimes in a perivascular distribution within granulation tissue, or within the inflammatory exudates.[7] Characteristic inclusions with virtually no associated inflammatory reaction may occur in severely immunocompromised patients.

As indicated by the name "cytomegalovirus," infected cells show both nuclear and cytoplasmic enlargement. Inclusions are preferentially found in endothelial cells, stromal cells, and macrophages, and rarely in glandular epithelial cells. Characteristic "owl's eye" intranuclear viral inclusions (**Fig. 4**) and basophilic granular intracytoplasmic inclusions (**Fig. 5**) may be seen on routine hematoxylin-eosin (H&E) preparations. Unlike adenovirus and herpes, CMV inclusions are often found deep within ulcer bases rather than at the edges of ulcers or in the superficial mucosa. In biopsy specimens, the diagnosis may

Table 1
Selected infectious mimics of chronic idiopathic inflammatory bowel disease and ischemic colitis

Mimics of Crohn Disease	Mimics of Ulcerative Colitis	Mimics of Ischemic Colitis
Cytomegalovirus	*Shigella* species	Cytomegalovirus
Salmonella species	*Salmonella* species, particularly nontyphoid	*Aspergillus*
Shigella species	*Entamoeba histolytica*	Zygomycetes
Yersinia	*Aeromonas* species	Enterohemorrhagic *Escherichia coli*
Mycobacterium tuberculosis	Rarely *Campylobacter*	*Clostridium difficile* (pseudomembranous colitis)
Aeromonas species		
Rarely *Campylobacter*		
Entamoeba histolytica		

be easily missed when only rare inclusions are present.

Of importance is that the gastrointestinal tract is also one of the most commonly affected organ systems in CMV vasculitis.[5,8,9] Histologic findings include endothelial viral inclusions with associated inflammation, necrosis, and thrombosis of the affected vessel (**Fig. 6**). Surrounding tissue shows associated mucosal ulceration, hemorrhage, and ischemic necrosis (**Fig. 7**). CMV inclusions alone within vascular endothelial cells are not diagnostic of vasculitis; the presence of associated inflammation of the vessel wall should be present, as well as thrombosis.

CYTOMEGALOVIRUS: DIFFERENTIAL DIAGNOSIS

The differential diagnosis of CMV infection is primarily other viral infections, particularly adenovirus. Adenovirus inclusions are usually crescent-shaped, located within surface epithelium, and exclusively intranuclear. CMV inclusions have an "owl's eye" morphology in the nucleus, are most often located within endothelial or stromal cells, and may be present within either the nucleus or cytoplasm. In addition, adenovirus does not usually produce significant macroscopic findings.

Fig. 1. Irregular, serpiginous ulcer with mucosal cobblestoning in the right colon of a patient with CMV colitis.

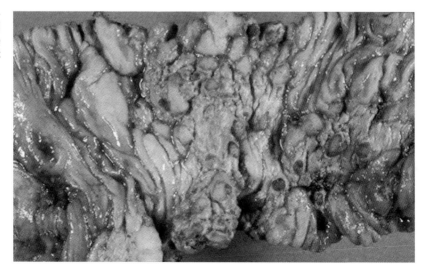

> ## △△ Differential Diagnosis
> ### INFECTIOUS DISEASES OF THE LOWER GASTROINTESTINAL TRACT
>
> Cytomegalovirus
>
> >Other viral infections
> >
> >Graft-versus-host disease
> >
> >Chronic idiopathic inflammatory bowel disease
> >
> >Ischemia
>
> Vasotropic fungi
>
> >Other infectious processes
> >
> >Ischemia
>
> Salmonella
>
> >Other infectious processes
> >
> >Chronic idiopathic inflammatory bowel disease
>
> Yersinia
>
> >Other infectious processes, particularly mycobacterial or fungal infection
> >
> >Crohn disease
>
> Enterohemorrhagic *E coli*
>
> >Ischemia
> >
> >Pseudomembranous colitis
>
> Amoebiasis
>
> >Other infectious processes
> >
> >>Nonpathogenic amoebae
> >>
> >>*Balantidium coli*
> >>
> >>Pseudomembranous colitis
> >
> >Chronic idiopathic inflammatory bowel disease
> >
> >Malignancy (amoeboma)

Distinction between CMV infection and graft-versus-host disease in bone marrow transplant patients may be particularly difficult, because the clinical and histologic features are very similar.[10] Immunohistochemistry or in situ hybridization studies should be employed to rule out CMV infection in this clinical setting, because failure to identify CMV infection could result in delay of antiviral therapy. Furthermore, these CMV infection and graft-versus-host disease

may coexist. Graft-versus-host disease is favored when there is abundant apoptosis associated with crypt necrosis and dropout, in the setting of minimal inflammation.

As mentioned, CMV infection can mimic chronic idiopathic inflammatory bowel disease and ischemia. CMV vasculitis with associated ischemia should be considered in any immunocompromised patient with bowel ischemia.[5,8,9] CMV infection should always be considered in the differential diagnosis of chronic idiopathic inflammatory bowel disease as well, because CMV can mimic Crohn disease and ulcerative colitis both grossly and microscopically.

In addition, secondary CMV infection may be superimposed on ulcerative colitis and Crohn disease.[11,12] In such cases, CMV superinfection is associated with exacerbations of the underlying disease, steroid-refractory disease, and a higher rate of complications. For this reason, some authorities recommend immunohistochemical evaluation for CMV as part of the routine evaluation of biopsies in steroid-refractory chronic idiopathic inflammatory bowel disease patients. The presence of CMV inclusions and acute inflammatory changes superimposed on well-developed features of chronicity, such as architectural distortion or neural hyperplasia, helps to establish a background of chronic idiopathic inflammatory bowel disease with superimposed CMV infection, rather than CMV infection alone.

CYTOMEGALOVIRUS: DIAGNOSIS

Examination of multiple levels, and use of immunohistochemistry, is extremely valuable in the diagnosis of CMV infection, particularly when inclusions are rare.[10,13] Other diagnostic aids include viral culture, polymerase chain reaction (PCR) assays, in situ hybridization, and serologic studies/antigen tests.[13] Isolation of CMV in culture, however, does not imply active infection, because virus may be excreted for months to years after a primary infection.

CYTOMEGALOVIRUS: PROGNOSIS

The prognosis is heavily dependent on the immune status of the patient. Antiviral therapy may be effective, but disseminated infection in severely immunocompromised patients may be fatal. As mentioned above, it is important to consider and exclude CMV in the context of colonic ischemia, graft-versus-host disease, and chronic idiopathic inflammatory bowel disease, so that there is no delay in antiviral therapy.

Fig. 2. (*A*) Deep fissuring ulcer in CMV colitis. (*B*) Numerous CMV inclusions are seen within stromal cells and macrophages at the base of the ulcer.

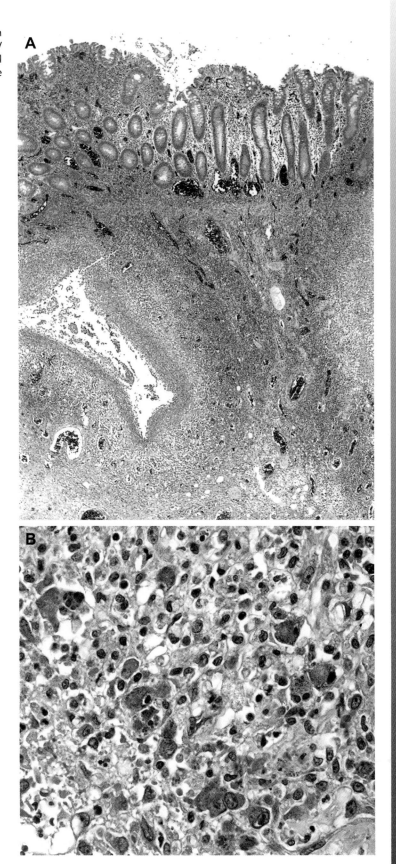

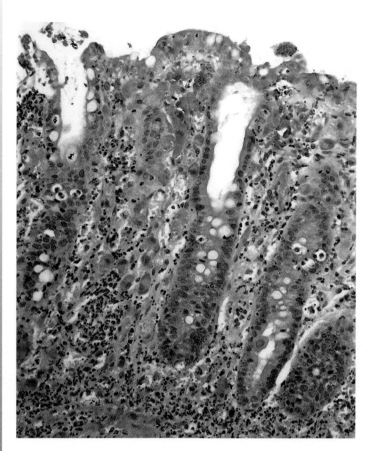

Fig. 3. CMV colitis featuring cryptitis, numerous apoptotic epithelial cells, a neutrophilic infiltrate in the lamina propria, and numerous inclusions within the endothelial and stromal cells.

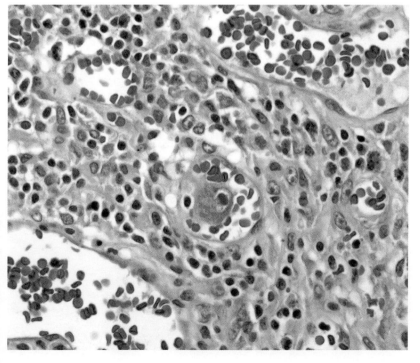

Fig. 4. The characteristic "owl's eye" inclusion of CMV within an endothelial cell at the base of a colonic ulcer.

Fig. 5. Granular, baso-
philic cytoplasmic CMV
inclusion in the base of
a colonic ulcer.

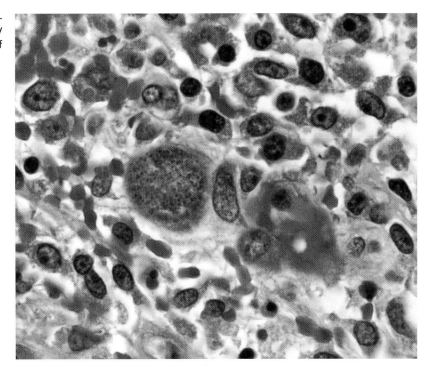

Fig. 6. CMV vasculitis,
featuring numerous endo-
thelial inclusions, acute
inflammation of the vessel
wall, and a fibrin
thrombus. (*Courtesy of* Dr
Margie Scott.)

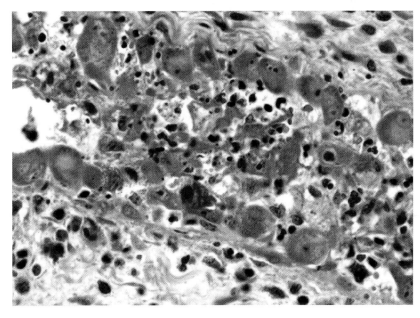

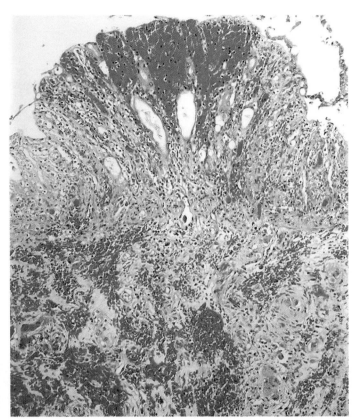

Fig. 7. Right colon ischemia associated with CMV vasculitis in a renal transplant patient.

VASOTROPIC FUNGI: *ASPERGILLUS* AND ZYGOMYCETES

VASOTROPIC FUNGI: OVERVIEW

Fungal infections of the GI tract are often a part of a disseminated disease process, but lower gastrointestinal symptoms and signs may be the presenting or dominant manifestations.[14-18] *Aspergillus* infection of the lower gastrointestinal tract occurs almost exclusively in immunocompromised patients, particularly those with prolonged neutropenia; therefore, bone marrow transplant recipients are at particular risk for infection.[19,20] The majority of patients with aspergillosis also have coexistent lung lesions. Gastrointestinal zygomycosis is relatively uncommon, and infection is associated with diabetes and other causes of metabolic acidosis, deferoxamine therapy, skin and soft tissue breakdown, intravenous drug use, neonatal prematurity, and malnourishment.[21-23] Signs and symptoms of lower gastrointestinal fungal infection include diarrhea, melena, frank GI bleeding, abdominal pain, and fever.[14-18,21-23]

VASOTROPIC FUNGI: GROSS FEATURES

The colon is the most frequent site of gastrointestinal involvement in aspergillosis, and is frequently involved in zygomycosis as well. Multiple sites of concomitant involvement are common.[15-19] The characteristic histologic lesion of aspergillosis is a nodular mucosal infarction ("target lesion") consisting of a central necrotic zone surrounded by a ring of hemorrhage (**Fig. 8**).[14-19] Ulcers are the most common gross manifestation of zygomycosis, and they are often large with rolled, irregular edges, mimicking malignancy.[21-24] These fungi may also superinfect preexisting ulcers.

VASOTROPIC FUNGI: MICROSCOPIC FEATURES

Aspergillus characteristically produces a nodular zone of ischemic necrosis centered on blood vessels containing fungi (**Fig. 9**).[14,25] Fungal hyphae often extend outward from the infarct in parallel or radial arrays (**Fig. 10**). The inflammatory response is variable and ranges from

Fig. 8. Characteristic gross "target lesion" of aspergillosis, with a central zone of necrosis and an outer zone of hemorrhage.

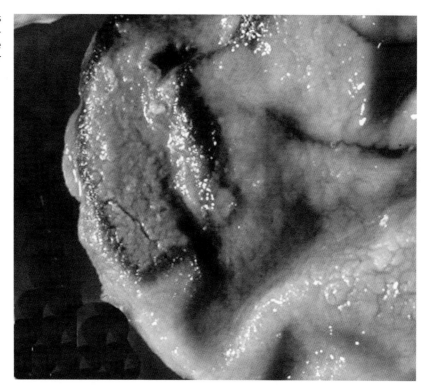

Fig. 9. Nodular zone of infarction at the ileocecal valve in a patient with aspergillosis. The central zone of necrosis is surrounded by acute inflammation and nuclear debris.

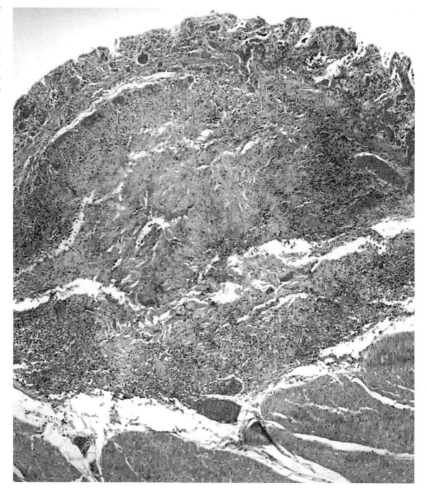

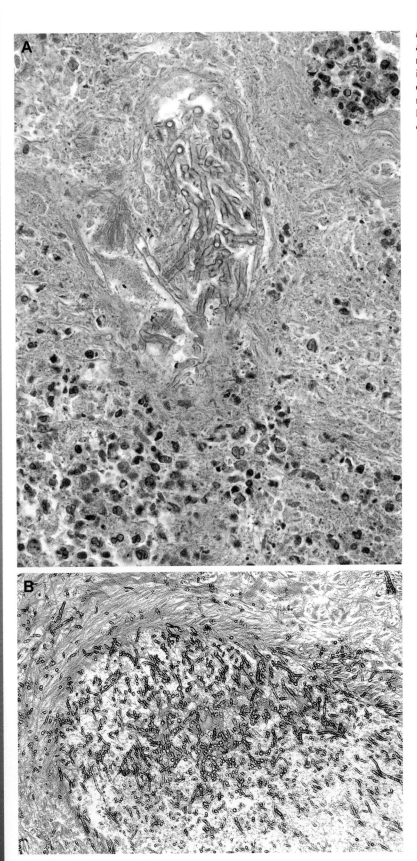

Fig. 10. (*A*) *Aspergillus* fills a vessel lumen, which is surrounded by necrosis, acute inflammation, and nuclear debris. (*B*) Gomori methenamine silver (GMS) stain highlights the fungi within an occluded vessel.

minimal to marked, with a prominent neutrophilic infiltrate. Granulomatous inflammation may occur as well. Transmural infarction of the bowel wall is common. The typical hyphae of *Aspergillus* are septate, have parallel walls, and branch at acute angles (**Fig. 11**).[14] The histologic lesions of zygomycosis are very similar to aspergillosis.[14,21–25] In contrast to *Aspergillus*, zygomycetes have broad, ribbon-like, pauciseptate hyphae with irregular walls, which branch randomly at various angles (**Fig. 12**).[14]

VASOTROPIC FUNGI: DIFFERENTIAL DIAGNOSIS

The differential diagnosis primarily includes other fungal infections, and microbiological culture may be required to distinguish between species.[14] Ischemia is also in the differential diagnosis.[18,19,25] Vasotropic fungal infection should be strongly considered in any immunocompromised patient with ischemic lesions of the gastrointestinal tract, and fungal stains should be employed to exclude this possibility.

VASOTROPIC FUNGI: DIAGNOSIS

Tissue biopsy remains one of the most important tools available in the diagnosis of fungal infections, especially because fungal cultures may require days to weeks for adequate growth and analysis.[14,25] Although organisms may be identifiable on H&E sections in heavy infections, GMS (Gomori methenamine silver) and PAS (periodic acid-Schiff) stains are invaluable diagnostic aids. Fungi often can be correctly classified in tissue sections based on morphologic criteria, but fungi exposed to antifungal therapy or ambient air may produce bizarre and unusual forms. Microbiological culture remains the gold standard for speciation, especially as antifungal therapy may vary according to the specific type of fungus isolated.

Helpful diagnostic aids, in addition to culture, include serologic assays, antigen tests, immunohistochemistry, and molecular assays, although the latter 2 methodologies are less widely available. Knowledge of the patient's geographic and/or travel history also may be helpful.

VASOTROPIC FUNGI: PROGNOSIS

The prognosis often depends on the immune status of the patient and the severity of the underlying illness. Antifungal therapy may be effective, but disseminated fungal infections are often fatal, especially in severely immunocompromised patients.

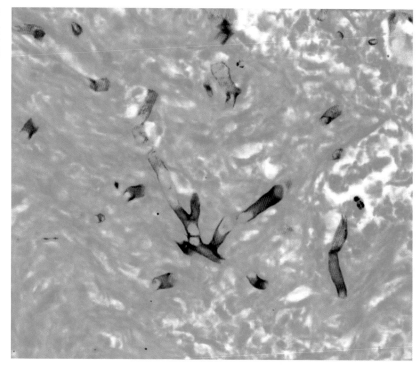

Fig. 11. The typical hyphae of *Aspergillus* are septate, have parallel walls, and branch at acute angles (GMS stain).

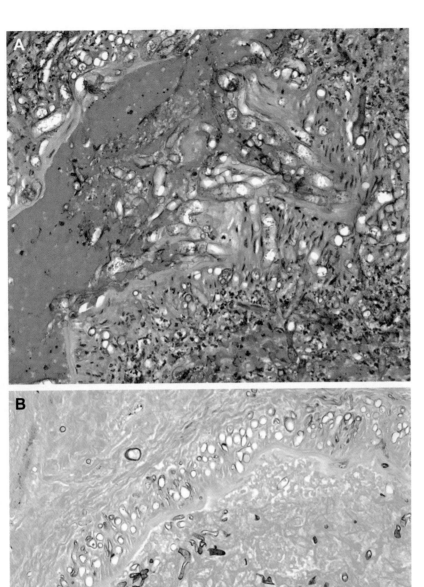

Fig. 12. (*A*) *Mucor* occlude a large vessel, with surrounding necrosis and hemorrhage. (*B*) GMS stain shows *Mucor* with broad ribbon-like, pauciseptate hyphae with irregular walls, which branch randomly at various angles.

SALMONELLOSIS

SALMONELLA: OVERVIEW

These gram-negative bacilli are transmitted through contaminated food and water, and are prevalent where sanitation is poor.[26–29] These bacilli are also an important cause of sporadic food poisoning in developed countries, as well as traveler's diarrhea. Patients with low gastric acidity are at increased risk of salmonellosis, and AIDS patients have a greater risk of Salmonella infection as well.[26–29] The discussion of Salmonella infection is generally divided into typhoid and nontyphoid serotypes or species. S typhi is the most common causative agent of typhoid fever, although other species rarely cause a similar clinicopathologic spectrum. Nontyphoid species (including S enteritidis, S typhimurium, S muenchen, S anatum, S newport, S paratyphi, and S give) usually cause a more self-limited gastroenteritis.[26–29]

Patients with typhoid fever typically present with fever, abdominal pain, and headache. Abdominal rash, delirium, hepatosplenomegaly, and leukopenia are common. The diarrhea begins in the second or third week of infection, and is initially watery but may progress to severe gastrointestinal bleeding and perforation.[26,27,29,30] Nontyphoid Salmonella species generally cause a less severe gastroenteritis with vomiting, nausea, fever, and watery diarrhea, presenting within 8 to 48 hours of ingesting contaminated food or water. Nontyphoid species are less likely to cause severe bloody diarrhea or significant sequelae.[26–29]

SALMONELLA: GROSS FEATURES

Any level of the alimentary tract may be involved in typhoid fever, but the characteristic pathology is most prominent in the ileum, appendix, and right colon.[26,29–34] Grossly, the bowel wall is thickened, and raised ulcerated nodules may be seen corresponding to hyperplastic Peyer patches. Linear ulcers, ovoid ulcers, or full-thickness ulceration and necrosis are common as the disease progresses. Perforation and toxic megacolon may complicate typhoid fever, and suppurative mesenteric lymphadenitis is variably present. Occasionally, the mucosa is grossly normal or only mildly inflamed and edematous.

The gross findings in nontyphoid Salmonella infection are often milder, including mucosal erythema, hemorrhage, ulceration, and exudation. Lesions can be focal, and occasionally the mucosa is grossly normal or only mildly hyperemic and edematous.[27–29]

SALMONELLA: MICROSCOPIC FEATURES

Following hyperplasia of Peyer patches, there is acute inflammation and ulceration of the overlying epithelium (**Fig. 13**), followed by obliteration of the lymphoid follicle by a predominantly mononuclear cell infiltrate (**Fig. 14**). Neutrophils are usually inconspicuous.[26,29–34] Necrosis begins in the Peyer patch and spreads to the surrounding mucosa, which eventually ulcerates. The ulcers are typically very deep, with the base at the level of the muscularis propria, and occasionally penetrate through it. Granulomas are rarely seen. Marked architectural distortion that may mimic ulcerative colitis or Crohn disease can be seen as well (**Fig. 15**).[26,29,31,33]

The histologic features of nontyphoid Salmonella infection are typically those of nonspecific acute infectious-type colitis,[27–29] including cryptitis, crypt abscesses, and a predominantly neutrophilic inflammatory infiltrate (**Fig. 16**). Severe cases may have mucus depletion, fibrinous exudates, and small microthrombi, and occasionally crypt distortion may be seen (**Fig. 17**). More recent descriptions of the pathology of Salmonella infection, however, have reported a fair amount of histologic overlap between the features of typhoid and nontyphoid species.[27,29,31,33]

SALMONELLA: DIFFERENTIAL DIAGNOSIS

The differential diagnosis of typhoid fever includes yersiniosis and other enteric bacterial pathogens, as well as ulcerative colitis and Crohn disease. There may be significant histologic overlap between salmonellosis and chronic idiopathic inflammatory bowel disease, particularly when significant architectural distortion is present. Typhoid fever often lacks neutrophils in comparison with other enteric pathogens as well as idiopathic inflammatory bowel disease, and granulomas are unusual in salmonellosis. Although significant crypt distortion has been reported in some cases of typhoid fever, it is generally more pronounced in ulcerative colitis. The differential diagnosis of nontyphoid Salmonella includes other causes of acute self-limited infectious colitis as well as chronic idiopathic inflammatory bowel disease.

Other food-borne bacteria that can produce architectural distortion, and thus mimic chronic idiopathic inflammatory bowel disease, include Shigella, Aeromonas, and rarely Campylobacter.

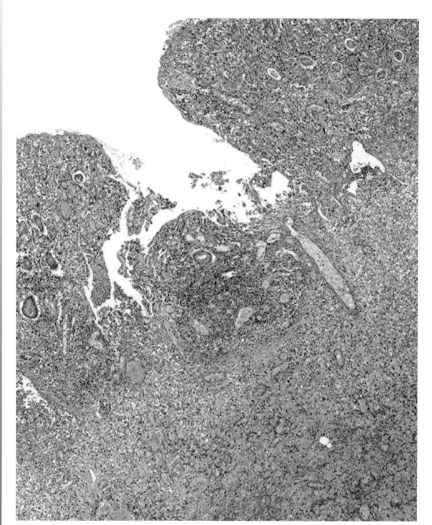

Fig. 13. The characteristic lesion of typhoid fever is a hyperplastic, ulcerated Peyer patch in the ileocecum. (*Courtesy of* Dr Brian West.)

SALMONELLA: DIAGNOSIS

Stool and/or blood cultures with appropriate biochemical tests for species identification may be invaluable in resolving the differential diagnosis in both typhoid fever and nontyphoid *Salmonella* infection.[27–29] In addition, the incubation period of *S typhi* infection is longer (10–15 days) than with other similar enteric pathogens.

SALMONELLA: PROGNOSIS

Although most *Salmonella* infections in developed countries resolve with antibiotics and supportive care, intestinal infection may progress to septicemia and death, particularly in the elderly, the very young, or patients with immune compromise or comorbid conditions.[26–29] Delayed treatment is associated with higher mortality, and antibiotics are particularly important for neonates, older patients, immunocompromised patients, and patients with cardiac valve abnormalities or indwelling prostheses.

YERSINIOSIS

YERSINIA: OVERVIEW

Yersinia is one of the most common causes of bacterial enteritis in western and northern Europe, and the incidence is rising in the United States. *Y enterocolitica* and *Y pseudotuberculosis* are the species that cause human gastrointestinal disease. These food- and water-borne gram-negative coccobacilli cause appendicitis (particularly granulomatous appendicitis), ileitis, colitis, and mesenteric lymphadenitis.[35–40]

Fig. 14. The inflammatory infiltrate in typhoid fever is mononuclear; neutrophils are often inconspicuous.

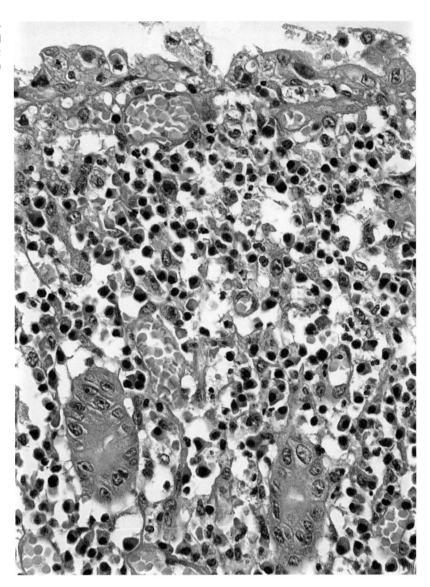

YERSINIA: GROSS FEATURES

Yersinia preferentially involves the ileum, right colon, and appendix.[36,40,41] Grossly, the bowel wall is thickened and edematous with nodular inflammatory masses centered on Peyer patches. Aphthoid and linear ulcers may be seen. Involved appendices are enlarged and hyperemic, similar to nonspecific suppurative appendicitis; perforation is often seen.

YERSINIA: MICROSCOPIC FEATURES

Both suppurative and granulomatous patterns of inflammation are common, and are often mixed.[36,40–42] There is significant overlap between the histologic features of *Y enterocolitica* and *Y pseudotuberculosis* infection, and either species may show epithelioid granulomas with prominent lymphoid cuffing (**Fig. 18**), lymphoid hyperplasia, transmural lymphoid aggregates (**Fig. 19**), mucosal ulceration, and lymph node involvement.[40] *Y enterocolitica* may also feature hyperplastic Peyer patches with overlying ulceration, necrosis, and palisading histiocytes rather than discrete granulomas.[36,40–42] *Y pseudotuberculosis* may show well-developed microabscesses within granulomatous inflammation (**Fig. 20**), almost always accompanied by mesenteric adenopathy.[36]

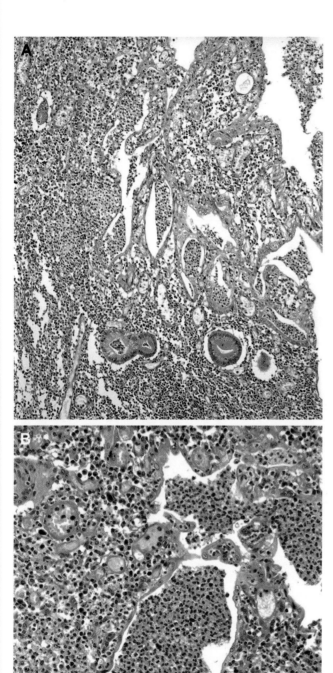

Fig. 15. (*A and B*) The marked architectural distortion in typhoid fever can easily mimic chronic idiopathic inflammatory bowel disease. (*Courtesy of* Dr Brian West.)

Fig. 16. Mucosal edema, cryptitis, a neutrophilic infiltrate in the lamina propria, and preserved architecture are more typical of nontyphoid *Salmonella* infection.

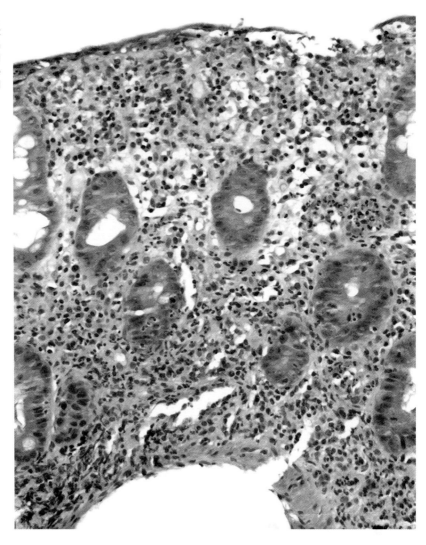

Fig. 17. Colon biopsy from nontyphoid *Salmonella* infection, showing crypt destruction and disorganization.

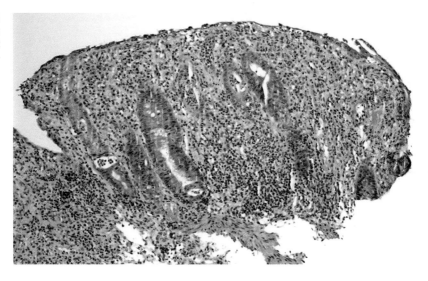

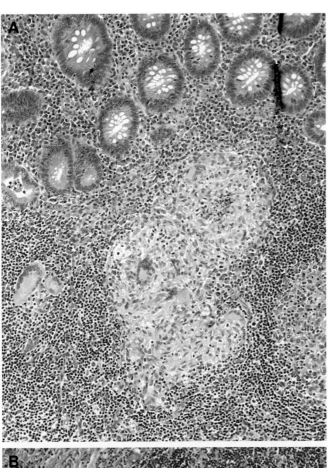

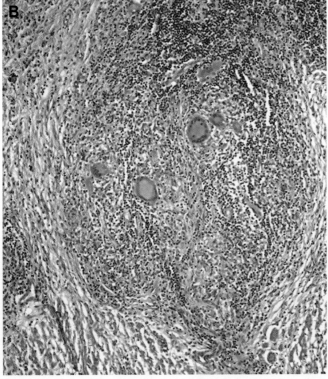

Fig. 18. (*A* and *B*) Granulomatous appendicitis due to *Yersinia enterocolitica* infection, showing epithelioid granulomas with a surrounding lymphoid cuff.

Fig. 19. Mural fibrosis and transmural lymphoid aggregates in *Yersinia* infection, mimicking Crohn disease.

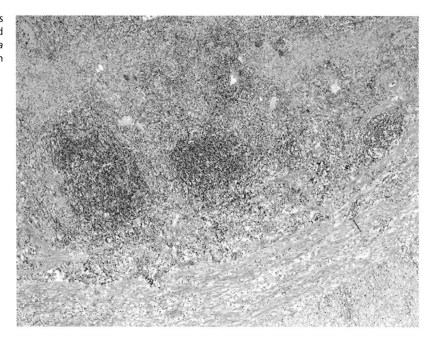

YERSINIA: DIFFERENTIAL DIAGNOSIS

The differential diagnosis often includes other infectious processes, particularly *Mycobacteria* and *Salmonella*. Acid fast stains and culture results help distinguish mycobacterial infection. The specific clinical features, and the presence of greater numbers of neutrophils, microabscesses, and granulomas, may help to distinguish yersiniosis from salmonellosis.

Crohn disease and yersiniosis may be very difficult to distinguish from one another and, in fact, *Yersinia* DNA has been found in some cases of Crohn disease.[43] Both disorders may show similar histologic features, including transmural lymphoid aggregates, skip lesions, and fissuring ulcers. In the past, isolated granulomatous appendicitis has frequently been interpreted as representing primary Crohn disease of the appendix. However, patients with granulomatous inflammation confined to the

Fig. 20. Yersinia pseudotuberculosis, featuring granulomatous inflammation with central abscess formation and overlying mucosal ulceration.

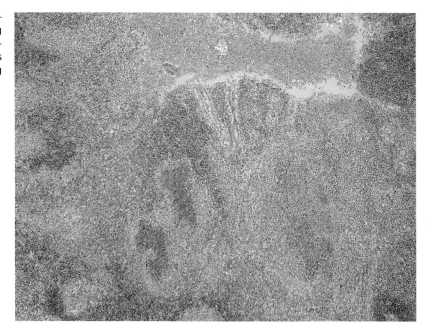

appendix rarely develop generalized inflammatory bowel disease.[38–40] Features that favor Crohn disease include cobblestoning of mucosa, presence of creeping fat, and histologic changes of chronicity including crypt distortion, thickening of the muscularis mucosa, and prominent neural hyperplasia. However, some cases are simply indistinguishable on histologic grounds alone. *Yersinia* should be considered in any initial diagnosis of Crohn disease, particularly if the patient has had the acute, sudden onset of symptoms, and if there are numerous granulomas.

YERSINIA: DIAGNOSIS

Gram stains are usually not helpful for the diagnosis of Yersinia, as the organisms are small, difficult to distinguish from other enteric flora, and often present in low numbers. Cultures, serologic studies, and PCR assays may be useful in confirming the diagnosis.[40,43]

YERSINIA: PROGNOSIS

Although yersiniosis is usually a self-limited process, occasional chronic infections (including chronic colitis) have been well documented. Immunocompromised and debilitated patients, as well as patients on deferoxamine or with iron overload, are at risk for serious disease.[35,36,44]

ENTEROHEMORRHAGIC *ESCHERICHIA COLI*

ENTEROHEMORRHAGIC *E COLI*: OVERVIEW

The most common strain of enterohemorrhagic *E. coli* (EHEC) is O157:H7. This bacterium gained national attention in the early 1990s when a massive outbreak in the western United States was linked to contaminated hamburger patties served at a fast-food restaurant. Although contaminated meat is the most frequent mode of transmission, infection may also occur through contaminated water, milk, produce, and

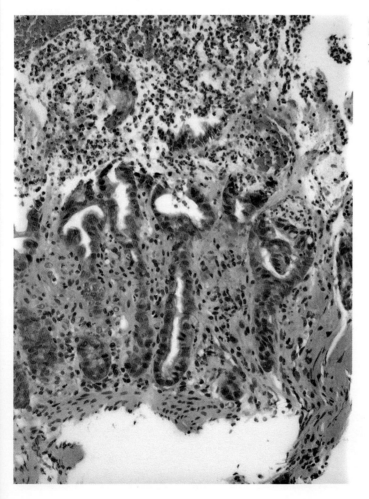

Fig. 21. Enterohemorrhagic *E coli* infection, featuring crypt withering, focal crypt necrosis, and overlying acute inflammation.

person-to-person contact. Gastrointestinal symptoms typically consist of bloody diarrhea with severe abdominal cramps and mild or no fever.[45–47] Nonbloody, watery diarrhea may occur in some cases. Only one-third of patients has fecal leukocytes.

ENTEROHEMORRHAGIC *E COLI*: GROSS FEATURES

Endoscopically, patients may have colonic edema, erosions, ulcers, and hemorrhage, and the right colon is usually more severely affected.[45–48] The edema may be so marked as to cause obstruction, and surgical resection may be required to relieve the obstruction or to control bleeding.

ENTEROHEMORRHAGIC *E COLI*: MICROSCOPIC FEATURES

The histologic features closely resemble ischemic colitis due to other causes, and include marked edema and hemorrhage in the lamina propria and submucosa, with associated mucosal acute inflammation, crypt withering (**Fig. 21**), lamina propria hyalinization (**Fig. 22**), and necrosis. Microthrombi may be present within small-caliber blood vessels, and abundant necroinflammatory exudate or pseudomembranes may be present as well (**Fig. 23**).[45,48]

ENTEROHEMORRHAGIC *E COLI*: DIFFERENTIAL DIAGNOSIS

The differential diagnosis for EHEC primarily includes ischemic colitis, from which EHEC may be histologically indistinguishable. History, including the specific clinical situation, possibility of consumption of contaminated food, age of the patient, and endoscopic findings may aid in distinguishing *E coli* infection from ischemia of other causes. Other organisms that produce pseudomembranous colitis are also in the differential diagnosis, including *Shigella* and particularly

Fig. 22. Marked crypt withering and lamina propria fibrosis in enterohemorrhagic *E coli* infection.

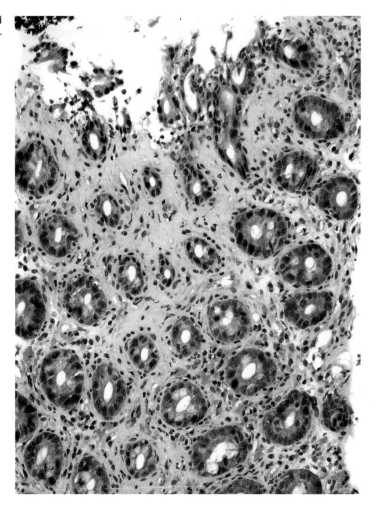

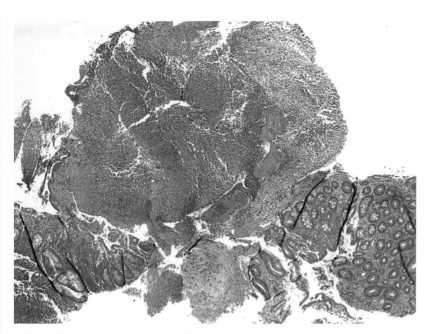

Fig. 23. Prominent overlying acute necroinflammatory debris in enterohemorrhagic *E coli* infection.

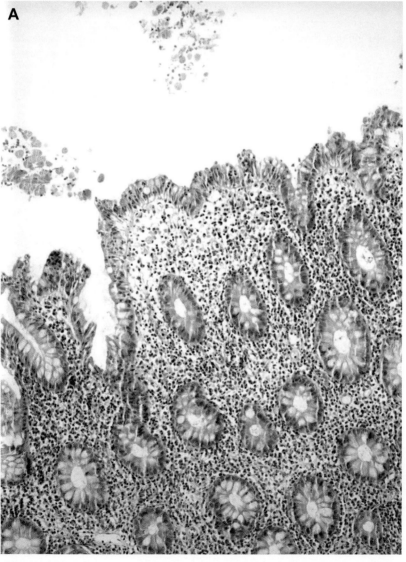

A

Fig. 24. (*A*) Minimal cryptitis and acute inflammation of the surface epithelium in noninvasive amoebiasis, with amoeba and necrotic debris at the surface of the biopsy.

Fig. 24. (*B*) Higher power view shows amoeba within the necrotic debris.

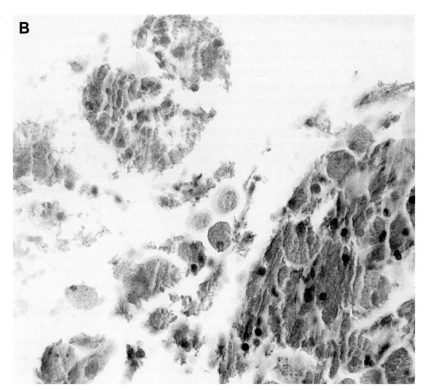

Clostridium difficile. The *C difficile* antigen test may be very helpful in distinguishing *C difficile*–related colitis from EHEC.

ENTEROHEMORRHAGIC *E COLI*: DIAGNOSIS

Stool culture may be invaluable in making the diagnosis. Routine stool cultures cannot distinguish 0157:H7 from normal intestinal flora, however, and microbiologic diagnosis requires screening on selective agar.[45–47] An immunohistochemical stain for this organism has recently been described as well,[49] and molecular assays exist but are not widely available.

ENTEROHEMORRHAGIC *E COLI*: PROGNOSIS

Supportive care is effective in most cases, and antibiotic therapy is generally not recommended. However, there are significant complications associated with EHEC, including intestinal obstruction, perforation, hemolytic-uremic syndrome, and thrombotic thrombocytopenic purpura.[45–47] Children and the elderly are at particular risk for grave illness.

ENTAMOEBA HISTOLYTICA

AMOEBIASIS: OVERVIEW

E histolytica is a motile protozoan that infects approximately 10% of the world's population, predominantly in tropical and subtropical regions. Infection is usually acquired through contaminated water or food, and can be spread by the fecal-oral route. Sexual transmission has been reported occasionally. Risk factors for symptomatic infection include pediatric age group, malnutrition, pregnancy, immunosuppression, and steroids. In the United States, this infection is most often seen in immigrants, overseas travelers, male homosexuals, and institutionalized persons.[50–55]

Many infected patients are asymptomatic. Symptomatic patients most commonly have diarrhea, abdominal cramps, and variable right lower quadrant tenderness; this is sometimes referred to as "nondysenteric" amoebiasis. Invasive disease, most often presenting as amoebic dysentery, reportedly occurs in less than 10% of infected persons. Amoebic dysentery presents suddenly, approximately 1 to 3 weeks after exposure, with severe abdominal cramps, tenesmus, fever, and diarrhea (which may be mucoid and/or bloody).[50–55]

AMOEBIASIS: GROSS FEATURES

The cecum is the most common site of involvement, followed by the right colon, rectum, sigmoid, and appendix. Colonoscopy may be normal in asymptomatic patients or those with mild disease. Early endoscopic findings include small ulcers, which may coalesce to form large, irregular geographic or serpiginous ulcers. Ulcers may undermine adjacent mucosa to produce the classic "flask-shaped" lesions, and there may be inflammatory polyps as well. The intervening mucosa is often grossly normal. Rare macroscopic findings include fulminant colitis resembling ulcerative colitis; pseudomembrane formation mimicking *C difficile*–related pseudomembranous colitis; and large inflammatory masses consisting of organisms and granulation tissue (amoebomas).

AMOEBIASIS: MICROSCOPIC FEATURES

Histologically, early lesions often show a mild neutrophilic infiltrate (**Fig. 24**), with concentration of the organisms at the luminal surface. In some cases, numerous organisms are present at the luminal surface with little associated inflammation. There is usually abundant associated amorphous eosinophilic necrotic material containing nuclear debris. In many cases, the abundant necrotic debris greatly exceeds the amount of associated inflammation that is present. In more advanced disease, ulcers are often deep, extending into the

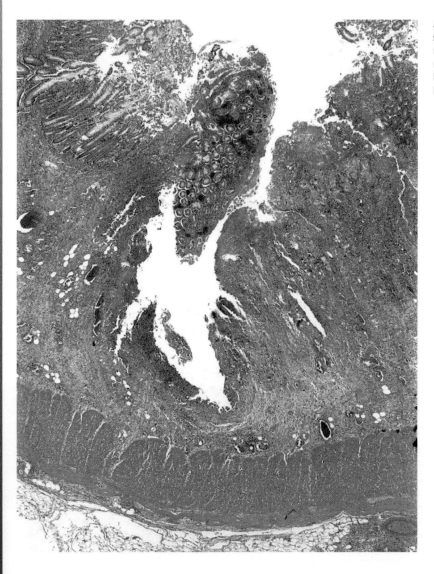

Fig. 25. Deep, flask-shaped ulcer with undermining of adjacent mucosa in invasive amoebiasis. (*Courtesy of* Dr David Owen.)

submucosa

submucosa (**Fig. 25**), with undermining of adjacent mucosa. The adjacent mucosa may be histologically normal, or may show gland distortion and inflammation that can mimic chronic idiopathic inflammatory bowel disease. Amoebae are found in ulcer beds, usually within the necrotic material (**Fig. 26**). Invasive amoebae are sometimes detected within the bowel wall (**Fig. 27**).[55–57]

Trophozoites (**Fig. 28**) have distinct cell membranes with foamy cytoplasm. The nuclei are round and eccentrically located, with peripheral margination of chromatin and a central karyosome.[56,57] The presence of ingested red blood cells is essentially pathognomonic of E histolytica, and helps to distinguish it from other amoebae (see later discussion). Distinction of trophozoites from macrophages within inflammatory exudates may be difficult, particularly in poorly fixed tissue sections. Amoebae are trichrome and PAS positive (**Fig. 29**); in addition, their nuclei are usually more rounded, paler, and have a more open nuclear chromatin pattern than those of macrophages.[57] Macrophages stain with CD68, α1-antitrypsin, and chymotrypsin, whereas amoebae do not.

AMOEBIASIS: DIFFERENTIAL DIAGNOSIS

E histolytica may be distinguished from most other amoebae by the presence of ingested red blood cells.[56,57] Two other species of amoeba, E dispar and E moshkovskii, which are histologically indistinguishable from E histolytica, have recently received attention because they have been recovered from the stool of patients with gastrointestinal symptoms.[52,58] To date, there is no convincing evidence that E dispar causes symptomatic gastrointestinal disease. There are rare reports of symptomatic infection with E moshkovskii, although many of these are also confounded by coinfection with E histolytica and other pathogens, and thus the true pathogenicity of this species also remains controversial. The rare ciliate Balantidium coli may mimic E histolytica histologically, but it is much larger, has a kidney-bean shaped macronucleus, and is ciliated.

The differential diagnosis of amoebiasis also includes chronic idiopathic inflammatory bowel disease, C difficile–related pseudomembranous colitis, and other types of infectious colitis.[55–57]

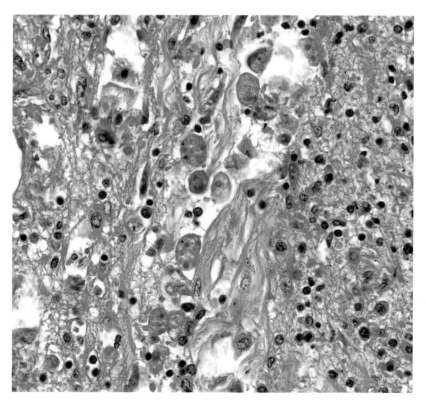

Fig. 26. Invasive amoeba containing erythrocytes in the bowel wall. (*Courtesy of* Dr David Owen.)

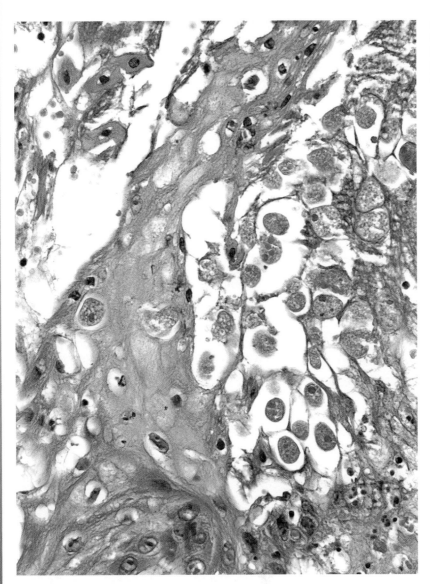

Fig. 27. Invasive amoeba within the anal squamous epithelium in an amoeboma. (*Courtesy of Dr David Owen.*)

Although amoebiasis can cause architectural distortion, the cryptitis, crypt abscesses, marked basal lymphoplasmacytosis, diffuse architectural distortion, and disease distribution typical of ulcerative colitis are not usually present in amoebiasis. Many of the characteristic features of Crohn disease are also absent in amoebiasis, including transmural lymphoid aggregates, mural fibrosis, granulomas, and neural hyperplasia. A careful search for trophozoites in unusual cases of inflammatory bowel disease or specimens from patients from endemic regions is warranted, however, as steroid administration can cause life-threatening complications if the diagnosis of amoebiasis is missed. Amoebomas can mimic carcinoma grossly and radiographically, and are often diagnosed only after biopsy or resection with tissue examination.[59,60]

AMOEBIASIS: DIAGNOSIS

In addition to the special stains and immunohistochemical stains discussed earlier, useful diagnostic tests for *E histolytica* include stool examination for cysts and trophozoites, stool culture, serologic tests, and PCR assays, although the latter are not widely available.[52,58,61]

AMOEBIASIS: PROGNOSIS

Symptomatic patients may be effectively treated with antiparasitic medications in most cases. Complications of intestinal amoebiasis include

Fig. 28. (*A* and *B*) Amoebae have distinct cell membranes with foamy cytoplasm, along with round and eccentrically located nuclei with peripheral margination of chromatin and a central karyosome. The presence of ingested red blood cells is essentially pathognomonic of *E histolytica.* Amoebae typically have more rounded nuclei with a more open chromatin pattern than macrophages.

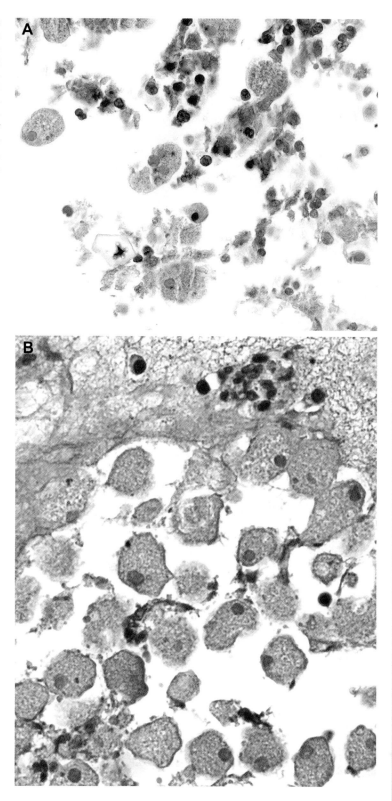

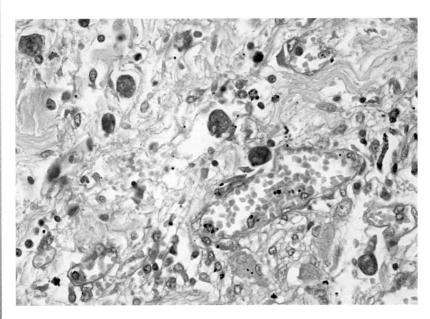

Fig. 29. PAS-positive amoebae within the bowel wall in a case of invasive amoebiasis. (*Courtesy of* Dr David Owen.)

bleeding; perforation; dissemination to other sites, particularly the liver; fistula formation between the intestine and the skin, peritoneum, and urogenital tract; and toxic megacolon. The

latter complication is often associated with corticosteroid use.[50–55,57]

 Pitfalls
INFECTIOUS DISEASES OF THE LOWER GASTROINTESTINAL TRACT

! Consider underlying infection (eg, CMV, vasotropic fungi) in any immunocompromised person who has ischemic colitis.

! Consider infectious colitis in the differential diagnosis of any patient with a new diagnosis of chronic idiopathic inflammatory bowel disease, especially cases in which features of chronicity are not well developed, or in which the symptoms were of sudden onset.

! Many infectious colitides can cause significant architectural distortion, mimicking chronic idiopathic inflammatory bowel disease.

! Many infections can be superimposed on chronic idiopathic inflammatory bowel disease; the diagnosis of one does not exclude the other.

! Viral inclusions and organisms may be rare and difficult to find; multiple levels and/or special studies may be required.

REFERENCES

1. Chetty R, Roskell DE. Cytomegalovirus infection in the gastrointestinal tract. J Clin Pathol 1994;47:968–72.
2. Francis ND, Boylston AW, Roberts AH, et al. Cytomegalovirus infection in gastrointestinal tracts of patients infected with HIV-1 or AIDS. J Clin Pathol 1989;42:1055–64.
3. Meiselman MS, Cello JP, Margaretten W. Cytomegalovirus colitis: report of the clinical, endoscopic, and pathologic findings in two patients with the acquired immunodeficiency syndrome. Gastroenterology 1985;88:171–5.
4. Buckner FS, Pomery C. Cytomegalovirus disease of the gastrointestinal tract in patients without AIDS. Clin Infect Dis 1993;17:644–56.
5. Crespo MG, Arnal FM, Gomez M, et al. Cytomegalovirus colitis mimicking a colonic neoplasm or ischemia colitis 4 years after heart transplantation. Transplantation 1998;66:1562–5.
6. Rich JD, Crawford JM, Kazanjian SN, et al. Discrete gastrointestinal mass lesions caused by cytomegalovirus in patients with AIDS: report of three cases and review. Clin Infect Dis 1992;15:609–14.
7. Greenson JK. Macrophage aggregates in cytomegalovirus esophagitis. Hum Pathol 1997;28:375–8.
8. Golden MP, Hammer SM, Wanke CA, et al. Cytomegalovirus vasculitis: case reports and review of the literature. Medicine 1994;73:246–55.

9. Keates J, Lagahee S, Crilley P, et al. CMV enteritis causing segmental ischemia and massive intestinal hemorrhage. Gastrointest Endosc 2001;53:355–9.

10. Kraus MD, Feran-Doza M, Garcia-Moliner ML, et al. Cytomegalovirus infection in the colon of bone marrow transplant patients. Mod Pathol 1998;11:29–36.

11. Dimitroulia E, Spanakis N, Konstantinidou AE, et al. Frequent detection of cytomegalovirus in the intestine of patients with inflammatory bowel disease. Inflamm Bowel Dis 2006;12:879–84.

12. Kambham N, Vig R, Cartwright CA, et al. Cytomegalovirus infection in steroid-refractory ulcerative colitis; a case-control study. Am J Surg Pathol 2004;28:365–73.

13. Fica A, Cervera C, Perez N, et al. Immunohistochemically proven cytomegalovirus end-organ disease in solid organ transplant patients: clinical features and usefulness of conventional diagnostic tests. Transpl Infect Dis 2007;9:203–10.

14. Chandler FW, Watts JC. Pathologic diagnosis of fungal infections. Chicago: ASCP Press; 1987.

15. Prescott RJ, Harris M, Banerjee SS. Fungal infections of the small and large intestine. J Clin Pathol 1992;45:806–11.

16. Smith JM. Mycoses of the alimentary tract. Gut 1969;10:1035–40.

17. Ellis M. Invasive fungal infections: evolving challenges for diagnosis and therapeutics. Mol Immunol 2001;38:947–57.

18. Cohen R, Heffner JE. Bowel infarction as the initial manifestation of disseminated aspergillosis. Chest 1992;101:877–9.

19. Young RC, Bennett JE, Vogel CL, et al. Aspergillosis: the spectrum of the disease in 98 patients. Medicine 1970;49:147–73.

20. Dictar MO, Maiolo E, Alexander B, et al. Mycoses in the transplanted patient. Med Mycol 2000;38(Suppl 1):251–8.

21. Gonzalez CE, Rinaldi MG, Sugar AM. Zygomycosis. Infect Dis Clin North Am 2002;16:895–914.

22. Lyon DT, Schubert TT, Mantia AG. Phycomycosis of the gastrointestinal tract. Am J Gastroenterol 1979;72:379–94.

23. Thomson SR, Bade PG, Taams M, et al. Gastrointestinal mucormycosis. Br J Surg 1991;78:952–4.

24. Hosseini M, Lee J. Gastrointestinal mucormycosis mimicking ischemic colitis in a patient with systemic lupus erythematosus. Am J Gastroenterol 1998;93:1360–2.

25. Schwarz J. The diagnosis of deep mycoses by morphologic methods. Hum Pathol 1982;13:519–33.

26. Boyd JF. Pathology of the alimentary tract in Salmonella typhimurium food poisoning. Gut 1985;26:935–44.

27. Edwards BH. Salmonella and Shigella species. Clin Lab Med 1999;19(3):469–87.

28. Goldsweig CD, Pacheco PA. Infectious colitis excluding E. coli 0157:H7 and C. difficile. Gastroenterol Clin North Am 2001;30(3):709–33.

29. Kelly JK, Owen DA. Bacterial diarrheas and dysenteries. In: Connor DH, Chandler FW, Schwartz DA, et al, editors. Pathology of infectious diseases. Stamford (CT): Appleton and Lange; 1997. p. 421–9.

30. Azad AK, Islam R, Salam MA, et al. Comparison of clinical features and pathologic findings in fatal cases of typhoid fever during the initial and later stages of the disease. Am J Trop Med Hyg 1997;56:490–3.

31. Kraus MD, Amatya B, Kimula Y. Histopathology of typhoid enteritis: morphologic and immunophenotypic findings. Mod Pathol 1999;12:949–55.

32. Mallory FB. A histological study of typhoid fever. J Exp Med 1898;3:611–38.

33. McGovern VJ, Slavutin LJ. Pathology of Salmonella colitis. Am J Surg Pathol 1979;3:483–90.

34. Sachdev HP, Chadha V, Malhotra V, et al. Rectal histopathology in endemic Shigella and Salmonella diarrhea. J Pediatr Gastroenterol Nutr 1993;13:33–8.

35. Baert F, Peetermans W, Knockaert D. Yersiniosis: the clinical spectrum. Acta Clin Belg 1994;49(2):76–84.

36. El-Maraghi NR, Mair N. The histopathology of enteric infection with Yersinia pseudotuberculosis. Am J Clin Pathol 1979;71:631–9.

37. Schapers RF, Renate R, Lennert K, et al. Mesenteric lymphadenitis due to Yersinia enterocolitica. Virchows Arch Pathol Anat 1981;390:127–38.

38. Dudley TH, Dean PJ. Idiopathic granulomatous appendicitis, or Crohn's disease of the appendix revisited. Hum Pathol 1993;24:595–601.

39. Huang JC, Appelman HD. Another look at chronic appendicitis resembling Crohn's disease. Mod Pathol 1996;9(10):975–81.

40. Lamps LW, Madhusudhan KT, Greenson JK, et al. The role of Y. enterocolitica and Y. pseudotuberculosis in granulomatous appendicitis: a histologic and molecular study. Am J Surg Pathol 2001;25:508–15.

41. Gleason TH, Patterson SD. The pathology of Yersinia enterocolitica ileocolitis. Am J Surg Pathol 1982;6:347–55.

42. Bradford ND, Noce PS, Gutman LT. Pathologic features of enteric infection with Yersinia enterocolitica. Arch Pathol 1974;98:17–22.

43. Lamps LW, Madhusudhan KT, Havens JM, et al. Pathogenic Yersinia enterocolitica and Yersinia pseudotuberculosis DNA is detected in bowel and mesenteric nodes from Crohn's disease patients. Am J Surg Pathol 2003;27(2):220–7.

44. Saebo A, Lassen J. Acute and chronic gastrointestinal manifestations associated with Yersinia enterocolitica infection: a Norwegian 10 year follow-up study on 458 hospitalized patients. Ann Surg 1992;215:250–5.

45. Griffin PM, Olmstead LC, Petras RE. *Escherichia coli* 0157:H7-associated colitis: a clinical and histological study of 11 cases. Gastroenterology 1990;99: 142–9.

46. Griffin PM. *E. coli* 0157:H7 and other enterohemorrhagic *E. coli*. In: Blaser MJ, Smith PD, Ravdin JI, et al, editors. Infections of the gastrointestinal tract. New York: Raven Press; 1995. p. 739–61.

47. Welinder-Olsson C, Kaijser B. Enterohemorrhagic *E. coli* (EHEC). Scand J Infect Dis 2005;37:405–16.

48. Kelly J, Oryshak A, Wenetsek M, et al. The colonic pathology of *E. coli* 0157:H7 infection. Am J Surg Pathol 1990;14:87–92.

49. Su C, Brandt LJ, Sigal SH, et al. The immunohistological diagnosis of *E. coli* 0157:H7 colitis: possible association with colonic ischemia. Am J Gastroenterol 1998;93:1055–9.

50. Li E, Stanley SL. Protozoa: amebiasis. Gastroenterol Clin North Am 1996;25(3):471–92.

51. Panosian CB. Parasitic diarrhea. Infect Dis Clin North Am 1988;2(3):685–703.

52. Ravdin JI. Amebiasis. Clin Infect Dis 1995;20: 1453–66.

53. Reed SL. Amebiasis: an update. Clin Infect Dis 1992;14:385–93.

54. Stanley SL Jr. Amoebiasis. Lancet 2003;361(9362): 1025–34.

55. Variyam EP, Gogate P, Hassan M, et al. Nondysenteric intestinal amebiasis: colonic morphology and search for *Entamoeba histolytica* adherence and invasion. Dig Dis Sci 1989;34:732–40.

56. Brandt H, Tamayo P. Pathology of human amebiasis. Hum Pathol 1970;1:351–85.

57. Braunstein H, Connor DH. Amebiasis-infection by *Entamoeba histolytica*. In: Connor DH, Chandler FW, Schwartz DA, et al, editors. Pathology of infectious diseases. Stamford (CT): Appleton and Lange; 1997. p. 1127–33.

58. Pillai DR, Keystone JS, Sheppard DC, et al. *Entamoeba histolytica* and *Entamoeba dispar*: epidemiology and comparison of diagnostic methods in a setting of nonendemicity. Clin Infect Dis 1999;29:1315–8.

59. Hardin RE, Ferzli GS, Zenilman ME, et al. Invasive amebiasis and ameboma formation presenting as a rectal mass: an uncommon case of malignant masquerade at a western medical center. World J Gastroenterol 2007;13:5659–61.

60. Ng DC, Kwok SY, Cheng Y, et al. Colonic amebic abscess mimicking carcinoma of the colon. Hong Kong Med J 2006;12:71–3.

61. Fotedar R, Star D, Beebe N, et al. Laboratory diagnostic techniques for *Entamoeba* species. Clin Microbiol Rev 2007;20:511–32.

PATHOLOGY OF GASTROINTESTINAL NEUROENDOCRINE TUMORS: AN UPDATE

Roger K. Moreira, MD[a], Kay Washington, MD, PhD[b],*

KEYWORDS

- Gastrointestinal • Neuroendocrine • Carcinoid

ABSTRACT

Gastrointestinal (GI) neuroendocrine tumors (NETs) are a heterogeneous group of relatively slow-growing neoplasms with marked site-specific differences in hormonal secretion and clinical behavior. Most are sporadic neoplasms, with only 5% to 10% arising in patients with hereditary disorders, most commonly in multiple endocrine neoplasia type 1. Although a uniform terminology is not universally accepted, use of the 4-category World Health Organization classification of these tumors is becoming more widespread, and recommendations for tumor grading and staging have been recently formulated. Most GI NETs are easily recognized on routine histologic examination; rarely, a limited panel of immunohistochemical markers may be useful in establishing the diagnosis. This article describes general and site-specific features of these tumors and outlines potential pitfalls in diagnosis.

GASTROINTESTINAL NEUROENDOCRINE TUMORS

OVERVIEW

The term gastrointestinal neuroendocrine tumor (GI NET) refers to a low-grade neoplasm arising from the diffuse neuroendocrine system scattered throughout the mucosa of the gut. Such tumors have historically been called carcinoid tumors, terminology that is recognized as archaic and ambiguous but still widely used in clinical practice and in tumor registries. Although not in universal usage, the term neuroendocrine is preferred rather than the term endocrine because of shared antigens between neural elements and these cells of the diffuse endocrine system in the GI tract, such as neuron-specific enolase, chromogranins, synaptophysin, and protein gene product 9.5.[1] The neuroendocrine cells that give rise to GI NETs are epithelial cells derived from the same stem cells as other epithelial cell lineages in the GI tract, such as enterocytes, Paneth cells, and goblet cells; at least 15 morphologically and functionally distinct GI neuroendocrine cell types producing different hormones have been identified.[2] In general, the differentiation pattern of GI NETs reflects the profile of neuroendocrine cells normally located in that part of the GI tract.

GI NETS arise as a result of molecular events in progenitor cells that are neuroendocrine committed but not necessarily terminally differentiated. This concept helps explain why certain NETs are more homogeneous, with a dominant hormonal secretory pattern reflecting that of normal neuroendocrine cells in the location in

Disclosures: This project was supported by grant number P50CA095103 from National Cancer Institute. The content is solely the responsibility of the authors and does not necessarily represent the official views of the NCI or NIH.

[a] Department of Pathology, Columbia University Medical Center, 630 West 168th Street, New York, NY 20032, USA

[b] Department of Pathology, Vanderbilt University Medical Center, 1161 21st Avenue South, Nashville, TN 32732, USA

* Corresponding author.

E-mail address: kay.washington@vanderbilt.edu

Key Features
GASTROINTESTINAL
NEUROENDOCRINE TUMORS

1. The most common sites for GI NETs are stomach, appendix, and rectum.

2. Many NETs are asymptomatic and are discovered incidentally.

3. Clinical behavior of GI NETs varies with tumor site; NETs of the appendix and rectum are usually benign; ileal and colonic NETs behave in a more aggressive fashion.

4. Histologic feature of low-grade GI NETs are similar in all sites, including various growth patterns (insular, trabecular, or solid, often with pseudorosette formation) and characteristic cytologic features (round, uniform nuclei, with salt-and-pepper type chromatin and small inconspicuous nucleoli). Poorly differentiated NETs may be more difficult to recognize as neuroendocrine and histologically resemble a poorly differentiated adenocarcinoma or extrapulmonary small cell adenocarcinoma.

5. Special types of NETs occur most often in the duodenum (periampullary somatostatinoma: prominent glandular formation, intraluminal mucin, psammoma bodies) and appendix (goblet cell carcinoids and tubular carcinoids).

6. Ancillary tests are rarely indicated but a panel of immunohistochemical markers (most commonly synaptophysin and chromogranin) may be useful in select cases.

which they arise, and others secrete multiple hormones or lack apparent hormonal functionality. For instance, enterochromaffin-like (ECL) cell NETs arise almost exclusively in the stomach, paralleling the normal distribution of ECL cells. Although GI NETs are derived from epithelial stem cells of the gut, investigations of the neoplastic progression for these tumors have shown that they do not share the same molecular alterations as GI adenocarcinomas, and infrequently show microsatellite instability or abnormalities of Wnt signaling.[3]

MOLECULAR EVENTS

Although only 5% to 10% of GI NETs are linked to hereditary syndromes (generally autosomal dominantly inherited syndromes resulting from mutations in tumor suppressor genes, **Table 1**), such cases have afforded important insights into molecular pathways involved in neuroendocrine neoplasia. For instance, the *MEN1* gene is mutated in up to 40% of sporadic GI and pancreatic NETs.[4] Molecular events seem to be different in GI NETs arising in different sites, with foregut tumors often showing loss of 11q, the site of MEN1, in contrast to hindgut tumors which often show losses on 18q.[5] Progress in understanding the molecular pathways involved has been hindered by the small number of cases studied and the complex and heterogeneous pathobiology of these tumors, but recent work suggests that CpG island methylation is an important pathway in sporadic GI NETs.[6]

EPIDEMIOLOGY

Analysis of more than 13,000 carcinoid tumors reported to the Surveillance, Epidemiology, and End Results (SEER) database from 1950 to 1999 suggests that the incidence of these tumors is increasing in the US population[7]; however, it is not clear if the marked increase in gastric and rectal carcinoids is related to changes in tumor registry reporting, improvements in diagnosis, or to a true increase in these tumor types. These tumors are relatively rare, with the incidence for all GI NETs estimated as 2.0/100,000 for men and 2.4/100,000 for women.[2] Average age for diagnosis for all carcinoid tumors was 61 years in the SEER data set. Rectal carcinoids are more prevalent among black and Asian populations in the United States. Five-year survival rates are best for appendiceal and rectal NETs.

CLINICAL FEATURES

The clinical behavior of GI NETs varies with their location in the GI tract. Small non–gastrin-secreting tumors are usually clinically silent and may be discovered only at autopsy or resection for other indications. When symptoms are attributable to GI NETs, they are caused by local tumor effects such as adhesions or abdominal fibrosis giving rise to abdominal pain or small bowel obstruction, or to secretion of bioactive substances such as serotonin, histamine, or gastrin. The carcinoid syndrome (cutaneous flushing of upper chest, neck and face; gut hypermotility with diarrhea) occurs in less than 10% of patients.[5] Diagnostic strategies for patients suspected of having GI NETs include biochemical testing for urinary 5-hydroxyindoleacetic acid or serum testing for increased chromogranin A levels, followed by localization of the tumor by octreoscan scintigraphy, positron emission tomography, or other radiographic imaging techniques.[5]

Table 1
Hereditary syndromes associated with GI NETs

Syndrome	Inheritance and Prevalence	Gene	Gene Product and Function	GI NETs	Major Tumor Sites
Multiple endocrine neoplasia type 1	Autosomal dominant; ~1:20,000 to 1:40,000	*MEN*; chromosome 11q13	Menin; controls cell growth and differentiation during development	Stomach and duodenum (gastrinomas); associated with Zollinger-Ellison syndrome; pancreas	Anterior pituitary, parathyroid, adrenal cortex, lung
Neurofibromatosis type 1	Autosomal dominant; ~1:4500	*NF1*; chromosome 17q11.2	Neurofibromin; tumor suppressor functions	1% of patients; usually duodenum/ampulla; express somatostatin but not associated with functional syndromes	Neurofibromas
Von Hippel-Lindau syndrome	Autosomal dominant; ~1:36,000	*VHL*, chromosome 3p25	VHL; multiple functions	Pancreatic NETs in 5% to 17%, usually nonfunctioning clear cell tumors	Renal cell carcinoma, hemangioblastoma, pheochromocytoma
Tuberous sclerosis complex	Autosomal dominant; 1:10,000	*TSC1*, 9q34 *TSC2*, 16p13.3	Hamartin Tuberin Tumor suppressor functions	Pancreatic NETs (rare)	Hamartomatous lesions in brain, skin, eye, heart, lung, kidney

Data from Toumpanakis CG, Caplin ME. Molecular genetics of gastroenteropancreatic neuroendocrine tumors. Am J Gastroenterol 2008;103(3):729–32.

GI NETs, most commonly ileal tumors, are asso-ciated with second primary tumors, usually discovered synchronously, in about 17% of patients. The most common site for second primary tumors is the GI tract, followed by genito-urinary tract and lung. These synchronous tumors are generally of higher grade than the GI NET, which may be discovered during staging workup of the associated second primary malignancy.[8]

TERMINOLOGY

There is no single unified terminology for GI NETS. Many pathologists in the United States still use the term carcinoid to describe all low-grade NETs, regardless of tumor site, and some use the term atypical carcinoid to refer to GI NETs with focal necrosis or increased mitotic activity. However, the atypical carcinoid has not been rigorously defined for GI tumors and this nomenclature is not in wide-spread use. The term carcinoid has fallen out of favor because of its failure to encompass the full biologic spectrum and site-specific heterogeneity of these tumors, as well as the narrow interpretation of this term to mean a serotonin-producing tumor associ-ated with carcinoid syndrome.[9] The World Health Organization, although retaining the carcinoid termi-nology in the 2000 publication on classification of tumors of the digestive system,[10] also outlines a 3-tier system[11] classifying these neoplasms as well-differentiated NETs of benign or uncertain malignant potential, well-differentiated neuroendocrine carci-noma, and poorly differentiated neuroendocrine

carcinoma. This system has gained more accep-tance among European pathologists and has the advantage of being more biologically oriented than the umbrella term carcinoid, although this termi-nology can be cumbersome to apply to individual cases.

GROSS FEATURES

GI NETs grossly are firm tan to pale yellow nodules located just beneath the mucosal surface. The muscularis propria may be thickened in the area of tumor, perhaps as a result of secretion of trophic factors by the tumor cells (**Fig. 1**). Dense fibrotic stroma associated with the tumor cells may produce annular strictures, and mesenteric fibrosis may be seen in small bowel NETs. Ischemic injury secondary to vascular sclerosis may also be seen in small bowel tumors (**Fig. 2**).[12] Extensive lymphatic involvement by tumor is manifested as small yellow nodules on the serosal surface. Multicentricity is common and is site-related; gastric and jejunoileal tumors (33%) are more commonly multiple, whereas multiplicity is rare with colonic or appendiceal NETs. Molecular studies have shown that most multiple GI NETs are independent primaries.[13]

MICROSCOPIC FEATURES

Most GI NETs are readily recognizable as low-grade NETs. They are composed of solid nests, cords, trabeculae, and glands of relatively uniform cells with round to oval nuclei with finely granular

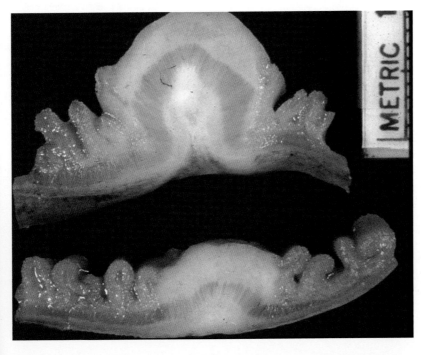

Fig. 1. Low-grade neuro-endocrine neoplasms of the GI tract grossly appear as yellow plaques; thick-ening of the bowel wall as a result of fibrosis and smooth muscle hyper-plasia may be seen, as in this example of an ileal tumor.

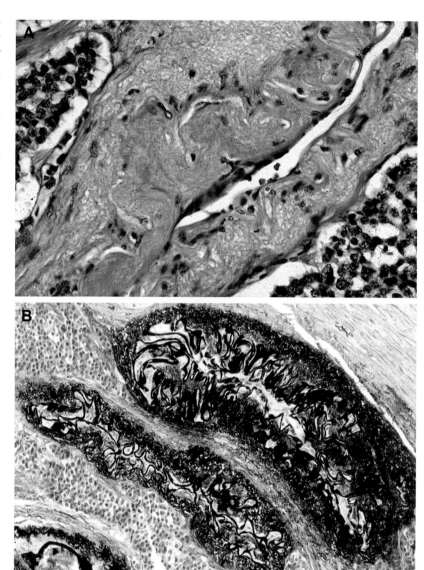

Fig. 2. Elastosis of mesenteric vessels, visible as acellular thickening of vessels walls (*A*) with duplication of the internal elastic lamina and adventitial elastosis on elastin stain (*B*) may cause bowel ischemia. These mesenteric vascular changes are primarily associated with ileal NETs.

chromatin and inconspicuous nucleoli (**Fig. 3**). Less commonly, cystic, tubular, or angiomatoid patterns may be seen. The cytoplasm is generally pale, but in some cases fine red granules are detectable (**Fig. 4**). Cytologic variants include clear cell NETs (generally found in the pancreas in patients with von Hippel-Lindau disease), and oncocytic and rhabdoid appearances. Large areas of tumor necrosis are uncommon and when present signify a higher-grade tumor, but punctate coagulative necrosis may be seen in larger low-grade tumors (**Fig. 5**). Perineural and lymphovascular invasion are associated with more aggressive behavior[14] (see **Fig. 5**B, C) and are generally not seen in small low-grade tumors.

PRECURSOR LESIONS

Endocrine cell hyperplasia is most commonly seen in the GI tract in the stomach in the setting of hypergastrinemia and chronic atrophic gastritis.[15] Duodenal gastrin-producing cells undergo a similar hyperplasia in patients with Zollinger-Ellison syndrome caused by multiple endocrine neoplasia (MEN) type 1. Hyperplastic lesions of the GI neuroendocrine system have been divided for research purposes into diffuse, linear, and nodular patterns; the distinction between nodular hyperplasia and dysplasia is made by size, with dysplastic (preinvasive) lesions measuring between 90 and 210 μm. Gastrin or somatostatin-producing lesions in the

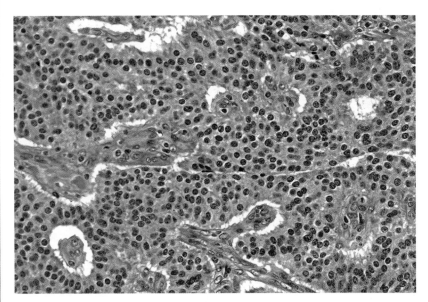

Fig. 3. Low-grade GI NETs are composed of cords, trabeculae, and solid nests of relatively uniform cells with oval finely granular chromatin, typical of neuroendocrine differentiation.

duodenum and measuring larger than 210 μm are classified as GI NETs; microinvasion is recognized by the identification of small clusters of neuroendocrine cells localized in the lamina propria between glands and associated with stromal alterations such as thickened collagen.[16] Although appendix, ileum, and rectum are common locations for GI NETs, endocrine cell hyperplasia and dysplastic lesions are rarely encountered in these sites, and in general sporadic NETs lack identifiable precursor lesions. Neuroendocrine cell hyperplasia and multiple GI NETs have been reported in the setting of ulcerative colitis[17] and Crohn disease, and are associated with epithelial dysplastic changes in some cases.[18]

DIFFERENTIAL DIAGNOSIS

Although most GI NETs do not present a diagnostic problem, tumors with a glandular growth pattern may be erroneously diagnosed as adenocarcinoma. Low-grade GI NETS should not be confused with high-grade neuroendocrine carcinoma or mixed high-grade adenocarcinoma/neuroendocrine carcinoma, both of which are associated with poor prognosis. In the rectum, locally invasive prostatic adenocarcinoma may be confused with an NET but knowledge of the clinical history and endoscopic appearance are helpful in avoiding this pitfall.

DIAGNOSIS

Most GI NETs do not require use of special stains or immunohistochemical studies for diagnosis. However, a panel of immunohistochemical

markers of neuroendocrine differentiation (**Table 2**) may be helpful in selected cases. Cytosolic markers such as neuron-specific enolase and CD56 are highly sensitive but relatively nonspecific for neuroendocrine differentiation. Synaptophysin,

⚠⚠ **Differential Diagnosis** OF **GI NETs**

- Gastric NETs

  - Type 1 and 2 (ECL) NETs

  - Sporadic (type 3)

  - Type 4 (high-grade neuroendocrine carcinoma)

- Duodenal and ampullary NETs

  - Gastrinoma

  - Somatostatinoma

  - Nonfunctioning NETs

- Appendiceal NETs

  - Goblet cell carcinoid

  - Tubular carcinoid

  - Adenocarcinoma

- Ileal NETs

- Colorectal NETs

Fig. 4. Red cytoplasmic granules are prominent in some GI NETs.

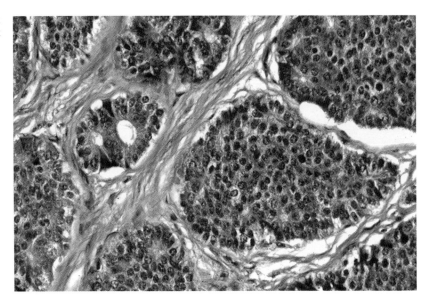

a marker associated with small vesicles, has the advantage of higher specificity, although retaining high sensitivity. The secretory granule marker chromogranin A is widely used and is highly specific for neuroendocrine differentiation (**Fig. 6**), but is not uniformly expressed among the different endocrine cell types, and is often negative in appendiceal and rectal NETs. Higher-grade NETs may be negative for chromogranin A expression, or display only focal positivity.

Immunohistochemical findings should be interpreted in the context of the overall microscopic appearance of the lesion, and it is advisable to use a panel of markers rather than a single marker. In practice, the most widely used panel is synaptophysin and chromogranin A, although in some instances low-grade NETs are negative for both markers. The pathologist may also be asked to determine likely sites of origin of NET metastatic to the liver; in such cases, octreoscan scintigraphy is superior to histopathologic assessment. However, expression of CDX2 has been reported in up to 80% of GI NETs, more commonly in tumors arising in the ileum and appendix, and seems to be a useful marker for NETs of GI origin,[19] although gastric NETs are frequently negative. Neuroendocrine secretory protein-55, a member of the chromogranin family of proteins found in dense core granules, has been reported to be expressed by NETs of the pancreas and adrenal medulla but not NETs of GI and lung origin.[20]

Cell-specific markers such as gastrin or somatostatin may be useful in subtyping GI NETs, but immunohistochemical expression of such hormones does not determine functional status of the tumor, which is defined by clinical manifestations. However, subtle clinical signs of overproduction of such hormones may be overlooked in the preoperative setting and only recognized retrospectively on diagnosis of a GI NET.

STAGING AND PROGNOSTIC MARKERS

According to the 2000 WHO classification,[11] GI NETs are classified into 4 categories, based on a combination of gross, histologic, and immuno-histochemical features (**Table 3**):

1. Well-differentiated NET of probable benign behavior
2. Well-differentiated NET of uncertain malignant behavior
3. Well-differentiated neuroendocrine carcinoma
4. Poorly differentiated neuroendocrine carcinoma.

Recently, TNM classification systems for foregut and hindgut NETs have been proposed by the European Neuroendocrine Tumor Society.[21,22] For foregut and hindgut NETs, the T category is assigned based on tumor size, depth of penetration into the bowel wall, and invasion of adjacent structures, according to specific tumor site (see Refs.[20,21] for details). In situ carcinoma (Tis) is recognized for gastric lesions less than 0.5 cm in this classification system. N and M categories are assigned based on the presence or absence of regional lymph node (N0–N1) or distant (M0–M1) metastases, respectively. A final stage is assigned according to the combination of T, N, and M categories.

The European Neuroendocrine Tumor Society[21,22] has also proposed a grading system (**Table 4**), in

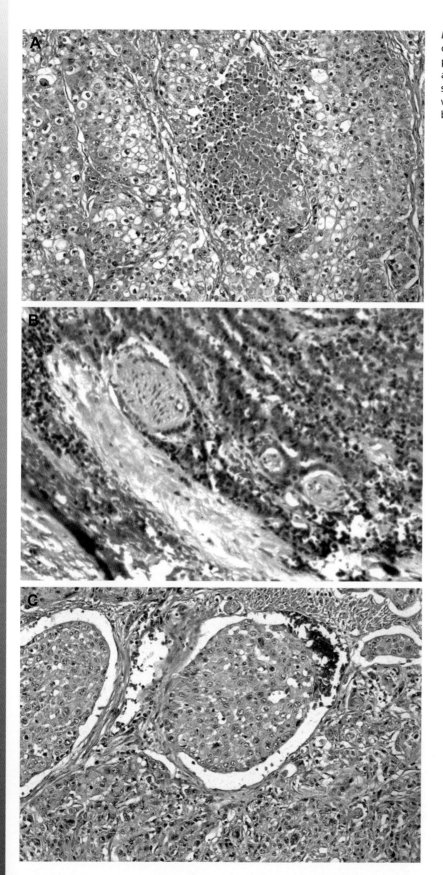

Fig. 5. Focal areas of coagulative necrosis (*A*), perineural invasion (*B*), and lymphovascular invasion (*C*) are associated with more aggressive behavior in GI NETs.

which GI NETs are classified in 3 different categories based on mitotic counts and/or Ki-67 tumor labeling index. G1 and G2 tumors usually correspond to well-differentiated NETs, whereas G3 indicates a poorly differentiated carcinoma.

Preliminary validation studies for this proposed staging system[23] using a data set of 202 patients have demonstrated prognostic relevance of staging and grading of lesions for foregut and pancreatic tumors. A recently proposed staging system using similar parameters (depth of tumor invasion, tumor size, lymph node metastases, and distant metastases) also seems to provide useful overall survival estimates when applied to a set of 108 GI NETs from all GI sites.[24]

SITE-SPECIFIC FEATURES

Gastric NETs

Gastric NETs form a relatively heterogeneous group of neoplasms because of the diverse population of native neuroendocrine cells in this organ. Tumors may arise from these cell types in a variety of clinical settings, and have been classified in 4 subtypes (Table 5). Types 1 and 2 tumors are ECL cell neoplasms that arise in the setting of hypergastrinemia. Type 1 tumors, by far the most common, are seen in patients with body-predominant atrophic gastritis and hypergastrinemia secondary to hypochlorhydria. These patients develop ECL cell hyperplasia (Fig. 7), which may progress to true NETs, often multifocal (Fig. 8).[25] The prognosis of type 1 tumors is usually favorable, and they can safely be resected endoscopically. In rare cases, more aggressive behavior and lymph node metastases are seen, usually associated with tumors larger than 2 cm and with infiltration of the gastric wall.[26] Type 2 tumors are seen in patients with hypergastrinemia caused by gastrin-producing tumors at other sites, such as the duodenum, pancreas, or porta hepatis region (gastrinomas), often in association with Zollinger-Ellison syndrome and MEN-1. Through similar mechanisms as for type 1 tumors, these patients will develop ECL cell hyperplasia and neuroendocrine neoplasms. Like type 1 tumors, type 2 neoplasms usually behave in a benign fashion. Metastatic disease occurs in approximately 10% of cases, usually in tumors larger than 2 cm and with invasion of the muscularis propria.[26] Type 3 tumors are defined as sporadic ECL cell neoplasms (ie, not associated with hypergastrinemia). As in types 1 and 2, type 3 tumors occur preferentially in the body and fundic regions, but tend to be solitary rather than multiple.[25] Type 3 tumors are frequently larger than 2 cm and carry a worse prognosis compared with types 1 and 2, especially if associated with muscularis propria infiltration and vascular invasion, in which case metastases are likely to be present. Type 4 tumors are poorly differentiated neuroendocrine carcinomas. These tumors are distributed throughout the

---

Table 2
Immunohistochemistry of GI NETs

	Foregut Tumors	Midgut Tumors	Hindgut Tumors
Site	Stomach, proximal duodenum	Jejunum, ileum, appendix, proximal colon	Distal colon, rectum
Immunohistochemistry			
Chromogranin A	86%–100% +	82%–92% +	40%–58% +
Neuron-specific enolase	90%–100% +	95%–100% +	80%–87% +
Synaptophysin	50% +	95%–100% +	94%–100% +
Serotonin	33% +	86% +	45%–83% +
Other immunohistochemical markers	Rarely, + for pancreatic polypeptide, histamine, gastrin, VIP, or corticotropin	Prostatic acid phosphatase + in 20%–40%	Prostatic acid phosphatase + in 20%–82%
Carcinoid syndrome	Rare	5%–39%	Rare

Abbreviation: VIP, vasoactive intestinal peptide.
Data from Refs.[55–61]

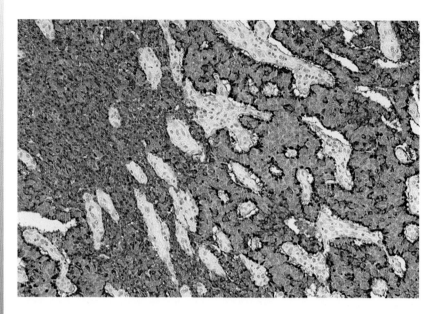

Fig. 6. Most low-grade GI NETs are strongly positive for chromogranin A, a component of neurosecretory granules, but roughly 50% of hindgut tumors are negative for this marker of neuroendocrine differentiation.

stomach, are more commonly diagnosed at a more advanced stage (>4 cm), and often present with extensive metastases.[2] The prognosis is, therefore, poor, with most patients dying within 1 year of diagnosis.[26] Like poorly differentiated neuroendocrine carcinomas elsewhere, type 4 tumors are positive for synaptophysin but often negative for chromogranin A by immunohistochemistry.

NETs of the Duodenum and Upper Jejunum

The percentage of duodenal and upper jejunal NETs in relation to all GI NETs ranges from 3% in

Table 3
WHO criteria for classification and assessment of the biologic behavior of GI NETs

Biologic Behavior	Metastasis	Invasion of Muscularis Propria	Histologic Differentiation	Tumor Size (cm)	Angio-Invasion	Ki-67 Index (%)	Hormonal Syndrome
Well-differentiated NET, probably benign	−	−	WD	≤1[a]	−	<2	−
Well-differentiated NET, uncertain behavior	−	−	WD	≤2	−/+	<2	−
Well-differentiated neuroendocrine carcinoma, low-grade malignant behavior	+	+[b]	WD	>2	+	>2	+
Poorly differentiated neuroendocrine carcinoma, high-grade malignant behavior	+	+	PD	Any	+	>30	−

Abbreviations: PD, poorly differentiated; WD, well differentiated.
[a] Exception: malignant duodenal gastrinomas are usually smaller than 1 cm and confined to the submucosa.
[b] Exception: benign neuroendocrine tumors of the appendix usually invade the muscularis propria.

Table 4
Grading of GI NETs

Grade	Mitotic Count (10 hpf)	Ki-67 Index (%)
G1	<2	≤2
G2	2–20	3–20
G3	>20	>20

Data from Rindi G, Kloppel G, Alhman H, et al. TNM staging of foregut (neuro)endocrine tumors: a consensus proposal including a grading system. Virchows Arch 2006;449:395–401; and Rindi G, Kloppel G, Couvelard A, et al. TNM staging of midgut and hindgut (neuro) endocrine tumors: a consensus proposal including a grading system. Virchows Arch 2007;451(4):757–62.

studies that included old tumor databases[7,27] to 22% in recent series.[28] These tumors show a slight male predominance (1.5:1) and usually affect patients in their fifth and sixth decade.[26]

Five distinct types of NETs are recognized in this location: gastrinomas, which account for approximately two-thirds of all NETs, followed by somatostatinomas, nonfunctioning (nonsyndromic) serotonin- and calcitonin-producing tumors,

poorly differentiated neuroendocrine carcinomas, and gangliocytic paragangliomas.[2]

Gastrinomas can either occur sporadically (75% of cases) or in association with MEN-1 (25% of cases).[29] By definition, gastrinomas are associated with increased serum levels of gastrin, and two-thirds of the patients present with Zollinger-Ellison syndrome. Although gastrinomas may occur in several different sites, they are usually located in the so-called gastrinoma triangle, and approximately 70% occur in the duodenum. Sporadic tumors are solitary and have no identifiable precursor lesions, whereas tumors arising in the setting of MEN-1 are usually multifocal and are believed to originate from an underlying precursor lesion (ie, G-cell hyperplasia).[16] Duodenal gastrinomas are usually small lesions, usually measuring less than 1 cm in diameter and located in the first portion of the duodenum. Histologically, they show a mixture of histologic growth patterns, often with a trabecular and pseudoglandular architecture.[26] In spite of their small size and lack of muscularis invasion, gastrinomas often have an aggressive behavior, with early regional lymph node metastases. Therefore, gastrinomas should be considered potentially malignant regardless of other features.

Table 5
Types of gastric NETs

	Type 1	Type 2	Type 3	Type 4
Frequency	70%–80% of cases	Rare	10%–15% of cases	Rare
Multiplicity	Multifocal	Multifocal	Solitary	Solitary
Size	0.5–1.0 cm	~1.5 cm or less	Variable; one-third larger than 2 cm	Large
Location	Corpus	Corpus	Any where in stomach	Anywhere in stomach
Associations	Hypergastrinemic states; chronic atrophic gastritis, ECL hyperplasia	Multiple endocrine neoplasia type 1, with Zollinger-Ellison syndrome	Sporadic	Sporadic
Clinical behavior	Usually benign	30% metastasize	71% of tumors >2 cm with muscularis propria and vascular invasion have lymph node metastases	High-grade carcinoma; metastases common; poor prognosis
Demographic profile	70%–80% are female, 50's-60's	Equally in men and women, mean age 50 years	More common in men, mean age 55 years	More common in men

Data from Graeme-Cook F. Neuroendocrine tumors of the GI tract and appendix. In: Odze RD, Goldblum JR, Crawford JM, editors. Surgical pathology of the GI tract, liver, biliary tract, and pancreas. Philadelphia: Saunders; 2004. p. 483–504; and Williams GT. Endocrine tumours of the gastrointestinal tract: selected topics. Histopathology 2007;50(1):30–41.

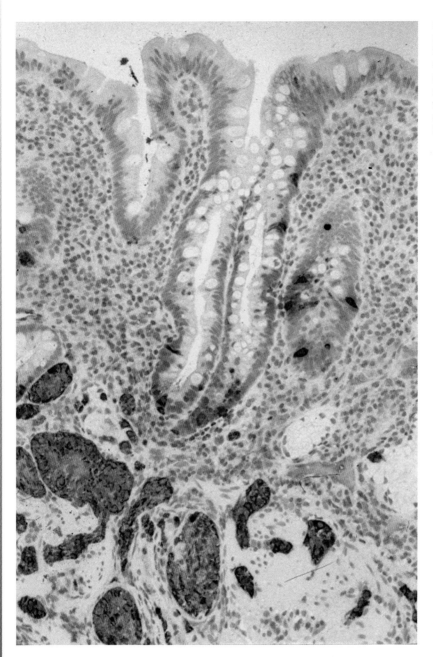

Fig. 7. ECL cell hyperplasia may be prominent in long-standing chronic atrophic gastritis associated with hypergastrinemia, and is best visualized with synaptophysin (shown) or chromogranin A immunohistochemistry.

Duodenal somatostatinomas represent 15% to 20% of duodenal NETs[26,30] and about 1% of all gastroenteropancreatic NETs.[31] They are predominantly located in the periampullary region, and are associated with type 1 neurofibromatosis (von Recklinhausen disease) in up to one-third of the cases, as well as with MEN-1.[32] Originally named glandular duodenal carcinoids, this tumor shows characteristic histologic findings that include prominent glandular architecture with intraluminal mucinous material, simulating an epithelial tumor, as well as the presence of psammoma bodies in most cases (**Fig. 9**). The cytologic features of a NET (ie, round, uniform nuclei, with salt-and-pepper chromatin, and abundant cytoplasm) are morphologic clues on sections stained with hematoxylin and eosin. Immunohistochemistry for somatostatin is positive in almost all cases, although associated somatostatin syndrome (diabetes, achlorhydria, cholelithiasis, and diarrhea) is rarely present. Muscularis propria invasion seems to be a poor prognostic feature, associated with lymph node metastasis. Duodenal/periampullary somatostatinomas do not seem to be related

Fig. 8. Type 1 gastric NETs arising in hypergastrinemia are usually small (<1 cm) (*A*) and multiple. Note linear ECL cell hyperplasia highlighted by immunohistochemistry for synaptophysin (*B*) in adjacent gastric mucosa.

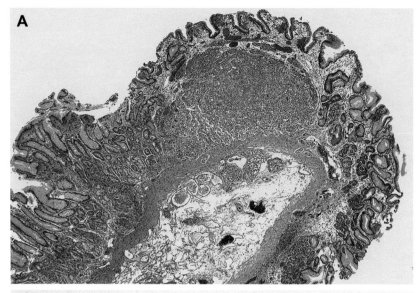

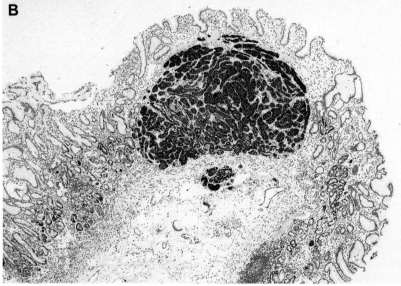

to pancreatic somatostatinomas, which are usually well-differentiated NETs that do not show any of the distinctive histologic features of their duodenal counterpart, and are sometimes associated with somatostatin syndrome.[9]

Nonfunctioning duodenal NETs can usually be shown to be formed by serotonin-producing cells or, less often, gastrin- and calcitonin-secreting cells. Hormonal syndromes, however, are not apparent. The prognosis of nonfunctioning NETs is significantly better than that of gastrinomas or somatostatinomas. In general, metastatic disease is not seen unless the tumor displays other unfavorable features such as extension beyond submucosa.[9]

Poorly differentiated duodenal carcinomas are hormonally inactive tumors that typically arise in the periampullary region of the duodenum. Histologically, they show an undifferentiated morphology, often with small cell features. Like poorly differentiated neuroendocrine carcinomas elsewhere in the GI tract, these tumors may show strong synaptophysin positivity; chromogranin A immunohistochemistry is negative or only weakly positive. The prognosis in generally poor, with early lymph node and liver metastases.[26]

Duodenal gangliocytic paragangliomas are rare neoplasms that, likewise, usually occur in the periampullary region. They have a polymorphous histologic appearance, with areas reminiscent of

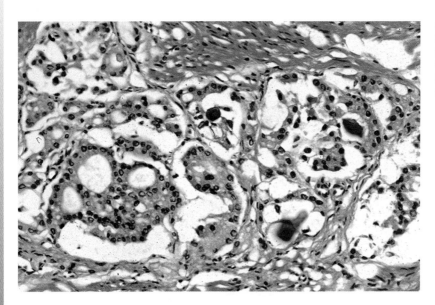

Fig. 9. Periampullary somatostatinomas display a glandular growth pattern with psammoma bodies and may be mistaken for adenocarcinoma.

a paraganglioma, carcinoid-like regions, ganglion cells, as well as Schwannian spindle cell elements. Immunohistochemical studies demonstrate the presence of somatostatin, serotonin, and pancreatic polypeptide in the endocrine cells, ganglion cells stain positively for neuron-specific enolase (NSE), and Schwann cells express S-100 and neurofilament.[33,34]

NETs of the Distal Jejunum and Ileum

Tumors in this location account for approximately 25% of all GI NETs, making this region the single most common site for NETs. Men and women are equally affected, with a peak incidence in the sixth decade.[7,30] The terminal ileum is the most common location. Histologically, tumors in the terminal ileum have a solid, nested, or trabecular architecture and are usually composed of cytologically bland cells. A background of densely fibrotic stroma is characteristic of ileal NETs. NETs of the ileum often present with small bowel stenosis, and are commonly associated with fibrosis of peritumoral tissues, peritoneal cavity, and retroperitoneum.[35] There is recent evidence that tumor-associated fibrosis may be caused by fibrogenic mediators such as tumor growth factor β and connective tissue growth factor (CTGF), via activation of intestinal stellate cells. These same mediators have been postulated to play a role in fibrotic processes in distant organs, such as heart and lungs, in the setting of carcinoid syndrome.[36] Immunohistochemically, these tumors may produce serotonin, substance P, and catecholamines.[9]

Ileal NETs generally pursue an aggressive clinical course, with frequent metastases to regional lymph nodes at the time of clinical presentation. Approximately 20% of patients present with liver metastases. Because serotonin is metabolized by the liver, only patients with metastatic disease (to liver or other distant organs) are at risk of developing carcinoid syndrome, characterized by flushing, diarrhea, bronchospasm, and endocardial fibrosis.[9]

NETs of the Appendix

Appendiceal NETs are among the most common in the GI tract and account for most appendiceal neoplasms. They are found in 0.32% to 0.6% of all surgically resected appendices, and occur primarily in the tip of the organ.[37] Most of these tumors are found incidentally, although some patients may present with appendicitis or recurrent abdominal pain. The peak incidence is during the fourth and fifth decades and women are affected more often than men.[9]

Most appendiceal NETs are believed to be enterochromaffin cell neoplasms, although rare examples of L-cell tumors occur. Histologically, appendiceal NETs usually demonstrate an insular, or, less commonly, a trabecular growth pattern. The cells are bland, with uniform, round nuclei, inconspicuous nucleoli, and abundant, pale, eosinophilic cytoplasm. Rare tumors demonstrate clear cell cytoplasm. These tumors have been called balloon cell carcinoids and are believed to be a variant of classic carcinoid tumors. They must be distinguished from goblet cell carcinoids, which contain true cytoplasmic mucin.[38] A fibrous background can also be seen in some cases, similar to that observed in ileal NETs. Immunohistochemically, appendiceal NETs are positive for synaptophysin, chromogranin A, and NSE, and may also express serotonin and substance P. S-100-positive sustentacular cells are typically present.[39]

Characteristically, these tumors infiltrate the muscularis propria and often extend into the periappendiceal fat. Although these features would predict an aggressive behavior in NETs elsewhere in the GI tract, appendiceal tumors have a much more favorable prognosis and lymph node metastases are uncommon. The frequency of metastatic disease, however, varies according to tumor size, being 0% for tumors less than 1 cm, 3% to 6.7% for 1- to 2-cm tumors, and 21% to 30% for tumors larger than 2 cm.[40,41] Many

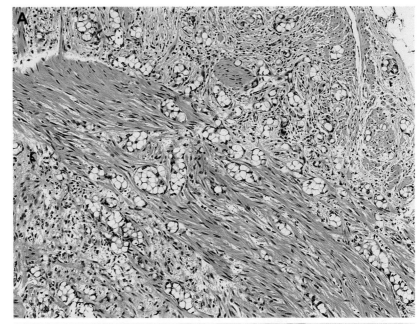
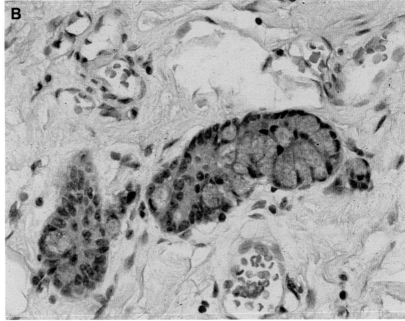

Fig. 10. Goblet cell carcinoid of the appendix consists of an admixture of goblet cells and often inconspicuous neuroendocrine cells (*A*). Mucicarmine stain highlights the mucin-containing goblet cells (*B*).

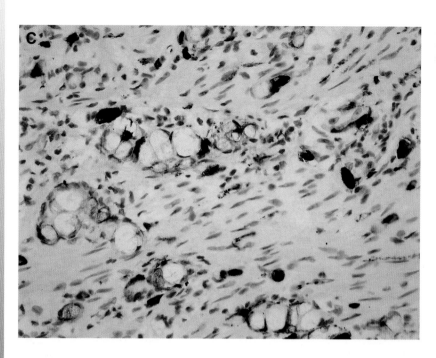

Fig. 10. Immunohisto-chemistry for synaptophy-sin (C) reveals scattered neuroendocrine cells.

other histologic parameters such as depth of invasion within the wall, location of the tumor within the length of the appendix, perineural invasion, lymphatic invasion, and presence of serosal tumor have been evaluated and found to be of no prognostic significance in several studies.[41–43] Conflicting results have been reported on the prognostic value of tumor invasion of the mesoappendix.[42,44,45]

Although most NETs of the appendix display classic carcinoid morphology, unusual subtypes in this location include goblet cell carcinoid, mixed carcinoid-adenocarcinoma, and tubular carcinoid.

Goblet cell carcinoids are unusual tumors that, like conventional carcinoids, tend to occur at the distal end of the appendix. However, they present grossly as diffuse areas of thickening of the appendiceal wall rather than as discrete masses. They occur most often during the fifth decade of life, and have an equal gender distribution. Although these tumors may be found incidentally, patients frequently present with appendicitis.

Histologically, goblet cell carcinoids are formed by small clusters of mucinous cells with a goblet cell–like appearance (**Fig. 10**), often admixed with a variable amount of endocrine and Paneth cells. In a minority of cases, small central lumina are present, giving the infiltrating glands an intestinal crypt appearance. Extensive invasion of the appendiceal wall by discrete and often inconspicuous nests of tumor cells is characteristic. Stromal reaction against infiltrating tumor is usually absent. Perineural and lymphatic invasion may be present

and presence of pools of extracellular mucin-containing tumor cells are not uncommon.[46] Cytologically, tumor cells are bland with cytoplasmic mucin staining positive with periodic acid-Schiff and Alcian blue. Immunohistochemically, goblet cell carcinoids are positive for keratin and carcinoembryonic antigen.[46,47] Synaptophysin and chromogranin highlight a variable number of neuroendocrine cells within the tumor nests.

Goblet cell carcinoid is considered by some to represent a form of low-grade adenocarcinoma,[37] partly because of the scarcity of neuroendocrine cells within the tumor. However, these neoplasms do not contain mutations commonly present in adenocarcinomas, such as K-ras, β-catenin or DPC-4, and certain chromosome losses (such as 11q, 16q, 18q) found in ileal carcinoids have been detected.[48] Electron microscopy studies demonstrated features of adenocarcinomas and carcinoid tumors, with the presence of cytoplasmic mucin and electron dense granules.[47] Although epithelial abnormalities such as disarray and nuclear enlargement of goblet cells and an association with mucinous neoplasms and appendicial carcinomas have been reported, a definite precursor lesion for goblet cell carcinoid has not been identified.

Traditionally, goblet cell carcinoids have been regarded as being more aggressive than conventional appendiceal carcinoids, but less aggressive than appendiceal adenocarcinomas.[49,50] Histologic features that have been found to have prognostic significance in these tumors include extension beyond the appendix, atypical histologic patterns, and more than 2 mitoses/10 high power fields.[50,51] Size is difficult to assess because of the infiltrative nature of these tumors and therefore is not a useful prognostic indicator. Perineural and lymphatic invasion do not seem to correlate with a worse outcome.[50] An important prognostic consideration in goblet cell carcinoids is the assessment of their growth pattern. Burke and colleagues[46] described atypical histologic features in goblet cell carcinoids that included fused/cribriform glands, solid growth, single filing of cells, diffusely infiltrating signet ring cells, compressed small glandular nests, as well as extracellular mucin pools containing fused glands lacking lumina, features collectively called carcinomatous growth patterns. Tumors containing greater than 50% carcinomatous growth pattern were likely to behave in an aggressive fashion. Conversely, tumors lacking a significant carcinomatous growth pattern were classified as goblet cell carcinoids and had a favorable prognosis.[38] More recently, Tang and colleagues[52] studied 63 appendiceal tumors with features of goblet cell carcinoids. The tumors were classified as typical goblet cell carcinoids or adenocarcinoma ex goblet cell carcinoids (based on the presence of atypical features such as large clusters of cells, signet ring cells, cellular atypia, areas of poor differentiated tumor, destructive growth within the appendiceal wall, among others). Irrespective of tumor stage, tumors classified as typical goblet cell carcinoids were associated with a 100% 5-year disease-specific survival, in contrast to 36%

and 0% survival for the subgroups showing atypical features. Therefore, if strict diagnostic criteria are used in the diagnosis of goblet cell carcinoids, these tumors almost invariably have a favorable prognosis, although atypical features indicate a much more aggressive behavior.

Tubular carcinoids are tumors composed of discrete small glandular structures lined by bland, cuboidal epithelium, which contain a small amount of luminal mucin.[39] The glandular structures show an infiltrative growth pattern in a background fibrotic stroma (**Fig. 11**). These neoplasms usually occur in the appendiceal tip and are almost always an incidental finding. Tubular carcinoids are derived from L cells and express enteroglucagon.[39] Chromogranin and synaptophysin staining is variable. These tumors in general behave in a benign fashion.

NETs of the Colon and Rectum

NETs of the colon are uncommon.[53] When they occur, these tend to be poorly differentiated tumors with aggressive behavior, usually associated with metastatic disease at the time of diagnosis. Chromogranin A is negative or only weakly positive because of the high-grade nature of the tumors.

NETs occur much more frequently in the rectum than in the colon, representing more than 27% of all GI NETs in large tumor registry databases.[7] Tumors in this location, as opposed to the colon, are generally small (<1 cm) well-differentiated neoplasms that present endoscopically as movable submucosal nodules. The prognosis is

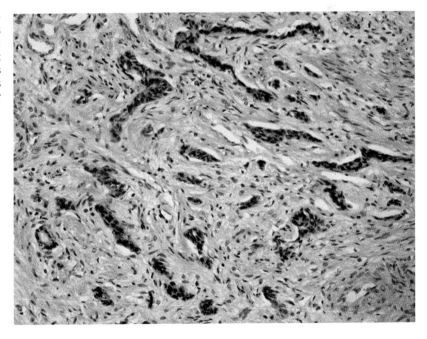

Fig. 11. Tubular carcinoid of appendix grows in infiltrative cords in a background fibrotic stroma. These tumors are composed of L cells and may be negative for chromogranin A.

favorable in most cases. High-risk features predictive of aggressive behavior include size greater than 2 cm, invasion into muscularis propria or deeper, lymphovascular invasion, and 2 or more mitoses per 50 high power fields.[54] Immunohistochemically, rectal NETs can be positive for glucagon and pancreatic polypeptide, and may express prostatic acid phosphatase; chromogranin A may be only weakly expressed (**Fig. 12**), leading to confusion with locally advanced prostate carcinoma. Poorly differentiated NETs in the rectum are uncommon, but when they occur, have a poor prognosis as in other GI sites.

In summary, GI NETs are relatively uncommon neoplasms in the GI tract compared with adenocarcinomas. They represent a morphologically and biologically heterogeneous group of tumors and are associated with genetic syndromes (most commonly MEN type 1) in approximately 5% to 10% of cases. Although no classification guidelines are universally accepted, the 4-category WHO scheme has gained increasing acceptance worldwide. TNM staging systems for GI NETs have also recently been proposed and are currently being evaluated. The existing guidelines emphasize that GI NETs should be assessed

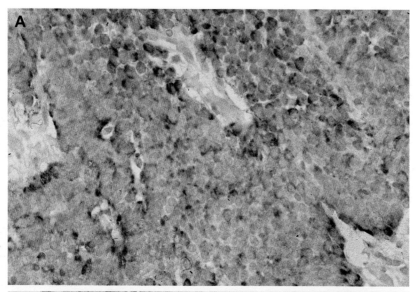

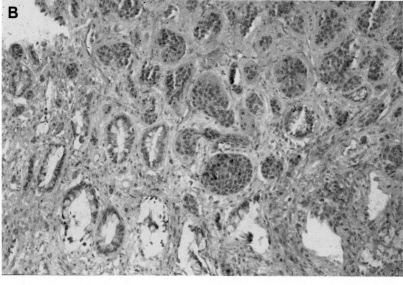

Fig. 12. Rectal NETs are often immunoreactive for prostatic acid phosphatase (*A*) and only weakly positive for chromogranin A (*B*), leading to diagnostic confusion with locally advanced prostate carcinoma.

Pitfalls
IN **GI NETs**

! Multifocal small NETs in the gastric body (type 1 gastric NETs) are commonly found in hyper-gastrinemic states and in chronic atrophic gastritis, and are generally clinically benign. Surgical resection is rarely indicated, and such lesions must be distinguished from solitary sporadic gastric NETs, which behave in a more aggressive fashion.

! GI NETS with a glandular growth pattern, most often seen in duodenal or ampullary somatostatin-producing NETs, may be confused with low-grade adenocarcinoma. Identification of psammoma bodies in a low-grade glandular neoplasm at this site should prompt consideration of somatostatinoma.

! Ileal NETs may be associated with extensive fibrosis and present clinically as localized areas of stenosis (mimicking Crohn disease). Mesenteric and retroperitoneal fibrosis may also be present.

! Strict criteria should be applied to diagnose typical goblet cell carcinoids of the appendix. Goblet cell carcinoids with atypical features usually behave aggressively.

! GI NETs, especially those arising in the appendix or rectum, may be negative for chromogranin A expression.

according to their location and site-specific morphologic features, reflecting their heterogeneous nature. Special types of GI NETs such as hypergastrinemia-associated gastric NETs, duodenal somatostatinomas, and gangliocytic paragangliomas, and appendiceal goblet cell carcinoids and tubular carcinoids should be recognized because of their particular biologic characteristics and clinical implications.

REFERENCES

1. Rindi G. Guidelines for the diagnosis and treatment of neuroendocrine gastrointestinal tumours: introduction. Neuroendocrinology 2004;80:395–6.
2. Kloppel G, Rindi G, Anlauf M, et al. Site-specific biology and pathology of gastroenteropancreatic neuroendocrine tumors. Virchows Arch 2007; 451(Suppl 1):S9–27.
3. Arnold CN, Sosnowski A, Schmitt-Graff A, et al. Analysis of molecular pathways in sporadic neuroendocrine tumors of the gastro-entero-pancreatic system. Int J Cancer 2007;120(10):2157–64.
4. Grotzinger C. Tumour biology of gastroenteropancreatic neuroendocrine tumours. Neuroendocrinology 2004;80(Suppl 1):8–11.
5. Modlin IM, Kidd M, Latich I, et al. Current status of gastrointestinal carcinoids [review]. Gastroenterology 2005;128(6):1717–51.
6. Perren A, Anlauf M, Komminoth P, et al. Molecular profiles of gastroenteropancreatic endocrine tumors. Virchows Arch 2007;451(Suppl 1):S39–46.
7. Modlin IM, Lye KD, Kidd M. A 5-decade analysis of 13,715 carcinoid tumors. Cancer 2003;97(4): 934–59.
8. Habal N, Sims C, Bilchik AJ, et al. Gastrointestinal carcinoid tumors and second primary malignancies. J Surg Oncol 2000;75(4):310–6.
9. Kloppel G, Perren A, Heitz PU. The gastroenteropancreatic neuroendocrine cell system and its tumors: the WHO classification. Ann N Y Acad Sci 2004;1014:13–27.
10. Hamilton SR, Aaltonen LA, editors. World Health Organization classification of tumours. Pathology and genetics of tumours of the digestive system. Lyon (France): IARC Press; 2000. p. 53–6.
11. Solcia E, Klöppel G, Sobin LH, editors. Histological typing of endocrine tumours. World Health Organization Edition. International histological classification of endocrine tumours. New York: Springer-Verlag; 2000. p. 175–208.
12. Qizilbash AH. Carcinoid tumors, vascular elastosis, and ischemic disease of the small intestine. Dis Colon Rectum 1977;20(7):554–60.
13. Katona TM, Jones TD, Wang M, et al. Molecular evidence for independent origin of multifocal neuroendocrine tumors of the enteropancreatic axis. Cancer Res 2006;66(9):4936–42.
14. Rorstad O. Prognostic indicators for carcinoid neuroendocrine tumors of the gastrointestinal tract [review]. J Surg Oncol 2005;89(3):151–60.
15. Rindi G, Solcia E. Endocrine hyperplasia and dysplasia in the pathogenesis of gastrointestinal and pancreatic endocrine tumors. Gastroenterol Clin North Am 2007;36:851–65.
16. Anlauf M, Perren A, Meyer CL, et al. Precursor lesions in patients with multiple endocrine neoplasia type 1-associated duodenal gastrinomas. Gastroenterology 2005;128(5):1187–98.
17. Gledhill A, Hall PA, Cruse JP, et al. Enteroendocrine cell hyperplasia, carcinoid tumours and adenocarcinoma in long-standing ulcerative colitis. Histopathology 1986;10(5):501–8.
18. Sigel JE, Goldblum JR, Sigel JE, et al. Neuroendocrine neoplasms arising in inflammatory bowel disease: a report of 14 cases. Mod Pathol 1998; 11(6):537–42.
19. Barbareschi M, Roldo C, Zamboni G, et al. CDX-2 homeobox gene product expression in neuroendocrine tumors: its role as a marker of intestinal

neuroendocrine tumors. Am J Surg Pathol 2004; 28(9):1169–76.

20. Srivastava A, Padilla O, Fischer-Colbrie R, et al. Neuroendocrine secretory protein-55 (NESP-55) expression discriminates pancreatic endocrine tumors and pheochromocytomas from gastrointestinal and pulmonary carcinoids. Am J Surg Pathol 2004;28(10):1371–8.

21. Rindi G, Kloppel G, Alhman H, et al. TNM staging of foregut (neuro)endocrine tumors: a consensus proposal including a grading system. Virchows Arch 2006;449:395–401.

22. Rindi G, Kloppel G, Couvelard A, et al. TNM staging of midgut and hindgut (neuro) endocrine tumors: a consensus proposal including a grading system. Virchows Arch 2007;451(4):757–62.

23. Pape UF, Jann H, Muller-Nordhorn J, et al. Prognostic relevance of a novel TNM classification system for upper gastroenteropancreatic neuroendocrine tumors. Cancer 2008;113(2):256–65.

24. Landry CS, McMasters KM, Scoggins CR, et al. Proposed staging system for gastrointestinal carcinoid tumors. Am Surg 2008;74:418–22.

25. Borch K, Ahren B, Ahlman H, et al. Gastric carcinoids: biologic behavior and prognosis after differentiated treatment in relation to type. Ann Surg 2005;242(1):64–73.

26. Kloppel G, Anlauf M. Epidemiology, tumour biology and histopathologic classification of neuroendocrine tumours of the gastrointestinal tract. Best Pract Res Clin Gastroenterol 2005;19(4):507–17.

27. Modlin IM, Sandor A, Modlin IM, et al. An analysis of 8305 cases of carcinoid tumors. Cancer 1997;79(4): 813–29.

28. Yao JC, Hassan M, Phan A, et al. One hundred years after "carcinoid": epidemiology of and prognostic factors for neuroendocrine tumors in 35,825 cases in the United States. J Clin Oncol 2008;26(18):3063–72.

29. Pipeleers-Marichal M, Donow C, Heitz PU, et al. Pathologic aspects of gastrinomas in patients with Zollinger-Ellison syndrome with and without multiple endocrine neoplasia type I. World J Surg 1993; 17(4):481–8.

30. Capella C, Solcia E, Sobin LH, et al. Endocrine tumors of the small intestine. In: Hamilton SR, Aaltonen LA, editors. World Health Organization classification of tumors. Pathology and genetics of tumours of the digestive system. Lyon (France): IARC Press; 2000. p. 77–82.

31. Nesi G, Marcucci T, Rubio CA, et al. Somatostatinoma: clinico-pathological features of three cases and literature reviewed. J Gastroenterol Hepatol 2008; 23(4):521–6.

32. Garbrecht N, Anlauf M, Schmitt A, et al. Somatostatin-producing neuroendocrine tumors of the duodenum and pancreas: incidence, types, biological behavior, association with inherited syndromes, and functional activity. Endocr Relat Cancer 2008; 15(1):229–41.

33. Bucher P, Mathe Z, Buhler L, et al. Paraganglioma of the ampulla of Vater: a potentially malignant neoplasm. Scand J Gastroenterol 2004;39(3): 291–5.

34. Scheithauer BW, Nora FE, LeChago J, et al. Duodenal gangliocytic paraganglioma. Clinicopathologic and immunocytochemical study of 11 cases. Am J Clin Pathol 1986;86(5):559–65.

35. Modlin IM, Shapiro MD, Kidd M, et al. Carcinoid tumors and fibrosis: an association with no explanation. Am J Gastroenterol 2004;99(12):2466–78.

36. Kidd M, Modlin IM, Shapiro MD, et al. CTGF, intestinal stellate cells and carcinoid fibrogenesis. World J Gastroenterol 2007;13(39):5208–16.

37. Misdraji J. Neuroendocrine tumours of the appendix. Curr Diagn Pathol 2005;11:180–93.

38. Li CC, Hirowaka M, Qian ZR, et al. Expression of E-cadherin, b-catenin, and Ki-67 in goblet cell carcinoids of the appendix: an immunohistochemical study with clinical correlation. Endocr Pathol 2002; 13(1):47–58.

39. Burke AP, Sobin LH, Federspiel BH, et al. Appendiceal carcinoids: correlation of histology and immunohistochemistry. Mod Pathol 1989;2:630–7.

40. Lauffer JM, Zhang T, Modlin IM, et al. Review article: current status of gastrointestinal carcinoids. Aliment Pharmacol Ther 1999;13(3):271–87.

41. Gouzi JL, Laigneau P, Delalande JP, et al. Indications for right hemicolectomy in carcinoid tumors of the appendix. The French Associations for Surgical Research. Surg Gynecol Obstet 1993; 176(6):543–7.

42. Glasser CM, Bhagavan BS, Glasser CM, et al. Carcinoid tumors of the appendix. Arch Pathol Lab Med 1980;104(5):272–5.

43. Moertel CG, Weiland LH, Nagorney DM, et al. Carcinoid tumor of the appendix: treatment and prognosis. N Engl J Med 1987;317(27):1699–701.

44. Rossi G, Valli R, Bertolini F, et al. Does mesoappendix infiltration predict a worse prognosis in incidental neuroendocrine tumors of the appendix? A clinicopathologic and immunohistochemical study of 15 cases. Am J Clin Pathol 2003;120(5):706–11.

45. Syracuse DC, Perzin KH, Price JB, et al. Carcinoid tumors of the appendix. Mesoappendiceal extension and nodal metastases. Ann Surg 1979;190(1): 58–63.

46. Burke AP, Sobin LH, Federspiel BH, et al. Goblet cell carcinoids and related tumors of the vermiform appendix. Am J Clin Pathol 1990;94(1):27–35.

47. Kanthan R, Saxena A, Kanthan SC, et al. Goblet cell carcinoids of the appendix: immunophenotype and ultrastructural study. Arch Pathol Lab Med 2001; 125(3):386–90.

48. Stancu M, Wu TT, Wallace C, et al. Genetic alterations in goblet cell carcinoids of the vermiform appendix and comparison with gastrointestinal carcinoid tumors. Mod Pathol 2003;16(12):1189–98.
49. McCusker ME, Cote TR, Clegg LX, et al. Primary malignant neoplasms of the appendix: a population-based study from the surveillance, epidemiology and end-results program, 1973–1998. Cancer 2002;94(12):3307–12.
50. Warkel RL, Cooper PH, Helwig EB, et al. Adenocarcinoid, a mucin-producing carcinoid tumor of the appendix: a study of 39 cases. Cancer 1978;42(6):2781–93.
51. Bak M, Asschenfeldt P, Bak M, et al. Adenocarcinoid of the vermiform appendix. A clinicopathologic study of 20 cases. Dis Colon Rectum 1988;31(8):605–12.
52. Tang LH, Shia J, Soslow RA, et al. Pathologic classification and clinical behavior of the spectrum of goblet cell carcinoid tumors of the appendix. Am J Surg Pathol 2008;32(10):1429–43.
53. Spread C, Berkel H, Jewell L, et al. Colon carcinoid tumors: a population-based study. Dis Colon Rectum 1994;37:482–91.
54. Fahy BN, Tang LH, Klimstra D, et al. Carcinoid of the rectum risk stratification (CaRRs): a strategy for preoperative outcome assessment. Ann Surg Oncol 2007;14(5):1735–43.
55. Bordi C, Yu JY, Baggi MT, et al. Gastric carcinoids and their precursor lesions. A histologic and immunohistochemical study of 23 cases. Cancer 1991;67(3):663–72.
56. Burke AP, Thomas RM, Elsayed AM, et al. Carcinoids of the jejunum and ileum: an immunohistochemical study of 167 cases. Cancer 1997;79:1086–93.
57. Cunningham JD, Aleali R, Aleali M, et al. Malignant small bowel neoplasms: histopathologic determinants of recurrence and survival. Ann Surg 1997;242:65–73.
58. Federspiel BH, Burker AP, Sobin LH, et al. Rectal and colonic carcinoids: a clinicopathologic study of 84 cases. Cancer 1990;65:135–40.
59. Kimura N, Sasano M. Prostate-specific acid phosphatase in carcinoid tumors. Virchows Arch A Pathol Anat Histopathol 1986;410:247–51.
60. Nash SV, Said JW. Gastroenteropancreatic neuroendocrine tumors. Am J Clin Pathol 1986;86:415–22.
61. Saclarides TJ, Szeluga D, Staren ED. Neuroendocrine cancers of the colon and rectum. Dis Colon Rectum 1994;37:635–42.

UPPER GASTROINTESTINAL TRACT IN INFLAMMATORY BOWEL DISEASE

Neal S. Goldstein, MD[a],*, Mitual Amin, MD[b]

KEYWORDS

- Inflammatory bowel disease • Crohn's • Ulcerative colitis • Esophagitis • Eosinophilic esophagitis
- Lymphocytic esophagitis • Nonspecific gastritis • Aphthoid ulcers

ABSTRACT

Involvement of the upper gastrointestinal tract by inflammatory bowel disease was long held to be a feature of Crohn's disease, whereas ulcerative colitis was considered to be limited to the colon. It is now recognized that ulcerative colitis associated inflammation can involve the upper gastrointestinal tract, primarily the stomach. In addition to aphthoid esophageal ulcers in Crohn's disease, eosinophilic esophagitis and so-called lymphocytic esophagitis occur in association with ulcerative colitis and Crohn's disease. Possible immune mechanisms behind these conditions are presented. The differential diagnosis of inflammation in each site is discussed.

Key Features
INFLAMMATORY BOWEL DISEASE

1. Upper gastrointestinal (GI) involvement is not a criterion for subtyping inflammatory bowel disease.

2. The diagnosis of Crohn's disease should not be based solely on active duodenitis.

3. Lower GI tract inflammatory bowel disease, focal lymphoplasmacytic inflammation accompanied by a granuloma is diagnostic of Crohn's disease, regardless of the level of active inflammation.

OVERVIEW

Involvement of the upper gastrointestinal tract (UGT) by inflammatory bowel disease (IBD) was long held to be a feature of Crohn's disease, whereas ulcerative colitis was considered to be limited to the colon and occasionally the distal ileum. For decades, it was dogmatically thought that ulcerative colitis did not involve the UGT to the extent that patients with IBD with otherwise classic ulcerative colitis were given a Crohn's disease diagnosis. Abundant evidence has accrued over the last 20 years that refute these tenets.

Not only have these canonical tenets been shed but the contemporary perspective of IBD has expanded with the understanding that the endoscopic appearance, pattern, and extent of inflammation shifts between the initial presentation and chronic disease state in Crohn's disease and ulcerative colitis. With improved medical therapy, patients with IBD come to endoscopy much earlier, shifting the activity level and extent of chronic changes seen in biopsy specimens. The morphology of Crohn's disease and ulcerative colitis at different stations along this temporal

[a] Advanced Diagnostics Laboratory, PLLC, 25241 Grand River Avenue, Redford, MI 483240, USA
[b] Department of Anatomic Pathology, William Beaumont Hospital, 3601 West 13 Mile Road, Royal Oak, MI 48073, USA
* Corresponding author.
E-mail address: nealgoldstein@AdvancedDiagnosticsLab.com

Surgical Pathology 3 (2010) 349–359
doi:10.1016/j.path.2010.05.004

road can differ between adults and pediatric patients. Contemporary IBD medical therapy can substantially alter the endoscopic appearance and morphology of both diseases with some medications acting systemically, whereas others target a specific area or region of the gastrointestinal (GI) tract. These superimposed alterations must be factored into contemporary pathologists' interpretation and be reflected in the semantics and phraseology of pathology reports. This article addresses the morphologic features of UGT inflammatory bowel disease, focusing on the clinicopathologic and temporal relationships that are commonly shared and those that are distinctive and unique to each disease.

DEFINITIONS

Contemporary IBD diagnoses and management are predicated on recent evidenced-based consensus and classification agreements.[1–4] Terminology and definitions used in this article reflect these publications. The importance of consensus terminology cannot be understated. Definitions pertinent to this article are listed in the following section.

Ulcerative colitis is a chronic inflammatory condition causing continuous mucosal inflammation of the colon without granulomas on biopsy, affecting the rectum and a variable extent of the colon in continuity, which is characterized by a relapsing and remitting course.

Colitis yet-to-be-classified is the term best suited for the minority of cases where a definitive distinction between ulcerative colitis, Crohn's disease, or other causes of colitis cannot be made after the history, endoscopic appearances, and histopathology of multiple mucosal biopsies and appropriate radiology have been taken into account.

Crohn's disease is a heterogeneous disorder with a variety of demographic, clinical, and phenotypic features. The diagnosis is established by a nonstrictly defined combination of clinical presentation, radiographic, endoscopic, or morphologic evidence of discontinuous and occasionally granulomatous inflammation.

Indeterminate colitis is a term reserved for pathologists to describe a colectomy specimen that has overlapping features of Crohn's disease and ulcerative colitis. It has distinct prognostic factors related to further surgery. It is not a synonym for IBD yet-to-be-classified.

UPPER GASTROINTESTINAL ENDOSCOPY

Upper GI endoscopy is performed to help establish a diagnosis of IBD, evaluate the extent of disease in patients, and evaluate the etiology of UGI symptoms in patients with known IBD. Gastroenterologists biopsy different regions of the UGI with specific questions in mind related to the underlying clinical scenario. The approach taken by the pathologist in evaluating UGI tissue biopsies differs between these situations. Pathologists need to structure their reports to reflect these scenarios to be clinically useful.

EPIDEMIOLOGY

Upper GI involvement in IBD is generally thought to be more common in pediatric patients than adult patients. This difference may be caused by the fact that adult gastroenterologists routinely perform upper GI endoscopy in asymptomatic patients with IBD less often than their pediatric counterparts. The prevalence of upper-GI involvement in ulcerative colitis and Crohn's disease is similar at initial disease presentation; esophageal inflammation in approximately 33% of patients, gastritis in 50%, and duodenitis in 20% (**Table 1**). Focally enhanced gastritis (FEG) was initially thought to be a useful morphologic marker of Crohn's disease in patients with colonic involvement; however, additional studies found the prevalence of focal active gastritis was sufficiently high in ulcerative colitis (12%–24%) and Crohn's disease (38/%–65%) and therefore not a reliable distinguishing marker.[5–11] Focally enhanced gastritis is common in patients without IBD. On its own, FEG should not be used as positive support that patients have IBD.

There are several important distinctions between ulcerative colitis and Crohn's disease:[2,12–23]

1. Most UGI inflammation in ulcerative colitis and Crohn's disease is accompanied by distal disease. Isolated UGI is the initial presenting site in approximately 10% of patients with Crohn's disease and extremely rare or does not occur in ulcerative colitis.

Table 1
Upper GI tract disease in IBD

Location	Prevalence at Initial Presentation	
	Ulcerative colitis	Crohn's disease
Esophagus	12%–50%	25%–72%
Stomach (nonspecific)	41%–69%	55%–92%
Duodenitis	15%–23%	23%–33%

2. Approximately 30% of patients with Crohn's disease have UGI involvement beyond the initial disease presentation setting, whereas UGI inflammation beyond the initial presentation in ulcerative colitis is extremely uncommon.

3. UGI erosions are extremely rare (0%–3%) in ulcerative colitis, whereas they occur approximately 10% in the esophagus, 20% in the stomach, and 33% in the duodenum of patients with Crohn's disease. Rare cases of active duodenitis with erosions occur in patients with ulcerative colitis, almost all of which are in the postcolectomy setting.[24–26]

4. Granulomas are not seen in ulcerative colitis and are diagnostic of Crohn's disease. Granulomas are seen in 10% to 40% of patients with Crohn's disease, most commonly in the stomach.[5,6,12–15,27] On its own, granulomatous inflammation should not be considered diagnostic of Crohn's disease.

MORPHOLOGY

ESOPHAGUS

Crohn's Disease

Esophageal Crohn's disease occurs in 5% to 10% of patients.[28] The most common lesions are sharply demarcated erosions or ulcers ranging in size from punctate aphthous to 3 mm (**Fig. 1**). Often submucosal inflammation causes erosion of the overlying mucosa (**Fig. 2**). The mucosa immediately surrounding the erosion or overlying the focal inflammation is typically normal. Aphthoid-sized erosions are most commonly caused by focally active inflammation that is of greater density than typically seen in gastric mucosa. Larger ulcers often have clusters of histiocytes or microgranulomas embedded within the granulation tissue ulcer base. When poorly formed or infiltrated by neutrophils, these can be easily overlooked as simply nonspecific fibrinopurulent

Fig. 1. Midesophagus. Crohn's disease. Nonspecific ulcer with abundant lymphoplasmacytic inflammation.

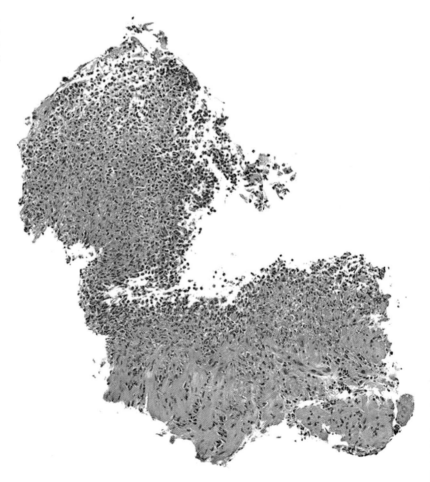

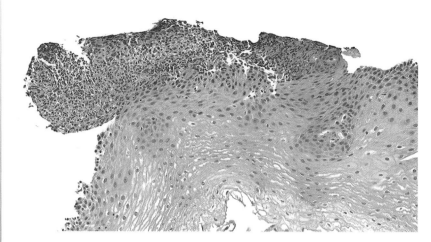

Fig. 2. Midesophagus. Crohn's disease. Mild focal submucosal inflammation composed of lymphohistiocytic and neutrophilic inflammation subjacent to normal squamous mucosa.

debris. Crohn's disease-associated active inflammation or microgranulomas almost always produce endoscopically seen lesions.

Two Crohn's disease alterations that typically produce microscopic esophagitis (endoscopically normal, histologically abnormal) are so-called lymphocytic and eosinophilic esophagitis. So-called lymphocytic esophagitis consists of a greater than normal density of intraepithelial lymphocytes (squiggle cells) (**Fig. 3**). It is not specific for Crohn's disease and has been seen in association with celiac disease, system disease, reflux esophagitis, and normal control patients. Aside from producing a distinctive histopathology, so-called lymphocytic esophagitis has no clinical associations or significance. Crohn's disease-related eosinophilic esophagitis can produce similar esophageal-related symptoms and have the identical range of morphologic alterations as allergic eosinophilic esophagitis (**Fig. 4**). Additionally, some Crohn's disease-related eosinophilic esophagitis appear to have less intraepithelial edema and basal hyperplasia than allergic-type eosinophilic esophagitis (**Fig. 5**). The underlying immunologic mechanism appears to differ between the two conditions. Increased eosinophils in Crohn's disease is predominantly a Th1-type response, whereas eosinophilic esophagitis is predominantly a Th2-type response[29–31] Crohn's disease-associated eosinophilic esophagitis is almost always accompanied by gastric,

duodenal, or lower-bowel Crohn's disease in the authors' experience.

Ulcerative colitis-associated esophageal inflammation consists of mild, lymphoplasmacytic inflammation without activity or granulomas. It is entirely nonspecific and includes cases of lymphocytic esophagitis (see previous discussion). Erosions or other endoscopically seen lesions are not a feature of ulcerative colitis-associated esophageal inflammation. Similar to Crohn's disease, some patients with ulcerative colitis have increased intraesophageal eosinophils.

DIFFERENTIAL DIAGNOSIS

When solitary, midesophageal Crohn's disease erosions are morphologically identical to pill-induced contact ulcers. However, multiple discrete erosions are characteristic of Crohn's disease.

STOMACH

The stomach is the most common UGI site of IBD-related inflammation. Crohn's disease can produce a range of morphologic alterations involving the antrum or fundic mucosa.[8–10,12–15,32–36] In the authors' experience, the most common pattern is mild, superficial chronic gastritis with activity that ranges from none to focal and mild (**Figs. 6 and 7**). Rarely is the density of chronic gastritis or activity of moderate intensity. When diffuse,

Fig. 3. Lower esophagus. Crohn's disease. So-called lymphocytic esophagitis. Increased intraepithelial lymphocytes.

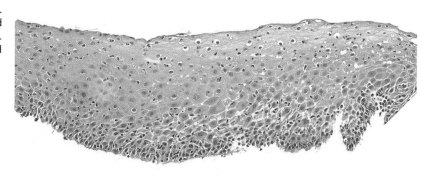

Fig. 4. Midesophagus. Crohn's disease-related eosinophilic esophagitis. Increased intraepithelial eosinophils, basal layer hyperplasia and slight intercellular edema.

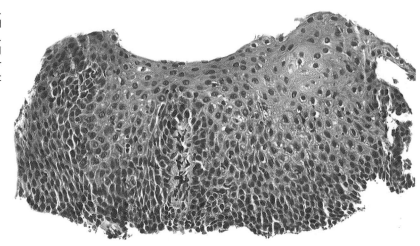

Fig. 5. Lower esophagus. Crohn's disease-related eosinophilic esophagitis. Increased intraepithelial eosinophils. Note the absence of basal layer hyperplasia and edema.

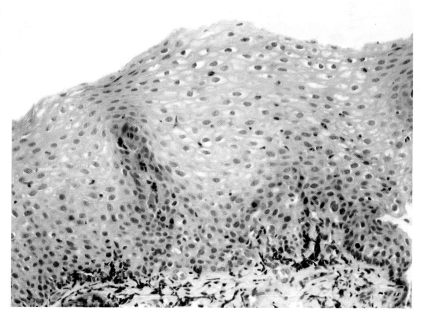

ΔΔ *Differential Diagnosis* DISEASES OF THE UPPER GI TRACT

1. Approximately one-third of patients with Crohn's disease have UGI inflammation beyond the initial presentation, whereas UGI inflammation beyond the initial presentation in ulcerative colitis is rare.

2. Endoscopic erosions with morphologic abnormalities are highly characteristic of Crohn's disease and extremely rare in ulcerative colitis.

3. Granulomas, in association with additional alterations, are diagnostic of Crohn's disease and are not seen in UGI-ulcerative colitis.

4. Active duodenitis with aphthoid erosions or endoscopic abnormalities is not a feature of ulcerative colitis. Crohn's enteritis or noninflammatory bowel diseases should be considered.

5. Solitary midesophageal Crohn's disease erosions are morphologically identical to pill-induced contact ulcers.

6. Multiple discrete midesophageal erosions are characteristic of Crohn's disease.

7. Helicobacter pylori gastritis is the principal lesion that can overlap extensively with Crohn's gastritis.

8. Focal chronic inflammation with mild activity that infiltrates and causes injury to glands or foveola, especially when multiple, can be seen in Crohn's disease-associated gastritis and is rare in ulcerative colitis-associated gastritis.

9. Focal lymphoplasmacytic inflammation with no or minimal activity not associated with gland or foveolar injury can be seen in Crohn's disease and ulcerative colitis and therefore cannot be used to distinguish between them.

Crohn's gastritis can be identical to Helicobacter pylori gastritis. Increased eosinophils, similar to the density seen in posteradication Helicobacter pylori gastritis, can heighten the morphologic mimicry.

Small inflammatory foci consisting of lymphocytes, macrophages, and clusters of neutrophils have been termed focally enhanced gastritis (**Fig. 8**). These foci can affect glands in the deeper mucosa (**Fig. 9**). When in the superficial region of the mucosa, the inflammation can involve the surface epithelium and produce an aphthoid erosion (**Fig. 10**). Granulomas are found in approximately 15% of gastric biopsies from patients with Crohn's disease.

Gastric inflammation in ulcerative colitis is typically focal, patchy, or diffuse mild superficial chronic gastritis with no or minimal activity (**Fig. 11**). This condition has been referred to as mild nonspecific gastritis and focal chronic gastritis by different authors.[5,9,14] Occasional lesions from ulcerative colitis patients with have mild activity that can infiltrate gland epithelium, usually without overt gland injury or inducing regenerative cytologic changes. Well-established activity that infiltrates foveola or glands is extremely rare in ulcerative colitis gastritis. Similar to Crohn's disease, when diffuse, ulcerative colitis gastritis can closely mimic Helicobacter pylori gastritis.

Focal chronic gastritis has gained the reputation of a useful morphologic feature for distinguishing between ulcerative colitis and Crohn's disease. In the authors' opinion, the specificity of focally enhanced gastritis as a marker of Crohn's disease depends on the users' definition of this entity. Small foci of lymphocytes and histiocytes, with no or minimal activity that does not involve glands or foveola, that are found in endoscopically normal mucosa is

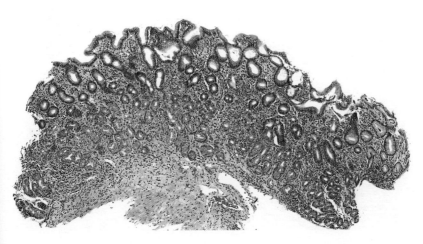

Fig. 6. Antrum. Crohn's disease. Superficial chronic gastritis.

Fig. 7. High magnification of **Fig. 6.** Increased eosinophils, simulating treated Helicobacter pylori gastritis.

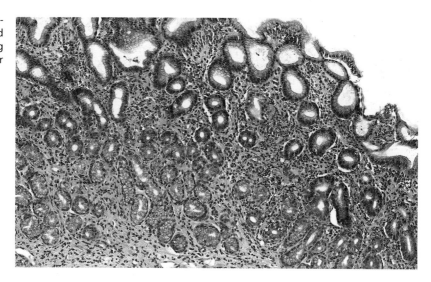

common in ulcerative colitis and Crohn's disease and should not be considered as a diagnostic marker of Crohn's disease. Conversely, well-established mild activity that infiltrates glands or foveola and is associated with epithelial injury is highly characteristic of Crohn's disease and extremely rare in ulcerative colitis. Whether the former is nonspecific gastritis and the latter is focally enhanced gastritis highlights the underlying semantic issues and the arbitrary nature of the line that separates minimal from mild activity.

Fig. 8. Focally enhanced gastritis. Panel shows spectrum of low-power magnification patterns of FEG.

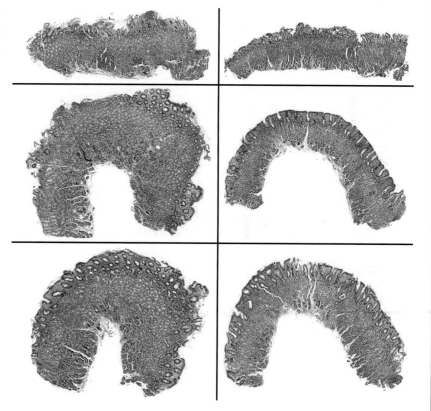

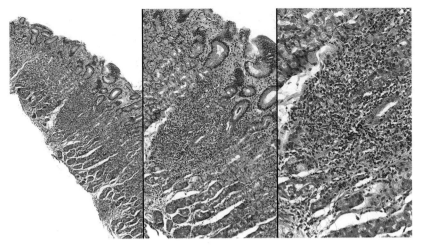

Fig. 9. Crohn's disease. Focally enhanced gastritis. Small cluster of lymphohistiocytic inflammation with neutrophils that surround and cause injury to several glands and foveola.

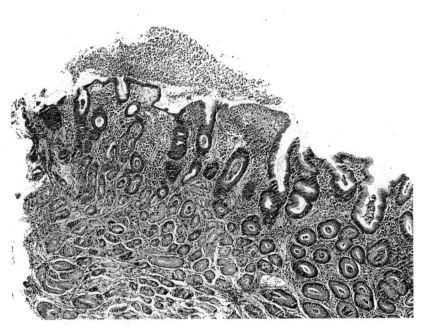

Fig. 10. Gastric antral mucosa with superficial focal active gastritis and an aphthoid erosion. The surface epithelium adjacent to the erosion is flattened and has regenerative changes.

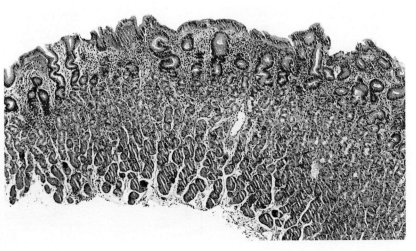

Fig. 11. Fundic mucosa. Ulcerative colitis-associated mild superficial chronic inactive gastritis, which has been referred to nonspecific gastritis.

Helicobacter pylori gastritis is the principal lesion that can overlap extensively with Crohn's gastritis. When the focally active inflammation is centered on the deep glands in the absence of superficial chronic gastritis, Crohn's disease should be considered. However, when the active inflammation is superficial or there is superficial chronic gastritis, the possibility of Helicobacter pylori infection should be considered and special stains should be applied to appropriately rule out this entity.

DUODENUM

Crohn's Disease

Most patients with duodenal Crohn's disease have gastric involvement.[37] Endoscopic abnormalities are most often seen in the duodenum compared with the stomach and esophagus in the authors' experience. The extent and pattern of Crohn's disease-related alterations in the duodenum are similar to those in the stomach; however, unlike the stomach, normal duodenal mucosa has mild to moderate lymphoplasmacytic inflammation and occasional lymphoid follicles, making it extremely difficult to distinguish between normal and mild Crohn's disease-related inflammation. Focal edema, often associated with dilated lymphatic vessels, causes pale areas in the lamina propria and villus architectural abnormalities, including focal flattening or leaflike shapes (**Fig. 12**). Regenerative changes of the surface epithelium surrounding aphthoid erosions produce a greater basophilic hue allowing low-magnification recognition of injured mucosa.

Ulcerative Colitis

Mild active duodenitis with endoscopically seen aphthoid erosions are not a feature of ulcerative colitis. As such, peptic, celiac, or Crohn's disease should be considered more likely disease entities.

Duodenitis

Peptic and viral duodenitis, especially in bulbar tissue, can closely mimic or produce the identical alterations as Crohn's enteritis. These lesions are much more common than Crohn's Disease in the general population. In contrast with these processes, most patients with Crohn's disease enteritis have disease elsewhere in the stomach, distal small bowel, or colon. Granulomas, although

Fig. 12. Duodenum. Crohn's disease. Patchy lamina propria edema causes pale areas in the mucosa and alterations of villus shape including blunted leaflike and focal flattening.

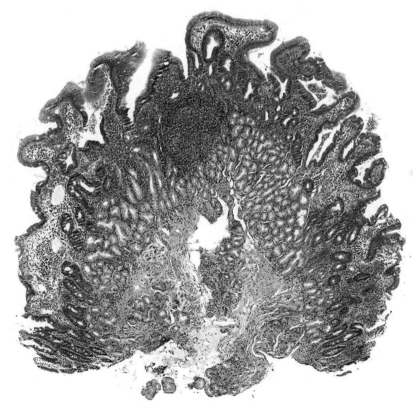

Pitfalls
DIAGNOSTIC REPORTING

! The content of the pathology report and diagnoses *must address the clinical questions*. Lack of attention to this issue can substantially devalue the pathologist's role.

uncommonly seen in Crohn's disease, are not a morphologic feature of peptic or viral duodenitis.

REFERENCES

1. Stange EF, Travis SPL, Vermeire S, et al. European evidence-based consensus on the diagnosis and management of ulcerative colitis: definitions and diagnosis. J Crohn's Colitis 2008;2:1–23.
2. Satsangi J, Silverberg MS, Vermeire S, et al. The Montreal classification of inflammatory bowel disease: controversies, consensus, and implications. Gut 2006;55:749–53.
3. Silverberg MS, Satsangi J, Ahmad T, et al. Toward an integrated clinical, molecular and serological classification of inflammatory bowel disease: report of a Working Party of the 2005 Montreal World Congress of Gastroenterology. Can J Gastroenterol 2005;19(Suppl A):5–36.
4. Gasche C, Scholmerich J, Brynskov J, et al. A simple classification of Crohn's disease: report of the Working Party for the World Congresses of Gastroenterology, Vienna 1998. Inflamm Bowel Dis 2000;6:8–15.
5. Kundhal PS, Stormon MO, Zachos M, et al. Gastral antral biopsy in the differentiation of pediatric colitides. Am J Gastroenterol 2003;98:557–61.
6. Parente F, Cucino C, Bollani S, et al. Focal gastric inflammatory infiltrates in inflammatory bowel diseases: prevalence, immunohistochemical characteristics, and diagnostic role. Am J Gastroenterol 2000;95:705–11.
7. Pascasio JM, Hammond S, Qualman SJ. Recognition of Crohn disease on incidental gastric biopsy in childhood. Pediatr Dev Pathol 2003;6:209–14.
8. Petrolla AA, Katz JA, Xin W. The clinical significance of focal enhanced gastritis in adults with isolated ileitis of the terminal ileum. J Gastroenterol 2008;43:524–30.
9. Sharif F, McDermott M, Dillon M, et al. Focally enhanced gastritis in children with Crohn's disease and ulcerative colitis. Am J Gastroenterol 2002;97:1415–20.
10. Xin W, Greenson JK. The clinical significance of focally enhanced gastritis. Am J Surg Pathol 2004;28:1347–51.
11. Kaufman SS, Vanderhoof JA, Young R, et al. Gastroenteric inflammation in children with ulcerative colitis. Am J Gastroenterol 1997;92:1209–12.
12. Ruuska T, Vaajalahti P, Arajarvi P, et al. Prospective evaluation of upper gastrointestinal mucosal lesions in children with ulcerative colitis and Crohn's disease. J Pediatr Gastroenterol Nutr 1994;19:181–6.
13. Abdullah BA, Gupta SK, Croffie JM, et al. The role of esophagogastroduodenoscopy in the initial evaluation of childhood inflammatory bowel disease: a 7-year study. J Pediatr Gastroenterol Nutr 2002;35:636–40.
14. Bousvaros A, Antonioli DA, Colletti RB, et al. Differentiating ulcerative colitis from Crohn disease in children and young adults: report of a working group of the North American Society for Pediatric Gastroenterology, Hepatology, and Nutrition and the Crohn's and Colitis Foundation of America. J Pediatr Gastroenterol Nutr 2007;44:653–74.
15. Tobin JM, Sinha B, Ramani P, et al. Upper gastrointestinal mucosal disease in pediatric Crohn disease and ulcerative colitis: a blinded, controlled study. J Pediatr Gastroenterol Nutr 2001;32:443–8.
16. Rutgeerts P, Onette E, Vantrappen G, et al. Crohn's disease of the stomach and duodenum: a clinical study with emphasis on the value of endoscopy and endoscopic biopsies. Endoscopy 1980;12:288–94.
17. Wagtmans MJ, Verspaget HW, Lamers CB, et al. Clinical aspects of Crohn's disease of the upper gastrointestinal tract: a comparison with distal Crohn's disease. Am J Gastroenterol 1997;92:1467–71.
18. Wagtmans MJ, van Hogezand RA, Griffioen G, et al. Crohn's disease of the upper gastrointestinal tract. Neth J Med 1997;50:S2–7.
19. Witte AM, Veenendaal RA, van Hogezand RA, et al. Crohn's disease of the upper gastrointestinal tract: the value of endoscopic examination. Scand J Gastroenterol Suppl 1998;225:100–5.
20. Hori K, Ikeuchi H, Nakano H, et al. Gastroduodenitis associated with ulcerative colitis. J Gastroenterol 2008;43:193–201.
21. Lemberg DA, Clarkson CM, Bohane TD, et al. Role of esophagogastroduodenoscopy in the initial assessment of children with inflammatory bowel disease. J Gastroenterol Hepatol 2005;20:1696–700.
22. Mehdizadeh S, Chen G, Enayati PJ, et al. Diagnostic yield of capsule endoscopy in ulcerative colitis and inflammatory bowel disease of unclassified type (IBDU). Endoscopy 2008;40:30–5.
23. Stange EF, Travis SP, Vermeire S, et al. European evidence based consensus on the diagnosis and management of Crohn's disease: definitions and diagnosis. Gut 2006;55(Suppl 1):i1–15.

24. Rubenstein J, Sherif A, Appelman H, et al. Ulcerative colitis associated enteritis: is ulcerative colitis always confined to the colon? J Clin Gastroenterol 2004;38:46–51.

25. Gooding IR, Springall R, Talbot IC, et al. Idiopathic small-intestinal inflammation after colectomy for ulcerative colitis. Clin Gastroenterol Hepatol 2008;6:707–9.

26. Ikeuchi H, Hori K, Nishigami T, et al. Diffuse gastroduodenitis and pouchitis associated with ulcerative colitis. World J Gastroenterol 2006;12:5913–5.

27. Maeng L, Lee A, Choi K, et al. Granulomatous gastritis: a clinicopathologic analysis of 18 biopsy cases. Am J Surg Pathol 2004;28:941–5.

28. Lenaerts C, Roy CC, Vaillancourt M, et al. High incidence of upper gastrointestinal tract involvement in children with Crohn disease. Pediatrics 1989;83:777–81.

29. Lucendo AJ. Immunopathological mechanisms of eosinophilic oesophagitis. Allergol Immunopathol (Madr) 2008;36:215–27.

30. Lucendo AJ, De RL, Comas C, et al. Treatment with topical steroids downregulates IL-5, eotaxin-1/CCL11, and eotaxin-3/CCL26 gene expression in eosinophilic esophagitis. Am J Gastroenterol 2008;103:2184–93.

31. Tella R, Gaig P, Lombardero M, et al. Allergic eosinophilic gastroenteritis in a child with Crohn's disease. J Investig Allergol Clin Immunol 2004;14:159–61.

32. Alcantara M, Rodriguez R, Potenciano JL, et al. Endoscopic and bioptic findings in the upper gastrointestinal tract in patients with Crohn's disease. Endoscopy 1993;25:282–6.

33. Meining A, Bayerdorffer E, Bastlein E, et al. Focal inflammatory infiltrations in gastric biopsy specimens are suggestive of Crohn's disease. Crohn's Disease Study Group, Germany. Scand J Gastroenterol 1997;32:813–8.

34. Oberhuber G, Puspok A, Oesterreicher C, et al. Focally enhanced gastritis: a frequent type of gastritis in patients with Crohn's disease. Gastroenterology 1997;112:698–706.

35. Wright CL, Riddell RH. Histology of the stomach and duodenum in Crohn's disease. Am J Surg Pathol 1998;22:383–90.

36. Yardley JH, Hendrix TR. Gastroduodenal Crohn's disease: the focus is on focality. Gastroenterolog 1997;112:1031–3.

37. Danzi JT, Farmer RG, Sullivan BH Jr, et al. Endoscopic features of gastroduodenal Crohn's disease. Gastroenterology 1976;70:9–13.

DRUG-INDUCED INJURY OF THE GASTROINTESTINAL TRACT

Ilyssa O. Gordon, MD, PhD[a], Vani Konda, MD[b],
Amy E. Noffsinger, MD[c],*

KEYWORDS

- Drug-induced injury • Gastrointestinal tract • Nonsteroidal antiinflammatory drugs
- Chemotherapeutic agents

ABSTRACT

The effects of drugs on the gastrointestinal (GI) tract are diverse and depend on numerous factors. Diagnosis is centered on histologic findings, with mostly nonspecific patterns of injury that must be interpreted in the correct clinical context. Nonsteroidal antiinflammatory drugs are a common cause of drug-induced GI injury, with effects primarily in the gastric mucosa but also throughout the GI tract. Another common class of drugs causing a variety of pathologic findings in the gut is chemotherapeutic agents. This article discusses the differential diagnosis of the various patterns of injury, including ischemic damage, and the histologic findings specific for certain drugs.

OVERVIEW

It is probable that gastrointestinal (GI) chemical injury often remains undiagnosed, because pathologists rarely have sufficient clinical information to make the diagnosis. Some of the nonspecific inflammation seen throughout the gut presumably results from chemical or drug exposure. However, some agents produce characteristic histopathologic changes, making it possible for the pathologist to suggest at least the possibility of drug-induced injury. Overall, it is estimated that from 2% to 8% of patients receiving drugs experience an adverse GI reaction, with GI bleeding accounting for the largest burden of adverse drug-related hospital admissions. Up to one-third of drug injuries affect more than a single GI site.

Chemicals injure the GI tract in numerous ways. Drug injuries result from the drugs themselves, their metabolites, or from by-products of food-drug (chemical) interactions. Host factors, specific meal composition and volume, and the drug or chemical type determine the nature of the interactions. Patients become exposed to chemical injury via several mechanisms including accidental ingestion, overdose as the result of suicidal intent, therapies for numerous diseases, their use as preventive agents, their use in diagnostic tests, consumption of foods that contain chemicals, and consumption of supplements or substances found at health food stores.

[a] Department of Pathology, University of Chicago Medical Center, 5841 South Maryland Avenue, MC 6101, Chicago, IL 60637, USA
[b] Section of Gastroenterology, Department of Medicine, University of Chicago Medical Center, 5841 South Maryland Avenue, MC 4076, Chicago, IL 60637, USA
[c] Department of Pathology, University of Cincinnati College of Medicine, 231 Albert Sabin Way, Cincinnati, OH 45267-0529, USA
* Corresponding author.
E-mail address: amy.noffsinger@uc.edu

Surgical Pathology 3 (2010) 361–393
doi:10.1016/j.path.2010.05.007

ESOPHAGUS

Esophagitis caused by drug injury occurs in approximately 3.9 people per 100,000 population per year, and can be caused by many different drugs, especially antibiotics.[1] Elderly patients are at increased risk because of decreased saliva production, altered esophageal motility, being on more drugs because of comorbid conditions, and spending more time in a reclining position.[2] Lower esophageal sphincter (LES) pressure may be decreased by some drugs, leading to reflux esophagitis, which can exacerbate damage caused by acidic drugs, as well as aspirin, iron, and tetracyclines.[2] Hiatal hernias, strictures, rings, webs, and esophageal compression from an enlarged heart, thyroid, or lymph nodes can prolong the amount of time that pills are in contact with the esophageal mucosa, thereby increasing the risk of injury.

STOMACH

Gastric erosions, ulcers, and hemorrhage can be caused by a variety of drugs, but the most common class of drugs implicated in gastric injury are nonsteroidal antiinflammatory drugs (NSAIDs). There is evidence that direct mucosal contact is not necessary for a drug to cause gastric injury, because intravenously administered agents can cause similar injuries to those administered orally. Patients on corticosteroids have an increased risk of gastric ulceration and upper GI bleeding with concomitant use of NSAIDs.[3,4]

SMALL INTESTINE

The effects of drugs on the small intestine may result from direct mucosal toxicity, alteration of motility, induction of ischemia, interference with micelle formation, alteration of the state of dietary ions or other drugs, and inhibition of mucosal enzymes.[5] Malabsorption is a common final pathway of small intestinal injury by a variety of drugs.

LARGE INTESTINE

Colitis caused by drug injury is likely underdiagnosed, and its true incidence is not known. The most common presentation is diarrhea, which can occur immediately or after the patient has been taking the drug for a long time, and accounts for 7% of all drug adverse events.[6] Drug injury to the colon can occur in a variety of ways, including ischemic, pseudo-obstructive, infectious, allergic, cytotoxic, or inflammatory mechanisms. Most drug-induced damage in the colon causes nonspecific histologic changes that are often indistinguishable from infectious colitis, ischemia, or idiopathic inflammatory bowel disease (IBD). Suppositories can cause nonspecific proctitis and rectal ulcers.[7]

NSAIDS

OVERVIEW

NSAIDs are widely prescribed[8] and commonly used in forms that are available over the counter. NSAIDs are commonly prescribed to treat joint diseases and to prevent cardiovascular and cerebrovascular thrombotic events. Patients taking NSAIDs have a threefold greater risk for the development of serious adverse GI events[3] and an increased risk of hospitalization for ulcer disease.[9,10] Aside from the commonly known complication of developing gastric and duodenal ulcers, which occurs in up to 25% of patients taking NSAIDs,[11] other significant gastroduodenal complications from NSAID use include GI bleeding, nonspecific small intestinal ulcers,[12] obstruction, perforation, and death.

Risk factors for complications from NSAID-related peptic ulcer disease include age greater than 60 years, history of previous ulcers, concurrent use of anticoagulants or corticosteroids, presence of systemic disorders, infection with *Helicobacter pylori*, and tobacco and alcohol use.[3,13–18] The type of NSAID also plays a role in the severity of GI injury.[19] Risk of NSAID-induced GI injury is also increased in the first month of use[9] and with increasing dose of the drug.[9,19–21] Sixty-five percent of patients on long-term NSAID therapy develop an enteropathy with bleeding, protein loss, and bile-acid malabsorption.[22,23]

CLINICAL PRESENTATION

About 50% of patients taking NSAIDs experience GI symptoms, including dyspepsia, heartburn, nausea, appetite loss, abdominal pain, or diarrhea.[24,25] However, symptoms do not necessarily predict the presence of endoscopically apparent GI damage.[26] Clinically silent small bowel damage occurs in about two-thirds of all patients on NSAIDs,[27] and about 50% of patients with NSAID-related peptic ulcer disease do not present clinically until complications occur.[11] Bleeding, which can occur anywhere along the GI tract, is a serious complication seen after long-term NSAID use.[3] NSAIDs can also cause ileal dysfunction, including malabsorption with changes in the mucosal and vascular permeability, protein loss, mucosal diaphragm disease, and iron deficiency anemia.[22,28] Effects on the colon include bleeding or perforation of colonic diverticula, relapse of IBD, microscopic colitis, strictures, obstruction, and bleeding from angiodysplasias.[27–31] Suppositories containing NSAIDs can cause anorectal erosions, ulcers, and stenosis.[32]

PATHOPHYSIOLOGY

The pathophysiology of NSAID damage in the GI tract is best understood for gastroduodenal lesions. In general, mucosal injury occurs because of inhibition of cyclooxygenase (COX) activity and reduction of mucosal prostaglandin synthesis. Most NSAIDs are nonselective, inhibiting the constitutively expressed COX-1 isoenzyme and the inducible COX-2 isoenzyme.[33] Therefore, although COX-2, which is rapidly induced in response to local inflammation, is the target for NSAIDs, suppression of COX-1, which is constitutively expressed in the GI mucosa, also occurs.[33] Selective COX-2 inhibitors are less ulcerogenic because they act only at sites of inflammation.[34,35]

NSAIDs also cause alterations in mucus and bicarbonate secretion, reductions in mucosal blood flow, adherence of neutrophils to the vascular endothelium, and neutrophil activation.[36,37] Cellular damage occurs as a result of luminal hydrogen ion and pepsin leakage into cells. Various inflammatory mediators, proteases, and procoagulants secreted by inflammatory cells contribute to the damage. NSAIDs also interfere with healing of preexisting ulcers by interfering with the action of mucosal growth factors, decreasing epithelial cell proliferation and angiogenesis, and slowing the maturation of granulation tissue.[37] Aspirin can damage the gastric mucosa directly at low pH by physically becoming embedded in the mucosa and causing erosions or ulcers. At higher pH, aspirin is solubilized by lipid, forming cytotoxic salicylates.

The mechanism of NSAID-related esophageal injury is less well understood, but may involve an increase in LES tone and impairment of cholinergic control of LES contraction, resulting in reflux esophagitis.[38–40]

In the small intestine, NSAIDs cause injury by damaging subcellular organelles.[28] This leads to nonspecific changes in the mucosa, resulting in increased permeability.[28] Decreased mucosal blood flow, decreased prostaglandin levels, and increased activity of neutrophils may also play a role in alterations that occur in GI barrier function.[36] Drug-enterocyte adducts may also form.[41]

Preexisting duodenal peptic ulcers caused by *H pylori* may become aggravated, and have a twofold increased risk of bleeding as a result of superimposed NSAID injury.[42]

GROSS AND ENDOSCOPIC FEATURES

Esophagus

NSAID-induced esophageal ulcers are typically discrete, large, shallow ulcers in the midesophagus surrounded by normal mucosa. Esophagitis and strictures may also be seen.

Stomach

Mild erythema, subepithelial or intramural petechial hemorrhages, erosions, and ulcers can be seen endoscopically. Erosions typically occur along the greater curvature and involve the full length of the stomach, including the antrum, and sometimes extending into the duodenum. Pyloric channel strictures may also be seen.

Small Intestine

Abnormalities can be seen by endoscopy as early as 2 weeks after starting NSAID therapy and include breaks in the mucosa, reddened folds, petechiae or red spots, denuded mucosa, and blood in the lumen without a visualized source.[43] Later findings include villous atrophy, ulcers, strictures, fibrosis, patchy hemorrhage and erosions, and perforation may be seen. Ulcers can be single or multiple and vary from small, discrete lesions on the tips of mucosal folds to large, deep ulcerations with central necrotic debris and fibrinous exudates. Although ulcers are more commonly seen in the distal small bowel,[44] duodenal ulcers are common in chronic NSAID users. Mucosal diaphragms, which are a specific type of stricture, are believed to be pathognomonic for NSAID injury in the small and large intestine.[45,46] Circumferential perforated membranes cause partial or complete luminal obstruction. Associated small serosal

**KEY PATHOLOGIC FEATURES
OF NSAID INJURY**

- Erosions or ulcers along GI tract
- Chemical gastropathy
- Acute erosive gastritis
- Mucosal diaphragms of the small or large intestine
- Colitis of various forms

constrictions may be seen on external examination. Circumferential linear ulcers may be a precursor of mucosal diaphragms.[47]

Large Intestine

Mucosal diaphragms, anorectal erosions, ulcerations, perforations, or strictures[48] may be seen, especially in patients taking NSAID suppositories. Patients with preexisting IBD and diverticulitis may have worsening of their disease.

MICROSCOPIC FEATURES

Esophagus

Mucosal inflammation, erosion, or ulceration may be present. Typical basal cell hyperplasia of reflux esophagitis may not be present because of the antiproliferative activity of NSAIDs.

Stomach

There are 3 major histologic types of NSAID-induced gastric injury: acute hemorrhagic gastritislike pattern, ulcers, and chemical gastropathy. In acute gastritis, there is edema and hemorrhage in the lamina propria, with minimal inflammation, and some damage of the overlying epithelium

(**Fig. 1**). Erosions and ulcers are small and sharply demarcated, and there is usually active inflammation consisting of neutrophils and eosinophils present in the surrounding mucosa. Changes of chemical gastropathy include foveolar tortuosity, pit elongation, mucin depletion, capillary dilatation with vascular congestion, mucosal villiform transformation, mucosal muscular stranding, and minimal mucosal inflammation, although increased eosinophils may be present (**Fig. 2**). Other findings include severe foveolar hyperplasia, edema, vascular ectasia, and features of H pylori gastritis. Reactive epithelial atypia may be severe in some cases. With chronic NSAID use, mucosal adaptation results in epithelial regeneration and decreased neutrophilic infiltrates.[49]

Small Intestine

Early lesions are characterized by patchy villous tip vacuolization, and focal villous blunting. There is inflammation of the lamina propria and intramucosal eosinophils and lymphocytes. Apoptotic bodies in the crypt bases are increased. Villous atrophy develops later. Erosions and ulcers develop in the tips of the mucosal folds, and there

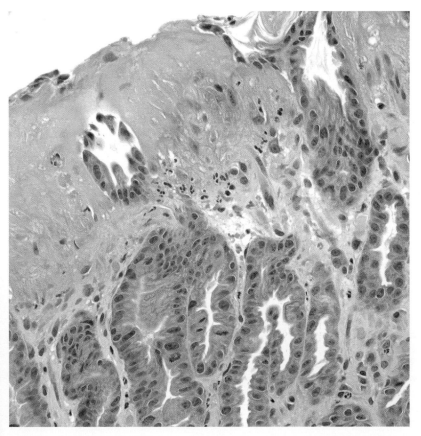

Fig. 1. Acute gastritis caused by NSAID injury. The surface epithelium is eroded, and there is a sparse infiltrate of neutrophils within the underlying lamina propria. The biopsy has an ischemic appearance with more extensive injury to the superficial gastric foveolae than to the deeper glands. The epithelium is mucin depleted and appears regenerative (H & E, ×200).

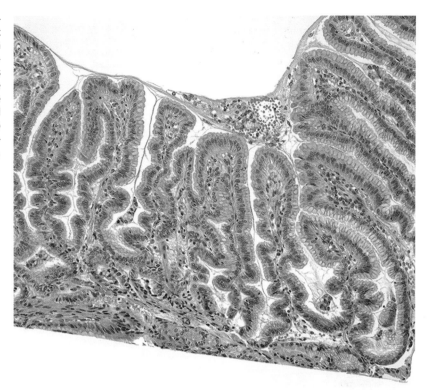

Fig. 2. Chemical gastropathy. The gastric mucosa has a villiform appearance and the foveolar epithelium is mucin depleted. Some of the gastric pits have a corkscrew or serrated appearance. There is no lamina propria inflammation present (H & E, ×100).

is typically a paucity of inflammatory cells in the ulcer bed. Histologic features of mucosal diaphragms consist of mucosal and submucosal fibrosis oriented perpendicular to the luminal surface. The overlying mucosa may be mildly inflamed with architectural distortion and varying degrees of villous atrophy. Pyloric metaplasia may be present, and is an indication of chronic mucosal ulceration. Densely hyalinized submucosal collagen may be present.

Large Intestine

Nonspecific mucosal ulceration is the most common type of colonic NSAID injury. In addition, a variety of forms of colitis can be seen, including pseudomembranous colitis, eosinophilic colitis, collagenous colitis, lymphocytic colitis, and ischemic colitis (**Fig. 3**). There may also be prominent epithelial apoptosis, especially in the bases of the crypts (**Fig. 4**).[50] Fenamates in particular cause a nonspecific colitis with features similar to ulcerative colitis.[51] Other findings may include nonspecific eosinophilia, pyloric metaplasia, and mucosal diaphragm disease. Granulomatous injury may be found in patients taking diclofenac.[52] Patients with preexisting IBD and diverticular disease may have exacerbation of their symptoms without other discrete histologic findings.

DIFFERENTIAL DIAGNOSIS

The GI changes seen in NSAID injury are not specific. They can also be seen in stress gastritis, duodenitis, and in many other forms of chemical injury, including alcohol ingestion and bile reflux. The histologic features may also overlap with ischemia. Focal colonic crypt injury with neutrophilic infiltrates producing cryptitis and crypt abscess occurs commonly in several diseases, including ischemia, infection, IBD, obstructive colitis, and NSAID injury. Intestinal strictures also occur in patients taking slow-release potassium preparations or with cystic fibrosis (CF) taking high-strength pancreatic supplements. However, concentric luminal diaphragmatic strictures are characteristic of NSAID injury. Diaphragm disease overlaps with findings found in neuromuscular and vascular hamartoma of the small bowel, and the latter may be the same entity as that seen in mucosal diaphragm disease. Mucosal eosinophilia can also be seen in patients with parasitic infections, allergies, IBD, eosinophilic gastroenteritis, connective tissue disorders and neoplasia.

DIAGNOSIS

NSAID injury in the GI tract is nonspecific, and should be considered whenever erosions or ulcers

DIFFERENTIAL DIAGNOSIS OF NSAID INJURY

- Stress gastritis
- Bile reflux gastritis
- Alcohol-induced gastropathy
- Peptic duodenitis
- Ischemia
- Infectious enterocolitis
- Parasitic infections
- Allergic injury
- Eosinophilic gastroenteritis
- Connective tissue disorders
- IBD
- Radiation or other strictures
- Neuromuscular and vascular hamartoma

are found. In the esophagus, there may be features of reflux esophagitis, but without significant basal cell hyperplasia. Acute erosive gastritis and chemical gastropathy can be seen in the stomach. However, foveolar hyperplasia is absent in up to 66% of NSAID users and prominent muscle stranding is absent in 53% of patients.[53] Nonspecific enteritis as well as any type of colitis can be caused by NSAID injury. Mucosal diaphragms in the small or large intestine are believed to be pathognomonic for NSAID injury.[46] Because of the overall nonspecific nature of the lesions caused by NSAIDs, the report of findings should be descriptive and NSAID use as a cause should be suggested to the clinician.

PROGNOSIS

Early recognition of NSAID injury is essential for prompting discontinuation or decrease in dosage of the offending agent. Switching to selective COX-2 inhibitors can dramatically decrease the risk of GI complications.[54,55] Buffered or enteric-coated formulations do not decrease the risk of serious GI complications.[56] Early lesions may heal if treated with antacids, H2 antagonists, prostaglandins, and sucralfate. Omeprazole can be used to treat or prevent gastroduodenal ulcers.[15,57] NSAID-induced colitis typically regresses with cessation of therapy.

The mortality attributable to NSAID-related GI toxicity is 0.19% to 0.22% per year, with an annual

PITFALLS IN NSAID INJURY

! The diagnosis of NSAID or any drug injury may be difficult if little or no clinical history is provided. The pathologist should always consider the possibility of drug injury when reviewing a GI biopsy, regardless of the history given.

relative risk of 4.21 compared with the general population not taking NSAIDs.[10,58] More than 10,000 deaths per year in the United States may be attributable to GI complications of NSAID use.[59,60]

CHEMOTHERAPEUTIC AGENTS

OVERVIEW

Many chemotherapeutic agents produce GI side effects, of which diarrhea and nausea are the most common. Between 15% and 20% of patients on 5-fluorouracil (5-FU) and leucovorin experience severe diarrhea.[61] These side effects can reduce patient compliance with chemotherapeutic regimens. Patients often develop pain and discomfort as a result of mucositis, which can affect the oral, esophageal, gastric, or intestinal mucosa. Other common presenting symptoms include stomatitis, nausea, vomiting, anorexia, abdominal pain, diarrhea, and ileus. These conditions may affect the patient's nutritional status indirectly, and there may also be direct effects of chemotherapy agents including decrease in nutrient absorption. Patients may rarely develop lactose intolerance.[62] Continuous infusion of 5-FU and cisplatin has been associated with the development and perforation of gastric and duodenal peptic ulcers and with perforation of chronic peptic ulcer.[63] Methotrexate can rarely cause toxic megacolon and malabsorption.[64]

KEY PATHOLOGIC FEATURES OF CHEMOTHERAPY INJURY

- Erosions/areas of ulceration
- Marked nuclear pleomorphism and cytologic atypia
- Atypical mitoses (ring forms common)
- Apoptotic bodies in crypt bases
- Withered crypts

Fig. 3. NSAID-associated collagenous colitis. (*A*) Low-power photomicrograph showing a prominent thickened subepithelial collagen band (H & E, ×40). (*B*) Higher-power view showing large numbers of lamina propria eosinophils. Many eosinophils are entrapped within the subepithelial collagen layer (H & E, ×200).

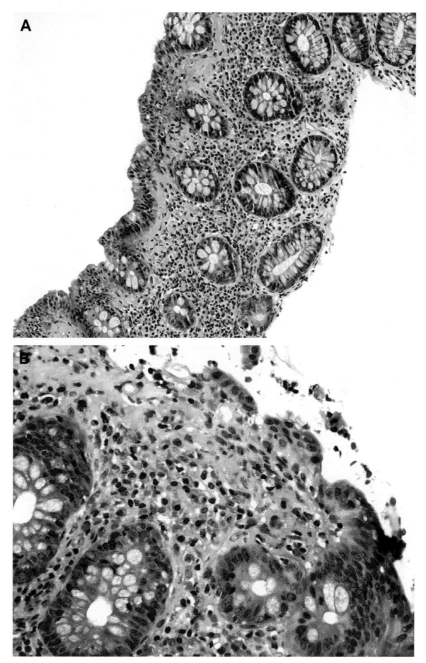

Patients taking cytosine arabinoside have a sequential pattern of injury affecting all segments of the GI tract, characterized by cellular atypia and maturation arrest, cellular necrosis, and cellular regeneration.[65] Colonic perforation has been associated with use of paclitaxel.[66] Other GI tract–related effects of chemotherapy agents include mucosal infections, ischemia, hemolytic uremic syndrome, enterocolitis, pseudomembranous colitis, and development of opportunistic infections including *Candida*, herpes, and cytomegalovirus (CMV).

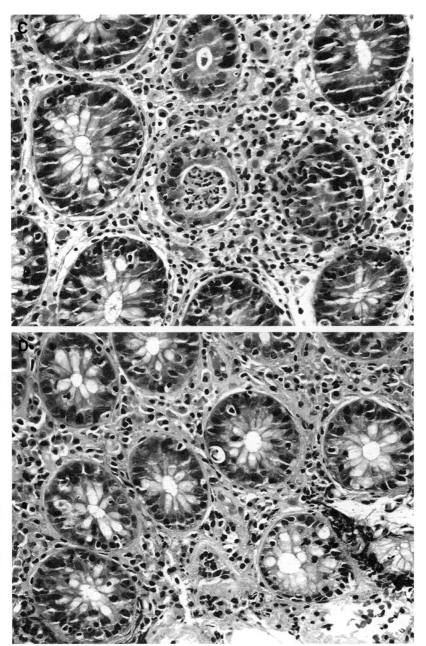

Fig. 3. (*C*) Focal active inflammation is present (H & E, ×200). (*D*) Apoptotic bodies are visible within many of the crypt bases (H & E, ×200).

PATHOPHYSIOLOGY

Direct Damage

The target of many systemic chemotherapeutic agents is mitotically active cells, which include tumor cells and cells in tissues with naturally rapid turnover, such as the GI epithelium. The result is mucosal inflammation (mucositis), ulceration, and crypt epithelial apoptosis. Interference with nucleic acid metabolism occurs with some agents, and may result in nuclear atypia and pleomorphism.

Indirect Damage

Some agents cause decreased disaccharidase activity in the small bowel, resulting in malabsorption and diarrhea. Decreased mucosal blood flow can result in decreased fibrinolytic activity, vasospasm, and ischemic necrosis. Secondary

Fig. 4. NSAID colonic injury. (*A*) This colonic crypt contains numerous basal apoptotic bodies, a nonspecific finding that can be seen in drug injury of many causes (H & E, ×200). (*B*) A different colonic crypt containing infiltrating eosinophils (H & E, ×200).

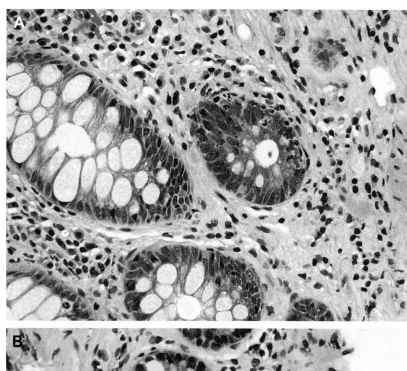

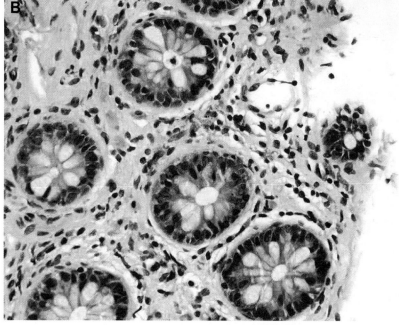

infection as a result of immunosuppression can lead to fungal or viral infections. Prolonged vomiting can result in Mallory-Weiss tears, intramural hematomas, and perforation. Indirect injury to the colon may manifest as infection, hemolytic uremic syndrome, pseudomembranous colitis, neutropenic colitis, and ischemia.

Damage to Nerves

Motility problems can also occur as a result of chemotherapeutic agent damage of the myenteric plexus. For example, vincristine, can damage the myenteric plexus and lead to pseudo-obstruction.

GROSS AND ENDOSCOPIC FEATURES

The esophagus is a commonly affected portion of the GI tract because of the effects of chemotherapeutic agents and radiation therapy used for malignancies arising in the chest. Endoscopic findings are nonspecific and include mucositis, erosions, ulcers, strictures, and fistulas in any part of the GI tract (**Fig. 5**). Gastric bezoars caused by myenteric plexus damage may be seen in patients on vinorelbine.[67] These cases may have an apparently unremarkable mucosa on endoscopic examination.

MICROSCOPIC FEATURES

Esophagus

Early damage is characterized by increased apoptotic bodies in the basal layer of the mucosa.

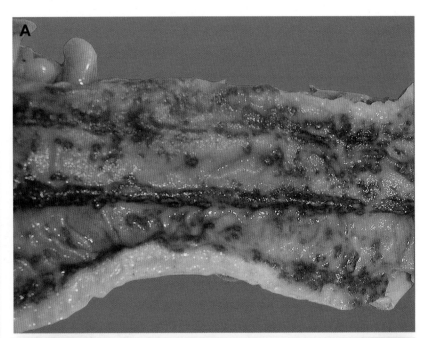

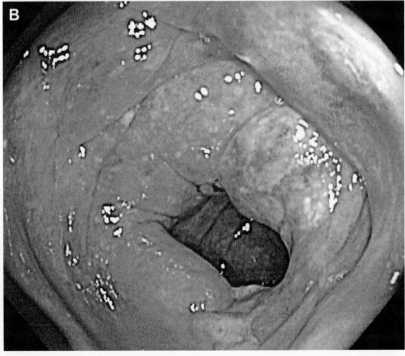

Fig. 5. Chemotherapeutic injury in the colon. (*A*) Taxane colitis. The mucosa shows multifocal erosion and ulceration. (*B*) Inflammation and erythema within the sigmoid colon secondary to chemotherapeutic drugs.

Erosions and ulcers may be seen later. Extensive mitotic arrest and ring-shaped mitotic figures can be seen in patients on taxol. Because of the dosing schedule of many chemotherapeutic agents, there may be cyclical damage and repair. Regenerative features include granulation tissue in healing ulcers, and enlarged and atypical squamous cells in intact epithelium. The basal layer may be thickened as a result of regeneration and may also contain atypical cells, sometimes with increased and atypical mitotic figures. Atypia may also be seen in cells in the underlying stroma, as well as in submucosal glandular cells. Barrett esophagus may be seen as a result of therapy with cyclophosphamide, methotrexate, or 5-FU.

Stomach

Gastric damage has been best described for hepatic arterial infusion chemotherapy (HAIC). Reactive glandular atypia with crowded, irregularly shaped glands lined by large, finely vacuolated, mucin-depleted cuboidal epithelial cells with abundant cytoplasm and bizarre, often multiple, nuclei may be present (**Fig. 6**).[68] The atypia is most prominent in the mucus neck and basal regions of the gastric glands, and is often more

bizarre than is typically seen in neoplastic processes. Mitotic figures may be absent or they may be numerous and atypical, including ringed forms. Necrotic and regenerative epithelium with reactive glandular atypia and finely vacuolated cytoplasm, in addition to an inflammatory infiltrate, can be seen in patients receiving floxuridine by HAIC.[69] Other findings include chemical gastropathy, erosions, ulcers, pyknotic nuclei, apoptotic bodies, and necrotic debris that can be found associated with the damaged epithelium or in the lumens of the underlying glands.

Small Intestine

The severity of the damage seen in the small intestine varies depending on the agent, but the small intestinal mucosa is the most sensitive portion of the GI tract to chemotherapeutic damage. Reduced mitotic activity can be seen in the small intestinal mucosa within 3 hours of drug exposure, and severe injury can occur within 24 hours and can persist until use of the chemotherapeutic agent is stopped.[70,71] The severity of the damage may be worse if multiple chemotherapeutic agents are used simultaneously.

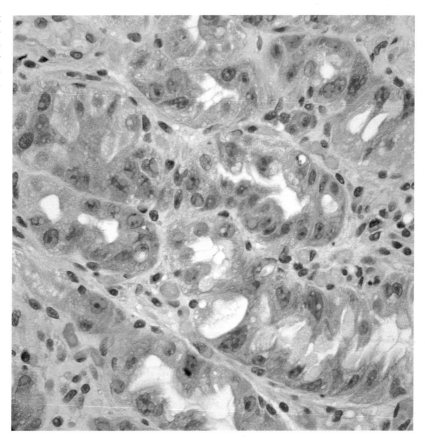

Fig. 6. Chemotherapeutic drug effects in the stomach. The gastric epithelium shows nuclear enlargement, mild pleomorphism, and prominent nucleoli (H & E, ×400).

Early changes include loss of brush borders, foamy cytoplasmic change, mucin depletion, and cuboidal epithelial cell shape. Nuclei may be pleomorphic with prominent nucleoli. In the bases of the crypts, nuclei lose polarity and apoptotic bodies are identifiable. These apoptotic bodies comprise karyorrhectic debris often surrounded by a clear or pale staining halo (so-called popcorn lesions). The drug-induced damage progresses upward from the crypt base, ultimately leading to mucosal necrosis, erosion, and ulceration. An infiltrate of lymphocytes and eosinophils in the lamina propria may be seen early, and may persist for months.

Villous blunting, with decreases in height and width, ranges from mild to complete atrophy, and is associated with decreased mitotic activity in crypts. Random epithelial cell atypia, including macrocytosis and prominent nucleoli, may be seen in crypts and villi, and there may be stromal cell atypia. Cystic dilatation occurs in glands containing cellular debris, apoptotic cells, and neutrophils.

When therapy is stopped, a regenerative phase ensues, lasting at least 2 weeks.[72] Hallmarks include numerous mitoses at all levels of the mucosa, including the tips of the villi, and nuclear pleomorphism. Persistent effects include inflammation and telangiectasia, although there may be depletion of normal inflammatory cells in the lamina propria and loss of Peyer patches.

Patients taking vitamin B12 and folate supplements during prolonged chemotherapy may have megaloblastic enterocyte nuclei. Therapy with anti–cytotoxic T lymphocyte antigen (anti-CTLA4) may lead to an autoimmune panarteritis with cryptitis, blunting of small intestinal villi, intraepithelial lymphocytosis of crypt bases, increased epithelial apoptosis, and an infiltrate of lymphoplasmacytic cells in the lamina propria.[73]

Large Intestine

The effects of chemotherapeutic agents on the large intestine are best described for 5-FU, with early changes of loss of nuclear polarity, nuclear pyknosis, karyorrhexis, and apoptosis.[74] Progression proceeds to the top of the crypts, resulting in mucosal necrosis and erosion.[75] Inflammation is present in the epithelium and in the lamina propria. After cessation of the offending agent, regenerative features can include cystic dilatation of crypts lined by pleomorphic epithelial cells or hyperplastic crypt epithelium with increased apoptotic bodies in the crypt bases, and there may be a prominent histiocytic infiltrate (**Fig. 7**).[75] Other cases may show only nonspecific colitis, cryptitis, inflammation, and ulceration. Irinotecan causes nonspecific changes in the colonic mucosa, including a moderate mononuclear infiltrate in the lamina propria, atrophic crypts, marked nuclear atypia of epithelial cells, multinucleation, and prominent nucleoli.[76]

In chemotherapeutic drug–associated neutropenic enterocolitis, the colon exhibits a severe necrotizing colitis with marked edema, vasculitis, and stromal hemorrhage with patchy to complete epithelial necrosis. Degenerated epithelial cells

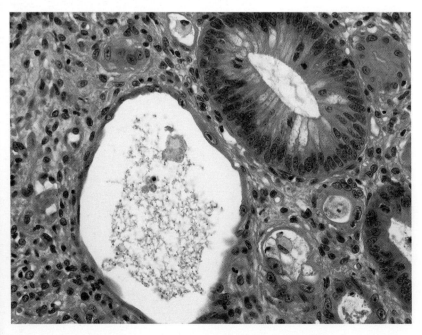

Fig. 7. Chemotherapeutic drug injury in the colon. Many of the colonic crypts appear withered as a result of extensive apoptosis of the epithelium. Other crypts appear regenerative with numerous mitotic figures (*upper right*) (H & E, ×200).

detach from the basement membrane and lie within dilated glandular lumens. The mucosa becomes variably ulcerated and a pseudomembrane containing fibrin and necrotic cellular debris covers the luminal surface. Vascular damage produces subtle or profuse intramural and intraluminal hemorrhage, and fibrin thrombi are often present in the submucosal vessels. Additionally, changes characteristic of chemotherapeutic injury, including prominent apoptosis in the crypts, focal crypt dropout, and glandular regeneration, are often present. There is a striking paucity of

inflammatory cells, despite the degree of mucosal damage, and neutrophils are absent (**Fig. 8**). The absence of neutrophils in the presence of significant cell injury allows the diagnosis of neutropenic enterocolitis.

DIFFERENTIAL DIAGNOSIS

Carcinoma may be suspected when there is cellular atypia and pleomorphism and increased mitotic activity anywhere along the GI tract. The main distinguishing feature is that these findings

Fig. 8. Neutropenic enterocolitis. (*A*) Low-power photomicrograph showing a deep ulcer extending into the intestinal wall (H & E, ×20). (*B*) Higher-power view of the adjacent mucosa showing prominent regenerative changes and a dense mononuclear infiltrate within the lamina propria. Note the absence of neutrophils (H & E, ×100).

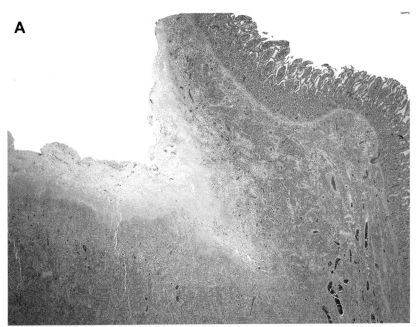

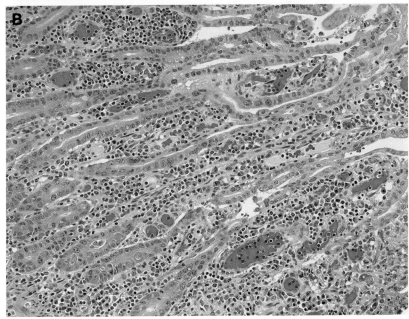

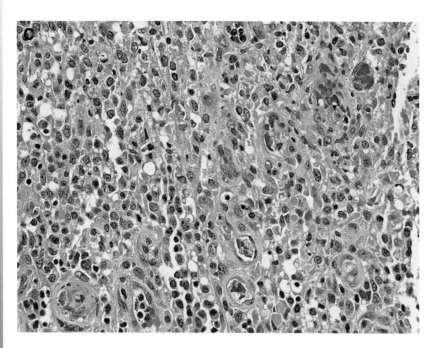

Fig. 8. (*C*) The granulation tissue within the ulcer bed contains no neutrophils as would normally be expected in a nonneutropenic patient (H & E, ×200).

are typically scattered throughout the mucosa, and do not form a localized lesion as would be seen in carcinoma. Mucosal atypia in carcinoma is usually in the foveolae and mucous neck region, whereas in chemotherapy injury atypia is more often in the glands. In addition, in chemotherapeutic injury, there is mucosal architectural preservation, stromal cell atypia, lack of infiltrative pattern, lack of desmoplastic stroma, and abundant cytoplasm with low nuclear/cytoplasmic ratio. In addition, the degree of epithelial cell atypia is often greater than that typically seen in carcinoma. Fewer overall mitotic figures and more ring mitoses favor chemotherapy injury rather than carcinoma.

IBD, CMV infection, and ischemia should be considered with focal or diffuse colonic erosions or ulcers, as well as when colonoscopy reveals erythema, friability, and edematous mucosal folds.

Colitis is nonspecific with many causes. Other causes of upper GI tract erosions and ulcers, including peptic and stress injury, should also be considered.

Decreased villous height and width may resemble villous blunting seen in celiac disease.

PROGNOSIS

Epithelial regeneration is usually complete 2 weeks after stopping the drug. A longer-term bleeding risk may be present as a result of the persistence of vascular ectasias and mucosal inflammation. Long-term complications rarely occur, but include the development of strictures and fistulas. Diarrhea is typically improved with opioid agonist or octreotide therapy. Alternative routes of nutrient replenishment may be required during the acute injury phase.

DIFFERENTIAL DIAGNOSIS OF CHEMOTHERAPY INJURY

- Neoplasia
- Infectious enterocolitis
- Ischemic enterocolitis
- IBD

PITFALLS IN DIAGNOSIS OF CHEMOTHERAPY INJURY

! Neutropenic enterocolitis following chemotherapy may be overlooked because relevant indicators are not present in a biopsy (neutrophils).

DRUG-INDUCED ISCHEMIC INJURY

OVERVIEW

Patients affected by ischemic injury are typically older with comorbid cardiovascular disease.[77] NSAIDs, potassium, and oral contraceptives are common drugs that cause ischemic injury, but many others may also induce ischemia (**Table 1**). Drug-induced ischemic injury occurs by a variety of mechanisms, depending on the agent responsible. Induction of vasospasm and decreased blood flow can be caused by various anesthetics, diuretics, interferon, NSAIDs, potassium chloride, cocaine, and amphetamines, among others. Ergotamines, which are used to treat migraines, can cause local vasoconstriction resulting in rectal ulceration when used as rectal suppositories.[82]

Vasculitis, which may be autoimmune in nature, can be caused by aspirin; antibiotics such as penicillin, erythromycin, and tetracycline; and thiazide diuretics. Thrombosis leading to ischemia is seen in patients taking oral contraceptives, potassium chloride, and vasopressin. Desmopressin, which is used in the treatment of diabetes insipidus, can cause ischemic enterocolitis as a result of mesenteric venous thrombosis and vasospasm with decreased blood flow.

Estrogen and progesterone in oral contraceptives and hormone replacement therapy cause ischemic injury by their thrombogenic activity in the mesenteric arteries or veins,[83–85] and can also cause malabsorption. Risk factors include smoking, and history of hypertension, diabetes, or hypercholesterolemia.[86]

Regardless of the mechanism of reduced blood flow to the intestines, the physiology of ischemic damage involves shunting of oxygen to the deeper mucosa through a countercurrent exchange mechanism, leaving the upper portions of the mucosa most vulnerable to the effects of hypoxia. The extent of ischemic damage is determined by a variety of factors, including duration and dose of the offending drug, collateral circulation, tissue resistance to hypoxia, autoregulatory mechanisms, and any underlying diseases.

CLINICAL PRESENTATION

The clinical presentation is nonspecific and includes abdominal pain, distension, nausea, and constipation. Elderly patients with preexisting cardiovascular disease may have rapid development of symptoms, usually starting with an episode of hypotension, followed by abdominal pain, nausea, vomiting, distension, diarrhea, and rectal bleeding.[87] Patients with reversible ischemic colitis can have crampy lower left quadrant pain, fever, leukocytosis, and tenesmus. Extensive ischemic damage can also lead to fever and leukocytosis, as well as ileus, motility disturbance, anorexia, and signs and symptoms of sepsis and shock.[77]

GROSS FEATURES

Gross findings of ischemic drug injury include segmental hemorrhage, hemorrhagic infarction, ischemic necrosis, ulcers, fibrosis, and strictures, often in the distal ileum or colon. The mucosal surface may be edematous and pale in the early stages, and there may be sloughing of the mucosa. Hemorrhage may be limited to the mucosa or extend to the submucosa, but the muscularis propria and deeper layers of the bowel wall are not involved until later. Eventually there is thinning of the intestinal wall, and the mucosa becomes friable with membranous exudates. The serosa may be

Table 1
Drugs that cause ischemic injury

Induce thrombosis	Estrogens[78] Oral contraceptives Potassium chloride Progesterone[78] DDAVP therapy in diabetes insipidus
Induce autoimmune vasculitis	Aspirin Erythromycin Penicillin Quinidine Some NSAIDs Tetracycline Thiazide diuretics
Induce vasculitis	Rutoside
Induce vasospasm or decreased blood flow	α-Adrenergic vasoconstrictors Alosetron[79] Amphetamines Anesthetics Cocaine Cyclosporine Digitalis Diuretics Ergotamine-related drugs High-dose IL2 therapy[80] α-Interferon[80] Neuroleptic and antipsychotics[81] NSAIDs Potassium chloride Sorbitol Desmopressin

unremarkable in the early stages, but later becomes dusky and dull, and perforations may be present. Patients with ischemic injury caused by estrogen and progesterone have thromboses of the superior mesenteric vein or, less commonly, the superior mesenteric artery. Enteric-coated potassium chloride can cause jejunal or ileal ulcers, ranging in size from 0.3 cm to 4 cm, with surrounding edema and hyperemia.[88]

The rich vascular network in the esophagus and stomach make drug-induced ischemic damage in these organs extremely rare. When present, damage occurs in the form of coagulative necrosis.

MICROSCOPIC FEATURES

The earliest changes from ischemic damage are seen in the epithelium, with intercellular edema being the earliest indicator of injury. At the basal site of enterocyte attachment to the basement membrane, membrane-bound cytoplasmic blebs mark the early changes, leading to detachment of the epithelium, which progresses from the tips of the villi to the bases of the crypts. The crypt cells may remain intact and unaffected in the early stages, and later become hypoplastic or withered. Associated crypt dilatation is often present. Isolated intramucosal degenerating goblet cells may be seen in subacute ischemia, usually in areas with extensive necrosis and epithelial sloughing. In cases of esophagitis from potassium chloride ingestion, there may be balloon cells, thickening of the stratum corneum, and subepithelial edema.[89,90]

With reperfusion, the lamina propria becomes edematous and hemorrhagic, compressing the crypts and causing crypt atrophy. With severe ischemia, there is crypt dropout and replacement by fibrosis. Fibrin thrombi may be present in mucosal capillaries. With subacute ischemia, edema and hemorrhage of the lamina propria occurs earlier, with telangiectatic capillaries and a prominence of neutrophils at the villous tips. The sloughed necrotic epithelium, fibrin, and neutrophils may create a pseudomembrane.

Features of regeneration, including epithelial atypia and increased mitotic activity, may be seen at the edges of ischemic damage or intermixed with degenerative features in smaller segments, as a result of blood flow from collateral vessels. Granulation tissue and fibrosis are also features of regeneration.

Enteric-coated potassium tablets cause erosions, deep ulcers, hemorrhage, edema, and strictures. Pyloric metaplasia may be present adjacent to areas of mucosal petechiae, crypt abscesses, and increased apoptotic bodies in crypt bases. Estrogen and progesterone typically cause villous atrophy with crypt hypoplasia or outright ischemia. A pseudodecidual reaction in the serosa or mesentery may be seen as a result of progesterone.

DIFFERENTIAL DIAGNOSIS

The differential diagnosis includes all forms of ischemic GI injury. Because the histologic changes of ischemia are the same regardless of the cause, the possibility of drug injury may be overlooked. Often, the diagnosis is made only in cases in which ischemia is unexpected, such as in the case of a young woman taking oral contraceptives.

PROGNOSIS

Regeneration of intestinal mucosa occurs with supportive therapy and restoration of blood flow, and the mucosa may appear histologically normal within 8 days of injury. Strictures can complicate the repair process, and may develop 2 to 8 weeks after the injury. Resection of affected portions of the bowel is needed for transmural necrosis and perforation. Without surgery, systemic acidosis, hypotension, shock, and secondary multiorgan failure can occur.

ANTIMICROBIAL DRUG INJURY

OVERVIEW

A variety of antibiotics can cause injury to the GI tract. The most common types of injury are

---

KEY PATHOLOGIC FEATURES
OF DRUG-INDUCED ISCHEMIC INJURY

- There are no specific features that differentiate drug-induced ischemic injury from other causes of GI ischemia
- The pathologist must have a high index of suspicion for drug injury, and must have knowledge of the clinical and drug history to establish the diagnosis

---

DIFFERENTIAL DIAGNOSIS OF
DRUG-INDUCED ISCHEMIC INJURY

- Other causes of GI ischemia
- Infectious colitis (eg, *Clostridium difficile*, enterohemorrhagic *Escherichia coli*)
- Mechanical injury (volvulus, intussusception)

esophagitis and *Clostridium difficile*–associated colitis. The most common class of antibiotics causing esophagitis is the tetracyclines, especially doxycycline.[1] Comorbid esophageal reflux may exacerbate injury caused by tetracyclines, which are acid in solution. Esophagitis may be pill induced, or a viral or fungal esophagitis may develop as a result of damaging effects of the antibiotic on the esophageal mucosa.

Erythromycin has been associated with the development of hypertrophic pyloric stenosis,[91] and can cause malabsorption and diarrhea with increased GI motor activity.

Malabsorption secondary to small intestinal injury may be caused by tetracycline, erythromycin, neomycin, and some antimalarial agents.[72] The pathophysiology of intestinal injury varies depending on the antimicrobial agent. The diarrhea seen with erythromycin use is caused by increased motility, inhibition of neutral amino acid absorption by enterocytes, inhibition of Na-K AT-Pase activity, and by inhibition of sodium-dependent sugar transport.[92] Flucytosine directly damages the intestinal mucosa, resulting in an ulcerative enterocolitis.[93]

C difficile infection and associated pseudomembranous colitis may be caused by almost any antibiotic, but clindamycin, ampicillin, and the cephalosporins are the most common. Penicillin and ampicillin cause a right-sided colitis that is not associated with *C difficile*. Penicillins and tetracyclines can cause a vasculitis and a hypersensitivity reaction resulting in Henoch Schonlein purpura secondary to a hypersensitivity reaction.

GROSS AND ENDOSCOPIC FEATURES

Pill-induced esophagitis may be present as a shallow lesion in the midesophagus near the aortic arch (**Fig. 9**). Candida esophagitis presents with white plaquelike lesions adherent to the esophageal mucosa. Patients with hypertrophic pyloric stenosis caused by erythromycin use have a thickened pylorus similar to that seen in the idiopathic form.[91] Colitis caused by *C difficile* is often associated with formation of pseudomembranes; white or yellowish plaques that are adherent to the colonic mucosa (**Fig. 10**). The intervening colonic mucosa is usually grossly and endoscopically unremarkable.

MICROSCOPIC FEATURES

Mucosal erosions and ulcers in the esophagus are indistinguishable from those with other causes. Spongiotic esophagitis may be seen in patients on tetracycline.[94] In cases with malabsorption caused by neomycin, there may be ballooning

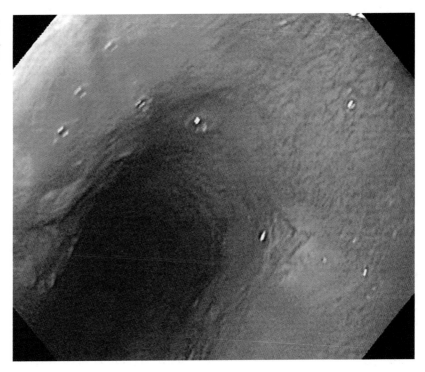

Fig. 9. Pill esophagitis. The esophageal mucosal surface showing the presence of erosions and crystalline pill fragments.

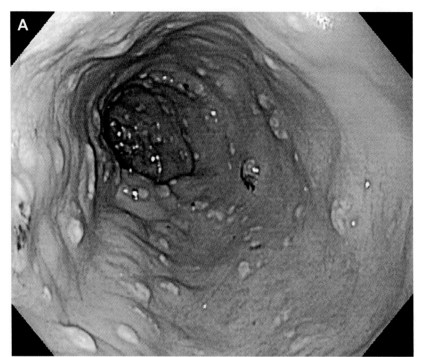

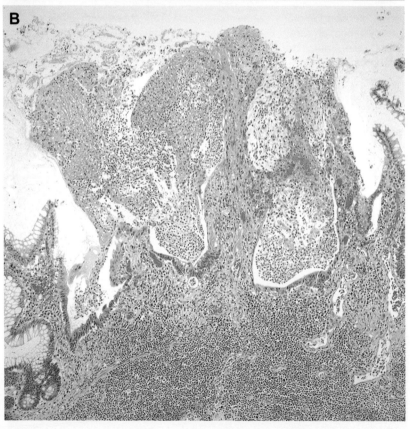

Fig. 10. Pseudomembranous colitis caused by *C difficile* infection. (*A*) Patchy whitish yellow pseudomembranes attached to the mucosal surface of the colon. (*B*) Low-power photomicrograph showing the characteristic volcanolike pseudomembranes that form in *C difficile* colitis. The pseudomembranes are composed of fibrin and neutrophils that appear to erupt from the eroded mucosal surface (H & E, ×100).

degeneration of small intestinal epithelial cells with villous atrophy, brush border fragmentation, and microvillous loss. In rare cases, there is an infiltrate of eosinophils, neutrophils, plasma cells, and periodic acid-Schiff (PAS)–positive macrophages in the lamina propria.

The histologic features of *C difficile* colitis reflect disease stage. *C difficile* can produce a wide range of mucosal appearances, with some patients exhibiting only congestion and edema or a nonspecific colitis. Only about 50% of patients with *C difficile* have classic pseudomembranous lesions. The earliest lesions consist of focal epithelial necrosis, neutrophilic infiltrates, and an edematous lamina propria. Pseudomembrane formation is initiated by epithelial breakdown with eruption of the exudate into the intestinal lumen. The linear deposition of neutrophils and gram-positive sporulating bacilli within the fibrin strands and mucus impart an almost pathognomonic appearance (see **Fig. 10**). The epithelial damage extends into the lower crypts as the process continues. The changes resemble those found in ischemic colitis. Fibrin thrombi may be found in superficial mucosal capillaries. Focal mushroom-shaped or volcanic pseudomembrane eruptions attach to the necrotic mucosa. The pseudomembranes contain epithelial debris, red blood cells, fibrin, mucus, and inflammatory cells. The changes are patchy in nature and the mucosa between the individual pseudomembranes often appears normal.

DIAGNOSIS

The endoscopic and histologic findings are usually nonspecific and the diagnosis is arrived at through clinicopathologic correlation. The differential diagnosis of esophageal ulceration includes other drugs such as NSAIDs, reflux, and malignancy. Celiac disease should be considered when villous atrophy or blunting is present, although in celiac disease there are also increased intraepithelial lymphocytes. Chronic intestinal infections such as giardiasis can cause an inflammatory infiltrate in the lamina propria. Pseudomembranous colitis may resemble ischemic colitis of any cause.

PROGNOSIS

Proven *C difficile* infection requires specific treatment. Most of the other described findings will regress with cessation of the offending antimicrobial agent.

IMMUNOSUPPRESSANT INJURY

OVERVIEW

Patients with IBD, autoimmune disease, or history of transplant may be on immunosuppressive therapies, some of which may lead to GI injury. Other conditions treated with immunosuppressive regimens include rheumatoid arthritis, obstructive lung diseases, chronic hepatitis, and connective tissue disorders.

Steroids are the most commonly prescribed immunosuppressant drug, and there is controversy as to whether they directly damage gut mucosa.[95,96] Underlying gastric mucosal injury, such as with *H pylori* infection, can be exacerbated by several effects of steroids, including G cell hyperplasia,[97] increased parietal cell acid production, inhibition of mucin secretion, decreased epithelial cell turnover, and inhibition of regeneration and repair. Immunosuppressive agents causing direct mucosal injury also predispose to infections by *Candida, Aspergillus,* herpes, CMV, *C difficile,* and microsporidia.

Cyclosporine is commonly prescribed to recipients of solid organ allografts, and can damage the intestinal microvasculature[98] or cause findings similar to graft-versus-host disease (GVHD), especially when the dose is being tapered.[99] Tacrolimus causes impaired intestinal absorption, increased permeability, and endotoxemia,[100] leading to nausea, vomiting, abdominal pain, distension, and diarrhea.[101,102] Mycophenolate mofetil causes abdominal pain, diarrhea, gastritis, esophagitis, anorexia, ulcers, GI hemorrhage, and perforation.[101,103,104] Mycophenolate also produces a colitis associated with prominent basal epithelial apoptosis resembling GVHD. A variety of agents can cause ulcers, hemorrhage, and perforation related to ischemia or infection.

GROSS AND ENDOSCOPIC FEATURES

Endoscopy may reveal nonspecific findings such as edema, decreased vascular pattern, patchy erythema, erosions, or ulcers.

MICROSCOPIC FEATURES

A hypocellular lamina propria, decreased Peyer patches with B cell depletion and a decrease of other mucosal-associated lymphoid tissue can be seen in patients taking steroids and azathioprine. Small erosions and necrosis of M cells predisposes to bacterial invasion and perforation.[105] Indomethacin may cause an eosinophilic infiltrate in the lamina propria, as well as neutrophilic infiltrate, necrosis of villi, and hemorrhage. Colonic necrosis, apoptosis, and regeneration may be seen in patients taking mycophenolate (**Fig. 11**).

DIAGNOSIS

Differential diagnosis includes other causes of mucosal erosion and ulcers, including ischemia, CMV infection, and opportunistic infection. The features of mycophenolate injury, including single cell apoptosis and features of regeneration in the colon, are indistinguishable from GVHD,[99] and an adequate clinical history is essential to accurate diagnosis.

PROGNOSIS

Cessation of the immunosuppressive agent leads to reversal of most GI injury. Octreotide can be helpful to alleviate diarrhea. Superficial ulcers may regress, but deeper ulcers may lead to perforation, especially in low birth weight neonates on high-dose steroid therapy.[106,107]

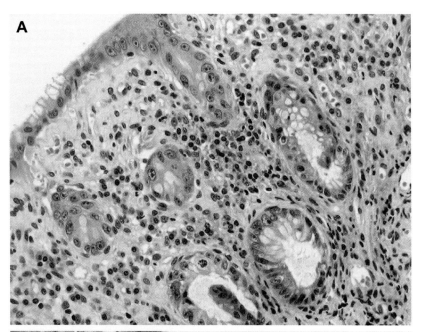

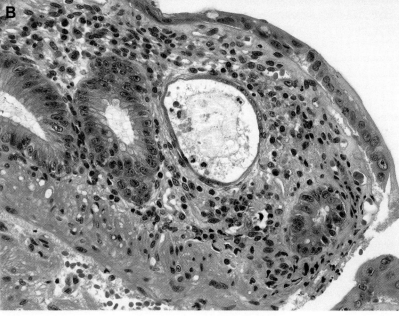

Fig. 11. Mycophenolate colonic injury. (*A*) The colonic mucosa appears regenerative and mucin depleted. Scattered apoptotic bodies are present in the bases of the colonic crypts (H & E, ×200). (*B*) Another patient's mucosa with more extensive injury. One crypt appears withered, and apoptotic debris is identifiable within the gland lumen (H & E, ×200).

KAYEXALATE-SORBITOL ENEMA INJURY

OVERVIEW

Patients with renal insufficiency may be on poly-styrene sulfonate (Kayexalate)-sorbitol enemas for treatment of hyperkalemia. Kayexalate is a cation exchange resin that acts in the large intestine. The resin releases sodium ions and picks up excess potassium ions. The resin and excess potassium are then eliminated in the stool. Kayexalate can cause constipation or impaction and is therefore administered together with sorbitol, an osmotic laxative. Vascular shunting as a result of the osmotic load, with mild colonic ischemia and colonic necrosis, occurs in a subset of patients with uremia. Patients may present with abrupt onset of severe abdominal pain shortly after receiving the enema. Upper or lower GI bleeding often prompts endoscopic examination.

GROSS AND ENDOSCOPIC FEATURES

In patients on Kayexalate-sorbitol enemas, lesions can be found throughout the GI tract, although they are most common in the colon. Eosphageal ulcers or erosions are often present,[108] and the distal esophagus may be dilated and thickened, with a cobblestone appearance.[108] Serpiginous ulcers of the stomach and terminal ileum may also be seen.[109] Severe cases show bowel necrosis. Rectal stenosis has been reported.[110]

MICROSCOPIC FEATURES

Withered hypoplastic crypts, erosions, ulcers, localized transmural coagulative necrosis with mild neutrophilic infiltrates, submucosal edema, pseudomembranes, and transmural inflammation may be seen.[108,111,112] Kayexalate crystals are usually present, adherent to the luminal surface of the epithelium or admixed with the inflammatory debris associated with ulcers.[108,112] A giant cell reaction to the crystals and necrosis may be seen in neonates with necrotizing enterocolitis caused by Kayexalate.[113] Kayexalate crystals appear as basophilic, nonpolarizable, PAS-positive, acid-fast–positive crystals forming a mosaic or fish-scale pattern (**Fig. 12**).

DIAGNOSIS

The differential diagnosis includes other causes of ischemia, erosions, and ulcers in the GI tract, including those caused by NSAIDs, stress, and carcinoma. Intestinal features, such as withered hypoplastic crypts and transmural necrosis, may

mimic acute ischemia without reperfusion. Kayexalate crystals may be confused with cholestyramine crystals, although the latter are bright orange-red and rhomboid on hematoxylin and eosin stain, and do not form a mosaic or fish-scale pattern.[112]

PROGNOSIS

Cessation of the enemas often allows for resolution of the GI tract damage. However, supportive therapy, including blood transfusion and even hemicolectomy, may be required.

COLCHICINE INJURY

OVERVIEW

Colchicine is used in the treatment of gout and acts as an antifibrosing agent in patients with certain types of cirrhosis and chronic liver disease. Colchicine acts by suppressing intestinal enzyme production and transport, by decreasing mucosal surface area and water transport, by retarding intestinal motility, and by causing hypothermia, all of which lead to intestinal malabsorption.[114,115]

CLINICAL FEATURES

Common side effects of colchicine include nausea, vomiting, abdominal pain, and diarrhea. Steatorrhea and megaloblastic anemia may also be seen. Therapeutic doses can cause gastroduodenal mucosal hyperemia and hemorrhagic gastroenteritis, whereas overdose can result in dysphagia, abdominal pain, mucoid and bloody diarrhea, and tenesmus, with marked mucosal inflammation.[116] Rarely, fatalities can occur, secondary to severe diarrhea and dehydration.

MICROSCOPIC FEATURES

The most striking feature of colchicine toxicity is mitotic arrest with absent mitotic spindles and bizarre chromatin patterns, including ring mitoses.[117] In the esophagus, these features are prominent in the basal layer of the squamous epithelium, whereas in the stomach, mitoses are frequent in the mucous neck region. Nuclear and cytoplasmic swelling of epithelial cells may also be present. Gastric foveolar cell hyperplasia with enlarged and crowded epithelial cells, loss of polarity, and epithelial pseudostratification can be seen, more in the antrum than in the body.[117,118] Villous atrophy and fusion with crypt hypoplasia develop secondary to the mitotic arrest in the small intestine (**Fig. 13**).

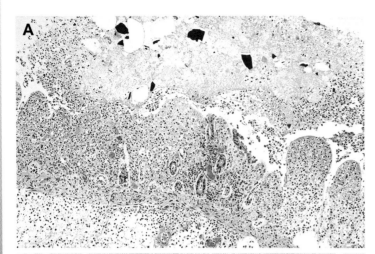

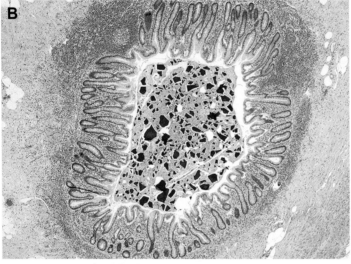

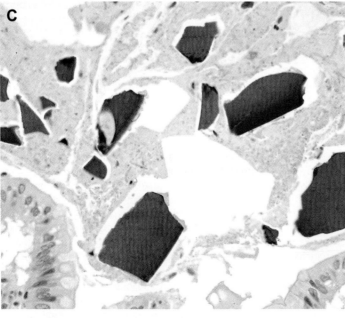

Fig. 12. Kayexalate injury in the colon. (*A*) Low-power photomicrograph showing findings typical of colonic ischemic injury. A few basophilic angulated crystals are present in the overlying debris within the colonic lumen (H & E, ×40). (*B*) Large numbers of Kayexalate crystals are identified in the lumen of the appendix (H & E, ×40). (*C*) The crystals have a characteristic mosaic or fish-scale appearance, deeply basophilic staining pattern, and are nonpolarizable (H & E, ×400).

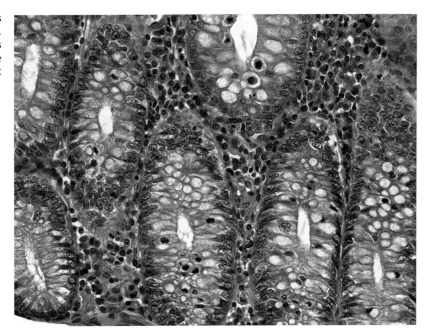

Fig. 13. Colchicine effects in the small bowel. Numerous mitotic figures arrested in metaphase are present in the crypt bases (H & E, ×200).

DIAGNOSIS AND DIFFERENTIAL DIAGNOSIS

Diagnosis is based on clinical suspicion and histologic findings on biopsy. The small and large intestine can be affected. Differential diagnosis includes other drug injury, especially chemotherapeutic agents such as taxol that can cause extensive mitotic arrest with ring-shaped mitotic figures. Dysplasia may also be considered in the differential diagnosis.

PROGNOSIS

The GI side effects of colchicine, as well as the associated histologic findings, regress on cessation of the drug.

PANCREATIC ENZYME INJURY/FIBROSING COLONOPATHY

OVERVIEW

Pancreatic enzyme insufficiency and intestinal malabsorption in patients with CF are treated with high-dose pancreatic enzyme supplements. There is a positive correlation between the dose of enzyme supplements and the development of fibrosing colonopathy.[119] Colonic strictures can develop after about a year of using high-dose pancreatic enzyme supplements.[120] In addition, the risk of developing fibrosing colonopathy is increased by the use of other drugs commonly used in this patient population, including corticosteroids, laxatives, and H2 blockers.[119]

Proposed mechanisms of colonic injury resulting from pancreatic enzyme supplementation are numerous, and most involve the slower colonic transit time in patients with CF.[121] Abnormally low small intestinal pH may contribute to the delayed dissolution of enteric coatings.[119] Colonic stasis and obstruction can also lead to loss of protective mucus and prolonged mucosal exposure. Once there is a breach of the mucosal barrier, a fibrosing reaction occurs in response to stromal exposure to the high concentrations of proteolytic and lipolytic enzymes contained in the pills.

The colonic fibrosis can be diffuse or patchy, and causes strictures, leading to the presenting complaint of abdominal pain and distension. Patients may also have ascites, watery stools, constipation, anorexia, and weight loss. Infants may develop an erythematous perianal rash.

GROSS AND ENDOSCOPIC FEATURES

The colon wall is thickened with narrowing of the luminal circumference, especially at the flexures, but normal external diameter. Rectal stenosis may be present, and flattened rugal folds, submucosal fibrosis, thickened muscularis propria, and subserosal hemorrhage are seen. Cobblestoned mucosa with ulcers may develop.

MICROSCOPIC FEATURES

In pediatric patients with CF and fibrosing colonopathy, an acute or chronic colitis with active cryptitis, erosions, and ulcers may be present.[121] Chronic inflammation is usually present in the lamina propria adjacent to areas of erosion. Edema in the lamina propria is prominent. Fraying and loss of the muscle fibers in the muscularis mucosa as a result of intervening collagen deposition may be severe and can lead to loss of the normal demarcation between mucosa and submucosa. An infiltrate of eosinophils and mast cells in the muscularis mucosa may also be seen. Mature dense collagen and thick hyalinized collagen bands are found in the submucosa, and may resemble keloidal scar tissue. Widening and fibrosis of the muscularis propria also occurs, predominantly in the inner circular layer. Severe attenuation and loss of the muscularis propria rarely occurs. Neural plexuses may be distorted, and ganglion cells are unusually prominent, especially in the deep mucosa near the bases of crypts.

DIAGNOSIS

The differential diagnosis includes other causes of colonic stenosis and obstruction unrelated to fibrosing colonopathy, including ischemia, radiation-induced strictures, and Crohn disease. Knowledge of the clinical history is vital to establishing the correct diagnosis.

PROGNOSIS

Fibrosis is irreversible, and surgery may be required for severe strictures and obstruction. Reduced incidence of fibrosing colonopathy is seen when pancreatic enzyme dosages of less than 10,000 units of lipase per kilogram body weight are used.[122]

BISPHOSPHONATE INJURY

OVERVIEW

Alendronate is the prototypical bisphosphonate, a class of drugs used in the treatment of osteoporosis. Serious esophageal injury, including ulceration,[123] may be seen in patients taking alendronate, usually along with other medications, including NSAIDs.[124] Patients typically taking alendronate are older and may have decreased esophageal motility, which can exacerbate damage caused by the pill being in contact with the esophageal mucosa (also called pill esophagitis).[125] Other factors contributing to bisphosphonate-associated esophagitis are taking the pill with too little water, and lying down too soon after taking the pill.[123] The common presenting complaint is dysphagia, retrosternal pain, and odynophagia.

Gastric mucosal damage, including ulceration and erosion, also occurs in most patients taking alendronate, and is severe in about 50% of patients.[126] Ulcers of the esophagus or stomach rarely lead to outright bleeding, but hospitalization may be required for some patients.[123] The injurious effects of alendronate do not seem to involve the duodenum.[126]

GROSS AND ENDOSCOPIC FEATURES

Endoscopy reveals erythema, ulcers, inflammatory exudates, and esophageal wall thickening, characteristic of an erosive esophagitis.[123] Ulcers in the esophagus may be deep and circumferential,[123] whereas those in the stomach tend to be more superficial.[126]

MICROSCOPIC FEATURES

Distal esophageal and gastric antral erosions and deep ulcers may be seen. The adjacent mucosa may show neutrophilic or eosinophilic intraepithelial infiltrates. Squamous cell nuclei may be enlarged and hyperchromatic, or even multinucleated, consistent with reactive atypia. Small intraepithelial vesicles may be seen. Clear refractile and polarizable crystals of alendronate are often present in the fibroinflammatory exudates associated with erosions and ulcers. Multinucleated foreign body giant cells may also be present.[125]

DIFFERENTIAL DIAGNOSIS

Differential diagnosis includes other causes of erosions and ulcers, including other drugs, stress, gastroesophageal reflux disease, and infection. Multinucleated epithelial cells can be mistaken for viral cytopathic effects produced by herpes or CMV.

PROGNOSIS

The injury heals with cessation of the offending agent.

PROTON PUMP INHIBITORS

OVERVIEW

Proton pump inhibitors (PPIs) are some of the most commonly prescribed drugs for acid reflux disease. Most patients treated for at least 1 year with typical daily doses will have some histologic changes that may be seen on gastric biopsy.

GROSS AND ENDOSCOPIC FEATURES

Fundic gland polyps are usually small sessile polyps seen in the fundus of the stomach. In patients on long-term high-dose PPI therapy, these polyps can be numerous, and may cover the gastric mucosal surface (**Fig. 14**).

MICROSCOPIC FEATURES

Diffuse, linear, or micronodular hyperplasia of G cells and ECL cells may be seen, with micronodular pattern of hyperplasia more common in patients with comorbid *H pylori* infections.[127] The normally tubular glandular lumens become serrated as a result of bulging protrusions of parietal cells that increase in size and number.[128] The antral mucosa may have increased apoptotic bodies.[129]

Small glandular cysts lined by flattened parietal and chief cells resembling fundic gland polyps may be found in some patients on long-term PPI therapy (**Fig. 15**).[128]

DIFFERENTIAL DIAGNOSIS

Differential diagnoses of parietal cell protrusions include *H pylori* gastritis, morbid obesity, Zollinger-Ellison syndrome, gastric ulcers, and gastric cancer.[130] G cell hyperplasia is characteristic of Zollinger-Ellison syndrome and can be seen with

steroid use.[97] Fundic gland polyps can also occur sporadically without associated PPI use.

PROGNOSIS

The histologic changes are usually incidental findings in gastric biopsies and are not known to impart any lasting damage to the mucosa.

LAXATIVES

OVERVIEW

Anthraquinones and other laxatives induce apoptosis of mucosal epithelium, resulting in melanosis coli, usually several months after beginning long-term therapy. Most patients are diagnosed with melanosis coli incidentally when undergoing endoscopy for chronic constipation or other reasons. History of unexplained chronic diarrhea or known laxative abuse is helpful.

The pigment in melanosis coli is a ceroid, containing melanin and glycoconjugates, which derive from the processing of apoptotic epithelial cells into lipofuscin and from anthranoids.[131,132]

Anthraquinones and other laxatives may work by stimulating neural tissue in the colon. However, evidence of nerve damage in the colon can also be seen, which may lead to cathartic colon. Patients with severe melanosis coli taking sennoside laxatives may have an increased risk of carcinogenesis as a result of delayed apoptosis,[133] although

Fig. 14. Multiple fundic gland polyps in the gastric mucosa of a patient taking PPIs.

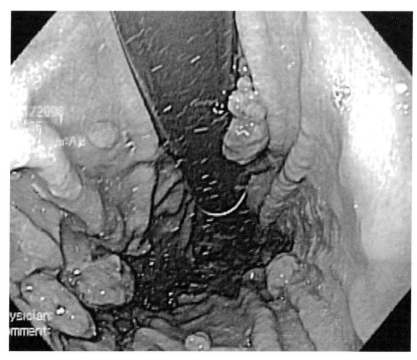

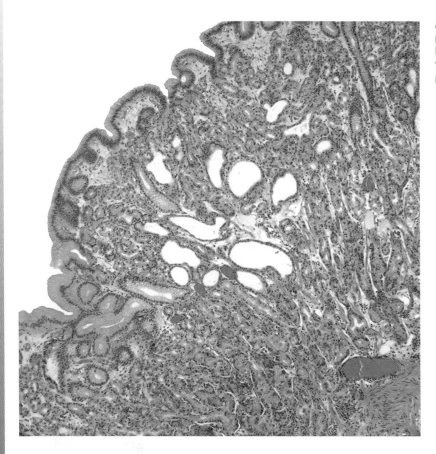

Fig. 15. Fundic gland polyp in a patient taking PPIs. Characteristic dilated fundic-type glands are present (H & E, ×100).

epidemiologic studies have not clearly established an association between sennoside laxatives and development of colon cancer.[134]

GROSS AND ENDOSCOPIC FEATURES

Patchy dark brown mucosal discoloration is more prominent in the right colon, and can cause a snakeskin appearance on endoscopy; a starry sky appearance may be seen as a result of sparing in areas of mucosal lymphoid tissue (**Fig. 16**).[135] Severe cases may extend to involve the left colon or diffusely involve the entire colon. Adenomas or colon cancers arising in pigmented areas are not usually pigmented.[135]

MICROSCOPIC FEATURES

A range of severity can be seen microscopically. The golden brown, refractile, and autofluorescent pigment is present in macrophages in the lamina propria (**Fig. 17**). In severe cases, pigmented macrophages populate the submucosa, and there are increased apoptotic bodies in the epithelium with superficial collections of debris, inflammation of the lamina propria, pigmented microgranulomas, and thickened muscularis mucosae.

Pigmented macrophages may be seen in draining mesenteric lymph nodes. PAS, acid-fast, Schmorl, and aniline blue sulfate are positive in the pigment, and iron and Perl reaction are negative.

Anthraquinone laxatives cause damage to neural and related tissue including axonal swelling and fragmentation, swelling of dendrites, proliferation of Schwann cells, and smooth muscle damage.[136]

DIFFERENTIAL DIAGNOSIS

Melanosis coli may occur in patients who have not used laxatives and who have generalized diarrhea or IBD.[137] The brown pigment can be mistaken for hemosiderin, which is larger, more refractile, and stains for iron. It is possible that any condition associated with increased apoptosis of the mucosal epithelium can cause melanosis coli.[138]

PROGNOSIS

The histologic changes of melanosis coli often regress within a year of stopping therapy, as the macrophages containing the pigment migrate to regional lymph nodes where they can persist.[131]

Fig. 16. Melanosis coli. (A) The colonic mucosa is brown with an irregular snakeskin pattern. (B) Another patient with melanosis coli showing the snakeskin appearance of the mucosa.

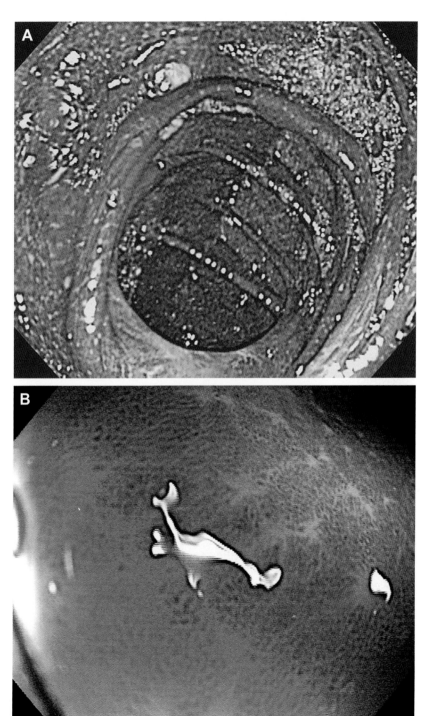

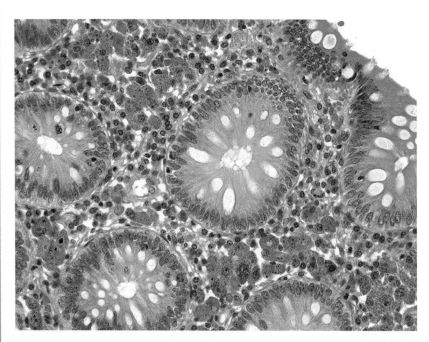

Fig. 17. Melanosis coli. The lamina propria contains numerous histiocytes containing gold-brown pigment (H & E, ×200).

SUMMARY

Many drugs produce GI side effects that may have a significant effect on the health and quality of life of the affected patient. However, GI drug injury is probably frequently overlooked by pathologists because they lack the appropriate clinical history or because the histologic changes induced by many drugs are nonspecific. The pathologist should be aware of possible drug effects, and consider this possibility in the differential diagnosis of almost any inflammatory or ischemic GI lesion. The pathologist should also develop an awareness of histologic findings that may be specific to certain forms of drug injury.

REFERENCES

1. Kikendall JW, Friedman AC, Oyewole MA, et al. Pill-induced esophageal injury. Case reports and review of the medical literature. Dig Dis Sci 1983; 28(2):174–82.
2. Stoschus B, Allescher HD. Drug-induced dysphagia. Dysphagia 1993;8(2):154–9.
3. Gabriel SE, Jaakkimainen L, Bombardier C. Risk for serious gastrointestinal complications related to use of nonsteroidal anti-inflammatory drugs. A meta-analysis. Ann Intern Med 1991;115(10): 787–96.
4. Piper JM, Ray WA, Daugherty JR, et al. Corticosteroid use and peptic ulcer disease: role of nonsteroidal anti-inflammatory drugs. Ann Intern Med 1991;114(9):735–40.
5. Ratnaike RN, Jones TE. Mechanisms of drug-induced diarrhoea in the elderly. Drugs Aging 1998;13(3):245–53.
6. Chassany O, Michaux A, Bergmann JF. Drug-induced diarrhoea. Drug Saf 2000;22(1):53–72.
7. Eckardt VF, Kanzler G, Remmele W. Anorectal ergotism: another cause of solitary rectal ulcers. Gastroenterology 1986;91(5):1123–7.
8. Walt R, Katschinski B, Logan R, et al. Rising frequency of ulcer perforation in elderly people in the United Kingdom. Lancet 1986;1(8479): 489–92.
9. Griffin MR, Piper JM, Daugherty JR, et al. Nonsteroidal anti-inflammatory drug use and increased risk for peptic ulcer disease in elderly persons. Ann Intern Med 1991;114(4):257–63.
10. Fries JF, Williams CA, Bloch DA, et al. Nonsteroidal anti-inflammatory drug-associated gastropathy: incidence and risk factor models. Am J Med 1991;91(3):213–22.
11. Naesdal J, Brown K. NSAID-associated adverse effects and acid control aids to prevent them: a review of current treatment options. Drug Saf 2006;29(2):119–32.
12. Allison MC, Howatson AG, Torrance CJ, et al. Gastrointestinal damage associated with the use of nonsteroidal antiinflammatory drugs. N Engl J Med 1992;327(11):749–54.
13. Papatheodoridis GV, Sougioultzis S, Archimandritis AJ. Effects of *Helicobacter pylori* and nonsteroidal anti-inflammatory drugs on peptic ulcer disease: a systematic review. Clin Gastroenterol Hepatol 2006;4(2):130–42.

14. Laine L, Bombardier C, Hawkey CJ, et al. Stratifying the risk of NSAID-related upper gastrointestinal clinical events: results of a double-blind outcomes study in patients with rheumatoid arthritis. Gastroenterology 2002;123(4):1006–12.

15. Hawkey CJ, Naesdal J, Wilson I, et al. Relative contribution of mucosal injury and *Helicobacter pylori* in the development of gastroduodenal lesions in patients taking non-steroidal anti-inflammatory drugs. Gut 2002;51(3):336–43.

16. Carson JL, Strom BL, Morse ML, et al. The relative gastrointestinal toxicity of the nonsteroidal anti-inflammatory drugs. Arch Intern Med 1987;147(6):1054–9.

17. Shorr RI, Ray WA, Daugherty JR, et al. Concurrent use of nonsteroidal anti-inflammatory drugs and oral anticoagulants places elderly persons at high risk for hemorrhagic peptic ulcer disease. Arch Intern Med 1993;153(14):1665–70.

18. Huang JQ, Sridhar S, Hunt RH. Role of *Helicobacter pylori* infection and non-steroidal anti-inflammatory drugs in peptic-ulcer disease: a meta-analysis. Lancet 2002;359(9300):14–22.

19. Langman MJ, Weil J, Wainwright P, et al. Risks of bleeding peptic ulcer associated with individual non-steroidal anti-inflammatory drugs. Lancet 1994;343(8905):1075–8.

20. Garcia Rodriguez LA, Jick H. Risk of upper gastrointestinal bleeding and perforation associated with individual non-steroidal anti-inflammatory drugs. Lancet 1994;343(8900):769–72.

21. Richy F, Bruyere O, Ethgen O, et al. Time dependent risk of gastrointestinal complications induced by non-steroidal anti-inflammatory drug use: a consensus statement using a meta-analytic approach. Ann Rheum Dis 2004;63(7):759–66.

22. Bjarnason I, Macpherson AJ. Intestinal toxicity of non-steroidal anti-inflammatory drugs. Pharmacol Ther 1994;62(1-2):145–57.

23. Davies NM, Saleh JY, Skjodt NM. Detection and prevention of NSAID-induced enteropathy. J Pharm Pharm Sci 2000;3(1):137–55.

24. Peura DA. Prevention of nonsteroidal anti-inflammatory drug-associated gastrointestinal symptoms and ulcer complications. Am J Med 2004; 117(Suppl 5A):63S–71S.

25. Wolfe F, Hawley DJ. The comparative risk and predictors of adverse gastrointestinal events in rheumatoid arthritis and osteoarthritis: a prospective 13 year study of 2131 patients. J Rheumatol 2000;27(7):1668–73.

26. Larkai EN, Smith JL, Lidsky MD, et al. Gastroduodenal mucosa and dyspeptic symptoms in arthritic patients during chronic nonsteroidal anti-inflammatory drug use. Am J Gastroenterol 1987;82(11):1153–8.

27. Fortun PJ, Hawkey CJ. Nonsteroidal antiinflammatory drugs and the small intestine. Curr Opin Gastroenterol 2007;23(2):134–41.

28. Bjarnason I, Hayllar J, MacPherson AJ, et al. Side effects of nonsteroidal anti-inflammatory drugs on the small and large intestine in humans. Gastroenterology 1993;104(6):1832–47.

29. Kaufmann HJ, Taubin HL. Nonsteroidal anti-inflammatory drugs activate quiescent inflammatory bowel disease. Ann Intern Med 1987;107(4):513–6.

30. Laine L, Connors LG, Reicin A, et al. Serious lower gastrointestinal clinical events with nonselective NSAID or coxib use. Gastroenterology 2003; 124(2):288–92.

31. Gibson GR, Whitacre EB, Ricotti CA. Colitis induced by nonsteroidal anti-inflammatory drugs. Report of four cases and review of the literature. Arch Intern Med 1992;152(3):625–32.

32. Gizzi G, Villani V, Brandi G, et al. Ano-rectal lesions in patients taking suppositories containing nonsteroidal anti-inflammatory drugs (NSAID). Endoscopy 1990;22(3):146–8.

33. Vane JR, Botting RM. Mechanism of action of nonsteroidal anti-inflammatory drugs. Am J Med 1998;104(3A):2S–8S [discussion: 21S–22S].

34. Mitchell JA, Akarasereenont P, Thiemermann C, et al. Selectivity of nonsteroidal antiinflammatory drugs as inhibitors of constitutive and inducible cyclooxygenase. Proc Natl Acad Sci U S A 1993; 90(24):11693–7.

35. Donnelly MT, Hawkey CJ. Review article: COX-II inhibitors–a new generation of safer NSAIDs? Aliment Pharmacol Ther 1997;11(2):227–36.

36. Scarpignato C. Nonsteroidal anti-inflammatory drugs: how do they damage gastroduodenal mucosa? Dig Dis 1995;13(Suppl 1):9–39.

37. Hawkey CJ. Non-steroidal anti-inflammatory drug gastropathy: causes and treatment. Scand J Gastroenterol Suppl 1996;220:124–7.

38. Cagossi M, Salgarello M, Patrignani P, et al. Effects of various prostaglandin synthesis inhibitors on the tone of the lower oesophageal sphincter in man. Eur J Clin Pharmacol 1992;43(3):303–5.

39. Sopena F, Lanas A, Sainz R. Esophageal motility and intraesophageal pH patterns in patients with esophagitis and chronic nonsteroidal anti-inflammatory drug use. J Clin Gastroenterol 1998;27(4): 316–20.

40. Bigard MA, Pelletier AL. [Esophageal complications of non steroidal antiinflammatory drugs]. Gastroenterol Clin Biol 2004;28(Spec No 3):C58–61 [in French].

41. Atchison CR, West AB, Balakumaran A, et al. Drug enterocyte adducts: possible causal factor for diclofenac enteropathy in rats. Gastroenterology 2000;119(6):1537–47.

42. Aalykke C, Lauritsen JM, Hallas J, et al. *Helicobacter pylori* and risk of ulcer bleeding among users of nonsteroidal anti-inflammatory drugs: a case-control study. Gastroenterology 1999; 116(6):1305–9.

43. Maiden L, Thjodleifsson B, Theodors A, et al. A quantitative analysis of NSAID-induced small bowel pathology by capsule enteroscopy. Gastroenterology 2005;128(5):1172–8.

44. Hayashi Y, Yamamoto H, Kita H, et al. Non-steroidal anti-inflammatory drug-induced small bowel injuries identified by double-balloon endoscopy. World J Gastroenterol 2005;11(31):4861–4.

45. Lang J, Price AB, Levi AJ, et al. Diaphragm disease: pathology of disease of the small intestine induced by non-steroidal anti-inflammatory drugs. J Clin Pathol 1988;41(5):516–26.

46. Zalev AH, Gardiner GW, Warren RE. NSAID injury to the small intestine. Abdom Imaging 1998;23(1):40–4.

47. Going JJ, Canvin J, Sturrock R. Possible precursor of diaphragm disease in the small intestine. Lancet 1993;341(8845):638–9.

48. Robinson MH, Wheatley T, Leach IH. Nonsteroidal antiinflammatory drug-induced colonic stricture. An unusual cause of large bowel obstruction and perforation. Dig Dis Sci 1995;40(2):315–9.

49. Konturek SJ, Brzozowski T, Stachura J, et al. Role of gastric blood flow, neutrophil infiltration, and mucosal cell proliferation in gastric adaptation to aspirin in the rat. Gut 1994;35(9):1189–96.

50. Lee FD. Importance of apoptosis in the histopathology of drug related lesions in the large intestine. J Clin Pathol 1993;46(2):118–22.

51. Price AB. Pathology of drug-associated gastrointestinal disease. Br J Clin Pharmacol 2003;56(5):477–82.

52. Baert F, Hart J, Blackstone MO. A case of diclofenac-induced colitis with focal granulomatous change. Am J Gastroenterol 1995;90(10):1871–3.

53. El-Zimaity HM, Genta RM, Graham DY. Histological features do not define NSAID-induced gastritis. Hum Pathol 1996;27(12):1348–54.

54. Bombardier C, Laine L, Reicin A, et al. Comparison of upper gastrointestinal toxicity of rofecoxib and naproxen in patients with rheumatoid arthritis. VIGOR Study Group. N Engl J Med 2000;343(21):1520–8 1522 p following 1528.

55. Silverstein FE, Faich G, Goldstein JL, et al. Gastrointestinal toxicity with celecoxib vs nonsteroidal anti-inflammatory drugs for osteoarthritis and rheumatoid arthritis: the CLASS study: a randomized controlled trial. Celecoxib Long-term Arthritis Safety Study. JAMA 2000;284(10):1247–55.

56. Kelly JP, Kaufman DW, Jurgelon JM, et al. Risk of aspirin-associated major upper-gastrointestinal bleeding with enteric-coated or buffered product. Lancet 1996;348(9039):1413–6.

57. Cullen D, Bardhan KD, Eisner M, et al. Primary gastroduodenal prophylaxis with omeprazole for non-steroidal anti-inflammatory drug users. Aliment Pharmacol Ther 1998;12(2):135–40.

58. Singh G, Triadafilopoulos G. Epidemiology of NSAID induced gastrointestinal complications. J Rheumatol Suppl 1999;56:18–24.

59. Ament PW, Childers RS. Prophylaxis and treatment of NSAID-induced gastropathy. Am Fam Physician 1997;55(4):1323–6 1331–1322.

60. Wolfe MM, Lichtenstein DR, Singh G. Gastrointestinal toxicity of nonsteroidal antiinflammatory drugs. N Engl J Med 1999;340(24):1888–99.

61. Buroker TR, O'Connell MJ, Wieand HS, et al. Randomized comparison of two schedules of fluorouracil and leucovorin in the treatment of advanced colorectal cancer. J Clin Oncol 1994;12(1):14–20.

62. Parnes HL, Fung E, Schiffer CA. Chemotherapy-induced lactose intolerance in adults. Cancer 1994;74(5):1629–33.

63. Liaw CC, Huang JS, Wang HM, et al. Spontaneous gastroduodenal perforation in patients with cancer receiving chemotherapy and steroids. Report of four cases combining 5-fluorouracil infusion and cisplatin with antiemetics dexamethasone. Cancer 1993;72(4):1382–5.

64. Atherton LD, Leib ES, Kaye MD. Toxic megacolon associated with methotrexate therapy. Gastroenterology 1984;86(6):1583–8.

65. Slavin RE, Dias MA, Saral R. Cytosine arabinoside induced gastrointestinal toxic alterations in sequential chemotherapeutic protocols: a clinicalpathologic study of 33 patients. Cancer 1978;42(4):1747–59.

66. Rose PG, Piver MS. Intestinal perforation secondary to paclitaxel. Gynecol Oncol 1995;57(2):270–2.

67. Ferrero JM, Francois E, Frenay M, et al. [Occurrence of gastric phytobezoar after chemotherapy with vinorelbine]. Presse Med 1993;22(13):638 [in French].

68. Petras RE, Hart WR, Bukowski RM. Gastric epithelial atypia associated with hepatic arterial infusion chemotherapy. Its distinction from early gastric carcinoma. Cancer 1985;56(4):745–50.

69. Doria MI Jr, Doria LK, Faintuch J, et al. Gastric mucosal injury after hepatic arterial infusion chemotherapy with floxuridine. A clinical and pathologic study. Cancer 1994;73(8):2042–7.

70. Trier JS. Morphologic alterations induced by methotrexate in the mucosa of human proximal intestine. I. Serial observations by light microscopy. Gastroenterology 1962;42:295–305.

71. Trier JS. Morphologic alterations induced by methotrexate in the mucosa of human proximal intestine. II. Electron microscopic observations. Gastroenterology 1962;43:407–24.

72. Lewis JH. Gastrointestinal injury due to medicinal agents. Am J Gastroenterol 1986;81(9):819–34.

73. Oble DA, Mino-Kenudson M, Goldsmith J, et al. Alpha-CTLA-4 mAb-associated panenteritis: a histologic and immunohistochemical analysis. Am J Surg Pathol 2008;32(8):1130–7.

74. Floch MH, Hellman L. The effect of five-fluorouracil on rectal mucosa. Gastroenterology 1965;48:430–7.

75. Milles S, Muggia A, Spiro H. Colonic histologic changes induced by 5-fluorouracil. Gastroenterology 1962;43:391–9.

76. Sandmeier D, Chaubert P, Bouzourene H. Irinotecan-induced colitis. Int J Surg Pathol 2005;13(2):215–8.

77. Boley SJ, Brandt LJ, Veith FJ. Ischemic disorders of the intestines. Curr Probl Surg 1978;15(4):1–85.

78. Tedesco FJ, Volpicelli NA, Moore FS. Estrogen- and progesterone-associated colitis: a disorder with clinical and endoscopic features mimicking Crohn's colitis. Gastrointest Endosc 1982;28(4):247–9.

79. Friedel D, Thomas R, Fisher RS. Ischemic colitis during treatment with alosetron. Gastroenterology 2001;120(2):557–60.

80. Sparano JA, Dutcher JP, Kaleya R, et al. Colonic ischemia complicating immunotherapy with interleukin-2 and interferon-alpha. Cancer 1991;68(7):1538–44.

81. de Silva P, Deb S, Drummond RD, et al. A fatal case of ischaemic colitis following long-term use of neuroleptic medication. J Intellect Disabil Res 1992;36(Pt 4):371–5.

82. Shpilberg O, Ehrenfeld M, Abramowich D, et al. Ergotamine-induced solitary rectal ulcer. Postgrad Med J 1990;66(776):483–5.

83. Voora D, Vijayan A. Mesenteric vein thrombosis associated with intravaginal contraceptives: a case report and review of the literature. J Thromb Thrombolysis 2003;15(2):105–8.

84. Hassan HA. Oral contraceptive-induced mesenteric venous thrombosis with resultant intestinal ischemia. J Clin Gastroenterol 1999;29(1):90–5.

85. Hoyle M, Kennedy A, Prior AL, et al. Small bowel ischaemia and infarction in young women taking oral contraceptives and progestational agents. Br J Surg 1977;64(8):533–7.

86. Tanis BC, Rosendaal FR. Venous and arterial thrombosis during oral contraceptive use: risks and risk factors. Semin Vasc Med 2003;3(1):69–84.

87. Abel ME, Russell TR. Ischemic colitis. Comparison of surgical and nonoperative management. Dis Colon Rectum 1983;26(2):113–5.

88. Watson MR, Mark JB. Ulceration of the small intestine. Relation to enteric-coated potassium. Am J Surg 1966;112(3):421–5.

89. Brewer AR, Smyrk TC, Bailey RT Jr, et al. Drug-induced esophageal injury. Histopathological study in a rabbit model. Dig Dis Sci 1990;35(10):1205–10.

90. Biedrzycki OJ, Arnaout A, Coppen MJ, et al. Isolated intramucosal goblet cells in subacute ischaemic enteritis: mimicry of signet ring cell carcinoma. Histopathology 2005;46(4):460–2.

91. Centers for Disease Control and Prevention (CDC). Hypertrophic pyloric stenosis in infants following pertussis prophylaxis with erythromycin–Knoxville, Tennessee, 1999. MMWR Morb Mortal Wkly Rep 1999;48(49):1117–20.

92. Navarro H, Arruebo MP, Alcalde AI, et al. Effect of erythromycin on D-galactose absorption and sucrase activity in rabbit jejunum. Can J Physiol Pharmacol 1993;71(3-4):191–4.

93. Cappell MS, Simon T. Colonic toxicity of administered medications and chemicals. Am J Gastroenterol 1993;88(10):1684–99.

94. Banisaeed N, Truding RM, Chang CH. Tetracycline-induced spongiotic esophagitis: a new endoscopic and histopathologic finding. Gastrointest Endosc 2003;58(2):292–4.

95. Conn HO, Poynard T. Corticosteroids and peptic ulcer: meta-analysis of adverse events during steroid therapy. J Intern Med 1994;236(6):619–32.

96. Messer J, Reitman D, Sacks HS, et al. Association of adrenocorticosteroid therapy and peptic-ulcer disease. N Engl J Med 1983;309(1):21–4.

97. Delaney JP, Michel HM, Bonsack ME, et al. Adrenal corticosteroids cause gastrin cell hyperplasia. Gastroenterology 1979;76(5 Pt 1):913–6.

98. Crane PW, Clark C, Sowter C, et al. Cyclosporine toxicity in the small intestine. Transplant Proc 1990;22(6):2432.

99. Papadimitriou JC, Cangro CB, Lustberg A, et al. Histologic features of mycophenolate mofetil-related colitis: a graft-versus-host disease-like pattern. Int J Surg Pathol 2003;11(4):295–302.

100. Gabe SM, Bjarnason I, Tolou-Ghamari Z, et al. The effect of tacrolimus (FK506) on intestinal barrier function and cellular energy production in humans. Gastroenterology 1998;115(1):67–74.

101. Maes BD, Dalle I, Geboes K, et al. Erosive enterocolitis in mycophenolate mofetil-treated renal-transplant recipients with persistent afebrile diarrhea. Transplantation 2003;75(5):665–72.

102. Fisher A, Schwartz M, Mor E, et al. Gastrointestinal toxicity associated with FK 506 in liver transplant recipients. Transplant Proc 1994;26(6):3106–7.

103. Akioka K, Okamoto M, Nakamura K, et al. Abdominal pain is a critical complication of mycophenolate mofetil in renal transplant recipients. Transplant Proc 2003;35(1):300–1.

104. Behrend M. Adverse gastrointestinal effects of mycophenolate mofetil: aetiology, incidence and management. Drug Saf 2001;24(9):645–63.

105. Roy MJ, Walsh TJ. Histopathologic and immunohistochemical changes in gut-associated lymphoid

tissues after treatment of rabbits with dexamethasone. Lab Invest 1992;66(4):437–43.

106. ReMine SG, McIlrath DC. Bowel perforation in steroid-treated patients. Ann Surg 1980;192(4):581–6.

107. O'Neil EA, Chwals WJ, O'Shea MD, et al. Dexamethasone treatment during ventilator dependency: possible life threatening gastrointestinal complications. Arch Dis Child 1992;67(1 Spec No):10–1.

108. Abraham SC, Bhagavan BS, Lee LA, et al. Upper gastrointestinal tract injury in patients receiving kayexalate (sodium polystyrene sulfonate) in sorbitol: clinical, endoscopic, and histopathologic findings. Am J Surg Pathol 2001;25(5):637–44.

109. Roy-Chaudhury P, Meisels IS, Freedman S, et al. Combined gastric and ileocecal toxicity (serpiginous ulcers) after oral kayexalate in sorbital therapy. Am J Kidney Dis 1997;30(1):120–2.

110. Chatelain D, Brevet M, Manaouil D, et al. Rectal stenosis caused by foreign body reaction to sodium polystyrene sulfonate crystals (Kayexalate). Ann Diagn Pathol 2007;11(3):217–9.

111. Gardiner GW. Kayexalate (sodium polystyrene sulphonate) in sorbitol associated with intestinal necrosis in uremic patients. Can J Gastroenterol 1997;11(7):573–7.

112. Rashid A, Hamilton SR. Necrosis of the gastrointestinal tract in uremic patients as a result of sodium polystyrene sulfonate (Kayexalate) in sorbitol: an underrecognized condition. Am J Surg Pathol 1997;21(1):60–9.

113. Rugolotto S, Gruber M, Solano PD, et al. Necrotizing enterocolitis in a 850 gram infant receiving sorbitol-free sodium polystyrene sulfonate (Kayexalate): clinical and histopathologic findings. J Perinatol 2007;27(4):247–9.

114. Venho VM, Koivuniemi A. Effect of colchicine on drug absorption from the rat small intestine in situ and in vitro. Acta Pharmacol Toxicol (Copenh) 1978;43(4):251–9.

115. Stemmermann GN, Hayashi T. Colchicine intoxication. A reappraisal of its pathology based on a study of three fatal cases. Hum Pathol 1971;2(2):321–32.

116. Hawkins CF. Gastrointestinal lesions causing macrocytic anemia. Proc R Soc Med 1965;58(9):717–21.

117. Iacobuzio-Donahue CA, Lee EL, Abraham SC, et al. Colchicine toxicity: distinct morphologic findings in gastrointestinal biopsies. Am J Surg Pathol 2001;25(8):1067–73.

118. Al-Daraji WI, Al-Mahmoud RM, Ilyas M. Gastric changes following colchicine therapy in patients with FMF. Dig Dis Sci 2008;53(8):2079–82.

119. Smyth RL, Ashby D, O'Hea U, et al. Fibrosing colonopathy in cystic fibrosis: results of a case-control study. Lancet 1995;346(8985):1247–51.

120. Smyth RL, van Velzen D, Smyth AR, et al. Strictures of ascending colon in cystic fibrosis and high-strength pancreatic enzymes. Lancet 1994;343(8889):85–6.

121. Pawel BR, de Chadarevian JP, Franco ME. The pathology of fibrosing colonopathy of cystic fibrosis: a study of 12 cases and review of the literature. Hum Pathol 1997;28(4):395–9.

122. FitzSimmons SC, Burkhart GA, Borowitz D, et al. High-dose pancreatic-enzyme supplements and fibrosing colonopathy in children with cystic fibrosis. N Engl J Med 1997;336(18):1283–9.

123. de Groen PC, Lubbe DF, Hirsch LJ, et al. Esophagitis associated with the use of alendronate. N Engl J Med 1996;335(14):1016–21.

124. Aki S, Eskiyurt N, Akarirmak U, et al. Gastrointestinal side effect profile due to the use of alendronate in the treatment of osteoporosis. Yonsei Med J 2003;44(6):961–7.

125. Abraham SC, Cruz-Correa M, Lee LA, et al. Alendronate-associated esophageal injury: pathologic and endoscopic features. Mod Pathol 1999;12(12):1152–7.

126. Graham DY, Malaty HM. Alendronate gastric ulcers. Aliment Pharmacol Ther 1999;13(4):515–9.

127. Klinkenberg-Knol EC, Nelis F, Dent J, et al. Long-term omeprazole treatment in resistant gastro-esophageal reflux disease: efficacy, safety, and influence on gastric mucosa. Gastroenterology 2000;118(4):661–9.

128. Cats A, Schenk BE, Bloemena E, et al. Parietal cell protrusions and fundic gland cysts during omeprazole maintenance treatment. Hum Pathol 2000;31(6):684–90.

129. Welch DC, Wirth PS, Goldenring JR, et al. Gastric graft-versus-host disease revisited: does proton pump inhibitor therapy affect endoscopic gastric biopsy interpretation? Am J Surg Pathol 2006;30(4):444–9.

130. Krishnamurthy S, Dayal Y. Parietal cell protrusions in gastric ulcer disease. Hum Pathol 1997;28(10):1126–30.

131. Walker NI, Bennett RE, Axelsen RA. Melanosis coli. A consequence of anthraquinone-induced apoptosis of colonic epithelial cells. Am J Pathol 1988;131(3):465–76.

132. Benavides SH, Morgante PE, Monserrat AJ, et al. The pigment of melanosis coli: a lectin histochemical study. Gastrointest Endosc 1997;46(2):131–8.

133. van Gorkom BA, Karrenbeld A, van der Sluis T, et al. Apoptosis induction by sennoside laxatives in man; escape from a protective mechanism during chronic sennoside use? J Pathol 2001;194(4):493–9.

134. Xing JH, Soffer EE. Adverse effects of laxatives. Dis Colon Rectum 2001;44(8):1201–9.

135. Freeman HJ. "Melanosis" in the small and large intestine. World J Gastroenterol 2008;14(27):4296–9.

136. Smith B. Effect of irritant purgatives on the myenteric plexus in man and the mouse. Gut 1968;9(2):139–43.

137. Pardi DS, Tremaine WJ, Rothenberg HJ, et al. Melanosis coli in inflammatory bowel disease. J Clin Gastroenterol 1998;26(3):167–70.

138. Byers RJ, Marsh P, Parkinson D, et al. Melanosis coli is associated with an increase in colonic epithelial apoptosis and not with laxative use. Histopathology 1997;30(2):160–4.

MUCINOUS NEOPLASMS OF THE VERMIFORM APPENDIX

Shu-Yuan Xiao, MD

KEYWORDS

• Mucinous neoplasms • Vermiform appendix • Appendiceal adenomas

ABSTRACT

Most epithelial neoplasms of the vermiform appendix are of mucinous type and can be stratified into 3 main diagnostic categories: (1) adenoma, (2) mucinous neoplasms of uncertain malignant potential or low-grade mucinous neoplasm, and (3) adenocarcinoma. Clinically, appendiceal mucinous adenomas and adenocarcinomas may present as right lower abdominal pain mimicking acute appendicitis, a mass, or pseudomyxoma peritonei. Nomenclature currently in use to describe and diagnose mucinous tumors of the appendix, particularly those of low morphologic grade, varies among surgical pathologists and centers, resulting in different histologic and clinical features being attributed to these entities in the literature. It may be of help, as already attempted by some investigators, to simply apply algorithmic parameters for such lesions (grade of the primary lesion, extensiveness and composite of extra-appendiceal involvement, and so forth), instead of adopting rigid classification categories. This approach allows for more objective data to be collected in hopes that it will provide a more nuanced understanding of the clinical behavior of the spectrum of mucinous appendiceal tumors. Remaining focused on histopathologic parameters of the primary and secondary sites of involvement may help in avoiding circular reasoning.

OVERVIEW

Epithelial neoplasms of the vermiform appendix, other than endocrine tumors, are uncommon; most of them are of mucinous type.[1] In a population-based study from The Netherlands, about 1% of all appendectomy specimens contained an epithelial tumor, with one-third of them being mucinous.[2] Appendiceal mucinous tumors can be stratified into 3 main diagnostic categories, namely, adenoma, mucinous neoplasms of uncertain malignant potential (UMP) (or low-grade mucinous neoplasm), and adenocarcinomas. All these tumor types may cause the development of periappendiceal or peritoneal mucin and/or epithelial cell deposits, as a result of rupture of a diverticulum, herniation through a thinned and hyalinized appendiceal wall, direct invasion through the wall, or other mechanisms yet to be determined.

Similar to conventional colonic adenomas, the adenomas occurring in the appendix can assume either tubular or villous morphology. Not surprisingly, sessile serrated polyps also occur. Although the gross configurations of appendiceal adenomas are similar to their colonic counterparts, appendiceal adenomas are more often circumferential owing to the small appendiceal diameter. Another unique feature, also related to the small lumen, is the susceptibility for mucosal herniation or diverticulum formation.[3] It is sometimes difficult to distinguish benign cystadenomas from more aggressive lesions. This difficulty is at least partially responsible for the high rate of aggressive serrated and villous appendiceal adenomas compared with colonic adenomas, as claimed by some investigators,[4] and also has led to controversies in diagnostic terminology.[5,6]

Clinically, appendiceal mucinous adenomas and adenocarcinomas may present as right lower abdominal pain mimicking acute appendicitis,

Department of Pathology, University of Chicago Medical Center, 5841 South Maryland Avenue, Chicago, IL 60637, USA
E-mail address: syxiao@uchicago.edu

Surgical Pathology 3 (2010) 395–409
doi:10.1016/j.path.2010.05.010

PATHOLOGIC KEY FEATURES BOX

- Most noncarcinoid appendiceal epithelial tumors are of mucinous type.

- Mucinous adenomas and cystadenomas are usually sessile, with segmental but circumferential mucosal involvement.

- Displacement of epithelium and mucin into submucosa or beyond may occur and should be distinguished from true invasion.

- Rupture of an appendiceal diverticulum may cause periappendiceal mucin extravasation in the absence of a mucinous appendiceal neoplasm.

- Although deposits of acellular mucin confined to the right lower quadrant may be rarely associated with benign cystadenomas, mucin accompanied by neoplastic epithelium is associated with increased risk of recurrent disease and wider peritoneal spread. The latter lesion should be placed into the low-grade adenocarcinoma category.

- Proper diagnosis requires consideration of the features of the primary tumor, as well the nature of any associated extra-appendiceal involvement. By this approach, a given tumor can be placed into one of these categories: adenoma (mucinous cystadenoma), mucinous cystic neoplasm of uncertain malignant potential (UMP), low-grade mucinous adenocarcinoma, and high-grade mucinous adenocarcinoma.

a mass, or pseudomyxoma peritonei (PMP). A primary appendiceal lesion is commonly identified in a surgical exploration for a peritoneal mucinous tumor. Rarely, a low-grade mucinous tumor of the appendix presents as a mucinous deposit in an inguinal hernia sac specimen.[7]

Risk factors that are associated with the development of appendiceal mucinous tumors appear to be similar to those implicated in the colon. For example, patients with inflammatory bowel disease who have synchronous colorectal dysplasia or cancer also have increased risk of developing appendiceal mucinous cystadenomas.[8,9] A synchronous appendiceal neoplasm can be seen in up to 4% of patients undergoing colorectal cancer surgery, prompting some

investigators to recommend appendectomy at the time of any colorectal cancer surgery.[10] However, genetic studies have shown that most of these tumors lacked microsatellite instability status or p53 gene overexpression, and DPC4 gene mutation is infrequently seen. Similar to the nonmucinous counterparts, mucinous adenocarcinomas of the appendix show frequent chromosome 18q loss (around 55%),[11] and K-ras (Kirsten rat sarcoma) mutations can be identified in 50% of cases.[12] It appears that K-ras mutations are more common in appendiceal adenomas with PMP than in appendiceal mucinous adenomas unassociated with PMP.[12,13] These and other similar studies also support the appendiceal origin of PMP in women, whereas ovarian origin had been postulated in the past.[13,14]

Nomenclature currently in use to describe and diagnose mucinous tumors of the appendix, particularly those of low morphologic grade, varies among surgical pathologists and centers. Despite numerous reports involving small or large series of cases, controversies in terminology and associated biologic behavior remain. These controversies are responsible for different histologic and clinical features being attributed to these entities in the literature. It may be of help, as already attempted by some investigators, to simply apply algorithmic parameters for such lesions (grade of the primary lesion, extensiveness and composite of extra-appendiceal involvement, and so forth), instead of adopting rigid classification categories. This approach allows for more objective data to be collected in the hope that it provides a more nuanced understanding of the clinical behavior of the spectrum of mucinous appendiceal tumors. Furthermore, remaining focused on histopathologic parameters of the primary and secondary sites of involvement may help in avoiding circular reasoning (using certain histologic features to define a diagnostic entity and then describing these entities with the same specific histologic features).

GROSS FEATURES

Mucinous neoplasms, including adenomas and adenocarcinomas, may take the form of a discrete sessile or polypoid lesion or produce a circumferential mucosal thickening. Mucin production by these tumors often leads to cystic dilation of the appendix, resulting in a mucocele (Fig. 1) and/or diverticulum formation. Because nonneoplastic processes can also cause this abnormality, mucocele should remain a clinical and descriptive term

Fig. 1. Appendiceal muco-cele caused by a mucinous cystadenoma (opened), with marked dilation and a diverticulum. The inside lining is smooth and shining, with residual clear luminal mucus.

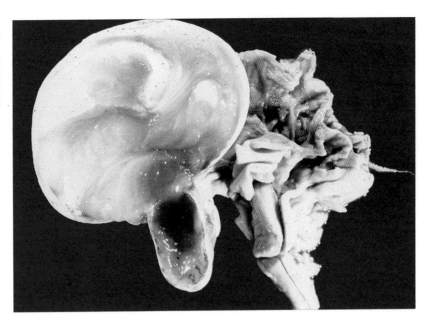

and never be used as a diagnostic label. Rupture of an appendiceal diverticulum in the setting of a mucinous appendiceal tumor can result in extravasation of mucin and/or neoplastic epithelium, resulting in an inflammatory reaction and fibrosis, and in the formation of a mass localized to the right lower quadrant.

The major significance of appendiceal mucinous neoplasms is the association with PMP, which is defined as grossly evident mucin accumulation in the peritoneal cavity. It is now well established that most cases of PMP develop from a primary appendiceal tumor with progressive dissemination in the peritoneal cavity of mucin-producing epithelial cells. Accumulation of the gelatinous mucin can cause bowel obstruction and extensive adhesions. High-grade appendiceal adenocarcinomas may also spread to the omentum and/or peritoneal surface as discrete metastatic tumor implants, without forming PMP.

MICROSCOPIC FEATURES

Appendiceal mucinous adenomas can be of serrated, tubular, or villous type, and usually display low-grade cytologic atypia (**Fig. 2**). With abundant mucin accumulation and increased intraluminal pressure, flattening of the neoplastic epithelium can occur (**Fig. 3**A, B), making the dysplastic, cytologic, and architectural features inconspicuous. There can be attenuation or complete loss of epithelium focally or extensively,

and mucin frequently dissects between the epithelial layer and the stroma (**Fig. 3**C). Atrophy or loss of the lymphoid tissue that normally underlies the appendiceal mucosa is not uncommon (see **Fig. 3**A, C). A concurrent diverticulum can be identified in up to 25% cases,[3,15] sometimes accompanied by acellular intramural or periappendiceal mucin extravasation (**Fig. 4**). Surgical pathologists should be aware that appendiceal diverticula are not uncommon and that rupture of such a diverticulum may result in mucin extravasation into the periappendiceal soft tissues, even when a mucinous neoplasm is not present. The epithelium lining the diverticulum may evert onto the serosal surface at the point of rupture, resulting in a histologic appearance resembling a mucinous adenocarcinoma.[16]

The clinical significance of the presence of periappendiceal mucin deposits associated with a low-grade epithelial lesion is a major source of diagnostic confusion and has led to a situation in which clinical outcome is regarded as unpredictable. Several diagnostic terms, such as "low-grade appendiceal mucinous neoplasm" (LGAMN) or "mucinous tumor of undetermined malignant potential" have been applied to lesions generally showing low-grade morphology but with additional worrisome findings. The lesional epithelium in these cases generally exhibits low-grade cytologic features (slight nuclear enlargement, hyperchromasia, mild nuclear stratification, few or no mitoses). In addition, careful examination may

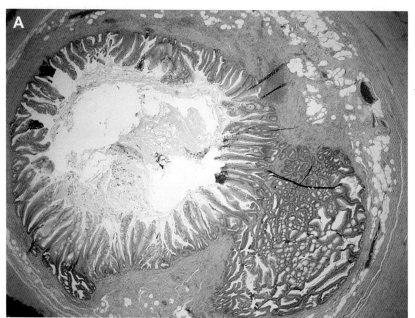

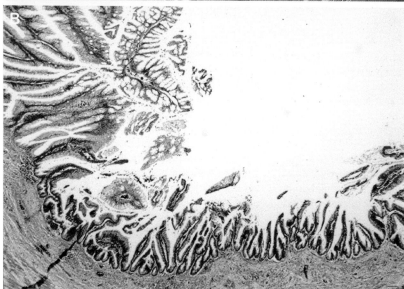

Fig. 2. A villous adenoma with cystic dilation and focal glandular herniation. (*A*) Note the villous architecture involving the mucosa circumferentially (H&E, ×2). (*B*) Higher magnification showing transition from a low villous to a tall villous area. Dysplasia is low grade (H&E, ×10).

reveal intramural or periappendiceal mucin deposits, with or without neoplastic epithelium. By definition, these lesions lack evidence of invasive growth, although herniation into or through a thinned and hyalinized wall may be evident in some cases. Proper diagnosis of these lesions is further described later in this article.

In contrast to adenomas, adenocarcinomas show more prominent cytologic atypia, increased mitosis, and architectural complexity. Adenocarcinomas are also characterized by frank mural invasion (**Fig. 5**). The vast majority of appendiceal adenocarcinomas are mucinous (the others being conventional gland-forming adenocarcinoma and signet-ring cell carcinoma). The key features that aid in the recognition of true invasion include irregularly shaped or angulated glands and/or clusters or individual cytologically malignant cells, infiltrating submucosa and beyond. Desmoplasia can be seen, although this can be difficult to recognize when the muscularis propria becomes densely collagenous as a result of pressure-induced compression. Not infrequently, the adjacent adenomatous component can be identified,

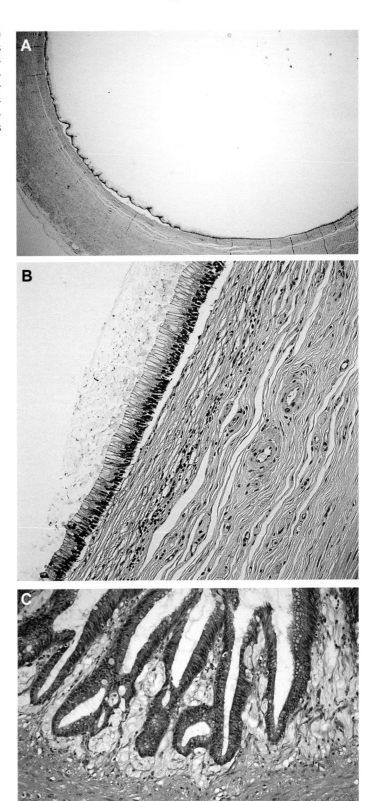

Fig. 3. Mucinous cystadenoma. (*A*) The lining epithelium is flattened as a result of intraluminal mucin accumulation (H&E, ×2). (*B*) The lining epithelial cells exhibit mucinous columnar cell morphology, with low-grade dysplasia (H&E, ×10). (*C*) Mucin extravasation has lifted the adenomatous epithelium (H&E, ×20).

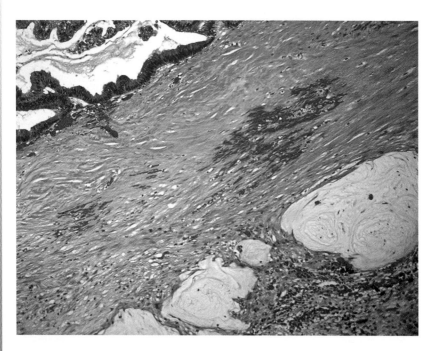

Fig. 4. Acellular mucin extravasation in a mucinous neoplasm of UMP. Note the inflammatory cell response to the mucin pools (H&E, ×20).

and a transition between the two may be evident. Nevertheless, some seemingly benign cystadenomas are associated with evident aggressive behavior (such as peritoneal adenomucinosis or carcinomatosis). In these cases, careful microscopic examination may reveal bland cytologic features and a broad pushing border, making the correct histologic classification of the primary lesion difficult.

Rarely, a mucinous tumor may also exhibit a component of goblet cell carcinoid (GCC); periappendiceal fat tissue and perineural invasion in these tumors are not uncommon.[17] Controversy exists on how to best classify these composite tumors,[18,19] and a designation of adenocarcinoma ex GCC has been proposed.[18] There are reports of appendiceal adenocarcinomas with bilateral ovarian metastases that exhibit a GCC-like pattern,[20] with documented focal chromogranin and/or synaptophysin positivity. These tumors demonstrate an aggressive clinical course with dismal long-term survival, similar to widely metastatic appendiceal adenocarcinoma without endocrine differentiation.

PMP is characterized by intra-abdominal deposits of pools of mucin with a variable amount of embedded neoplastic epithelium (**Fig. 6**A). The embedded neoplastic epithelium may be in the form of isolated or small clusters of cells, strips of epithelium, or glandular elements (**Fig. 6**B). The most widely used classification scheme stratifies PMP into disseminated peritoneal adenomucinosis (DPAM), peritoneal mucinous carcinomatosis (PMCA), and an intermediate or discordant feature group (PMCA-I/D), based on the degree of cellularity, cytologic and histologic atypia, and invasiveness of the PMP and the associated primary appendiceal tumor.[21] Distinction between DPAM and PMCA is based on the prevailing microscopic features of the peritoneal lesions. The defining microscopic feature of DPAM is the presence of only scant mucinous epithelium, with little cytologic atypia or mitotic activity. In contrast, PMCA is characterized by more abundant embedded epithelium with the architectural and cytologic features of carcinoma. The PMCA-I/D designation is used in 2 separate situations. PMCA-I is used when the bulk of the peritoneal disease is of the DPAM type, but focally, there is neoplastic epithelium with high-grade cytologic features. DPAM-D is diagnosed when there is discordance between the peritoneal deposits, which exhibit low-grade features typical of DPAM, but the appendiceal primary is an obvious adenocarcinoma.

Immunohistochemically, appendiceal mucinous adenocarcinomas are reactive for CK20, CEA, CDX-2, MUC2, and MUC5AC. Rarely, tumors arising from a mature cystic teratoma of the ovary exhibit the same immunoprofile.[22,23] Tumor cells in PMP often express MUC2 and MUC5AC.[24]

Fig. 5. High-grade invasive adenocarcinoma. (*A*) The tumor exhibits a complex glandular architecture and infiltrates the muscle wall (H&E, ×20). (*B*) High-grade tumor cells float in mucin pools present within the mesoappendiceal fat (H&E, ×20).

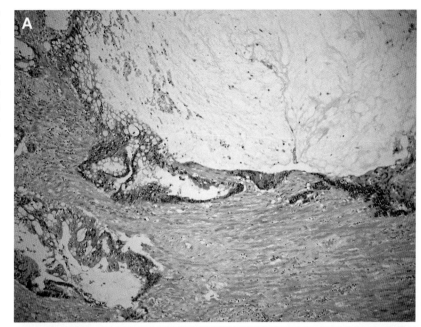

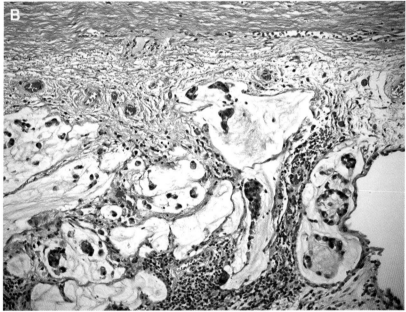

DIFFERENTIAL DIAGNOSIS

The main differential diagnostic issues are (1) distinction among mucinous neoplasms of different stages (benign, UMP or low-grade, and carcinoma) and (2) mucinous adenocarcinomas involving other abdominal organs or the peritoneum of unknown primary. The first issue is discussed in the following section. Much knowledge

has been gained over the past 2 decades on the nature, origin, and the relationship among appendiceal mucinous neoplasms, ovarian mucinous neoplasms, and PMP. Challenges still remain; for example, metastatic carcinomas from the gastrointestinal (GI) tract, pancreaticobiliary system, breast, and other organs account for about 5% of all ovarian malignancies. When these metastases are first presented as an ovarian tumor,

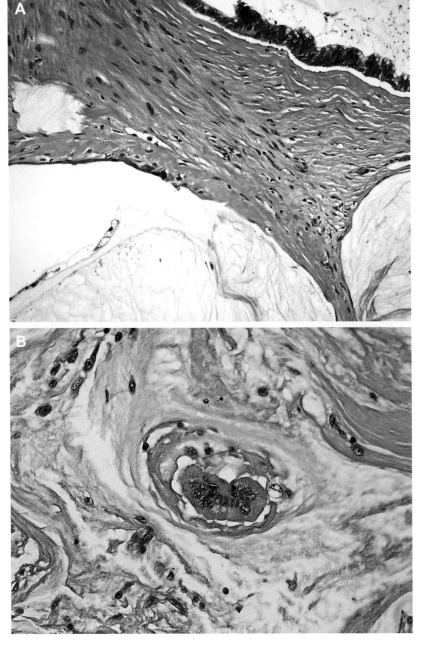

Fig. 6. PMP. (*A*) Abundant strips of high-grade neoplastic epithelial cells infiltrate the peritoneal soft tissues, diagnostic of peritoneal mucinous carcinomatosis. In this case, there was an associated appendiceal mucinous cystadenocarcinoma (H&E, ×40). (*B*) Clusters of neoplastic epithelial cells floating in a mucin pool (H&E, ×40).

they pose a differential challenge because an appropriate chemotherapy regimen has to be tailored to the specific primary.

For unilateral ovarian tumors, a simple algorithm using tumor size (≥13 cm indicating primary) has been shown to be diagnostically useful.[25] Ovarian mucinous tumors that exhibit goblet cell differentiation are usually of metastatic origin, although rare primary ovarian mucinous tumors can harbor goblet cells as well.[26] The presence of a unilateral tumor of low stage that lacks surface tumor deposits, a nodular growth pattern, and lymphovascular invasion is usually of primary ovarian origin. Immunohistochemically, metastatic appendiceal tumors are usually CK7 negative, whereas primary ovarian mucinous borderline tumors are uniformly CK7 positive. When there is a synchronous appendiceal mucinous tumor, ovarian

- Mucocele (due to an inflammatory process causing luminal obstruction)
- Ruptured appendiceal diverticulum with extravasation of mucin
- Mucinous adenoma or cystadenoma
- Mucinous neoplasm of UMP
- Low-grade mucinous adenocarcinoma
- High-grade mucinous adenocarcinoma
- PMP caused by mucinous tumors from a non-appendiceal site (colon, ovary, stomach, small bowel, urinary bladder, and so forth)
- PMP caused by spread from an appendiceal mucinous neoplasm

mucinous carcinoma (particularly of high stage), and PMP and if the CK7 immunostain is negative, it is almost certain that the primary lies in the appendix. Conversely, if the tumors are CK7 positive and CDX2 negative, an ovarian primary is more likely.[27] Nevertheless, it should be noted that a significant number of primary ovarian mucinous tumors exhibiting intestinal differentiation are positive for CDX2 as well (from 36% to 40%).[28] A more recently described immuno-marker, guanylyl cyclase C, may be of help in this regard. It is a brush border membrane receptor for the endogenous peptides, guanylin, and uro-guanylin, and has been found to be positive in most colorectal and appendiceal tumors but negative in ovarian mucinous tumors (only 2 of 27 were positive in one study).[29] Another marker, meprin α, may also aid in the distinction between a primary ovarian and a metastatic tumor from the GI tract, because it is expressed in a lower frequency in ovarian cancers.[30]

In considering the origin of an intra-abdominal or pelvic metastatic mucinous adenocarcinoma, the possibility of an urachal adenocarcinoma should also be considered in addition to ovarian, upper GI tract, and pancreaticobiliary primaries, particularly when immunohistochemical stains show an overlapping pattern. Urachal mucinous adenocarcinoma can metastasize to the ovaries and should be considered if an appendiceal primary is not evident. Recently, a rare type of collision tumor was reported in which an appendiceal mucinous adenocarcinoma metastasized to a peritoneal mesothelioma.[31] Other rare primary tumors may cause PMP, including mucinous borderline tumor

of the renal pelvicalyceal system.[32] Lymph node metastasis of appendiceal mucinous adenocarcinoma, although rare, does occur.[33] It is usually also accompanied by widespread peritoneal disease.

DIAGNOSIS

Critical to accurate diagnosis of an appendiceal mucinous neoplasm is meticulous processing of the appendectomy specimen, and careful gross and microscopic examination. All grossly dilated or enlarged appendixes should be well fixed and then serially sectioned and completely submitted for histologic examination, taking care to separately identify the proximal surgical margin of resection. The rationale for this practice includes

1. High-grade cytologic and/or architectural features can be quite focal and are important to recognize.
2. Invasion can be focal.
3. Extra-appendiceal spread needs to be fully evaluated for cellularity.

Because 48% cases of appendixes with a diverticula harbored a neoplasm in one reported study, such cases should also be submitted entirely.[15]

The diagnosis of a benign cystadenoma or a frankly invasive adenocarcinoma is generally straightforward. The main diagnostic challenge is with the lesions variously described as UMP or LGAMN. There is much confusion and inconsistency regarding proper labeling of these tumors. For example, it is not uncommon to identify acellular mucin pools dissecting within the hyalinized wall of the appendix associated with a benign cystadenoma. However, when low-grade neoplastic epithelium accompanies the mucin within the appendiceal wall, some investigators regard this finding as diagnostic of invasive adenocarcinoma,[34] whereas others prefer to label such cases as LGAMN[5] or UMP.[33,35] Likewise, in some cystadenomas, dissection of acellular mucin through the appendiceal wall and into the periappendiceal soft tissues occurs. Although this may be the consequence of rupture of a benign mucinous cystadenoma (sometimes through a diverticulum), the possibility of a lesion of higher grade also exists. These cases are regarded as UMP by most investigators,[33–35] although the term LGAMN is preferred by others.[5] A thorough search must be made for the presence of neoplastic epithelium within the mucin deposits. If neoplastic epithelium is identified, then a diagnosis of low-grade adeno-carcinoma is warranted,[34] although some prefer the term "low malignant potential."[33,35] This term is applicable even if the primary appendiceal lesion exhibits low-grade cytologic features indistinguishable from a cystadenoma without periappendiceal extension. These initially localized tumors limited to the right lower quadrant may recur as fully-fledged PMP.[5]

In addition, for cases of otherwise typical adenoma but with a positive proximal surgical margin, some investigators advocate the use of the label "UMP" because it is impossible "to know what is left beyond the margin," and it is difficult to predict the clinical outcome of such cases. When a benign colonic adenoma is excised but the polypectomy margin is positive, it is not designated as UMP but it is noted that the adenoma is incompletely excised.

A microscopically "bland" appendiceal mucinous tumor without a frankly invasive growth pattern can be associated with peritoneal spread in the form of PMP. Although, classically, PMP is slowly progressive with a relatively high 5-year survival rate, most patients ultimately succumb to tumor. Therefore, it is logical that appendiceal mucinous tumors with concurrent PMP be diagnosed as adenocarcinoma (albeit often low grade). However, this diagnosis is problematic in that a histologically identical appendiceal primary tumor without PMP could be diagnosed as UMP.

From the preceding discussion, it can be seen that a uniform diagnostic scheme for appendiceal mucinous tumors does not exist at present. In daily practice, it is necessary to provide the clinician with a full description of the histologic features present in the appendiceal specimen, including the presence or absence of periappendiceal disease in the form of acellular or cellular deposits, and a separate description of any peritoneal disease if such specimens are provided. The diagnostic terms and microscopic features are summarized in the following sections.

ADENOMA

Adenomas include circumferential lesions (mucinous cystadenoma) and discrete sessile or polypoid lesions (which can be further specified as villous, sessile serrated, and so forth) (see **Figs. 2** and **3**). By definition, the tumor is confined to the appendix, with no mural invasion on thorough examination. There should be no periappendiceal mucin deposits. However, if focal periappendiceal mucin deposits can be unequivocally shown to be related to the rupture of an appendiceal diverticulum, then a diagnosis of mucinous cystadenoma may still be rendered. If the proximal resection margin involves the adenomatous lesion it should be noted in the report, but the diagnosis remains unchanged. These lesions correspond to the group 1 lesions, as described by Pai and colleagues,[6] and are clinically benign.

MUCINOUS APPENDICEAL NEOPLASM OF UMP

Three distinct lesions should be placed in this category:

- Mucinous cystadenoma with extension into the muscular wall with a distinctly pushing border that is suspicious but not diagnostic for

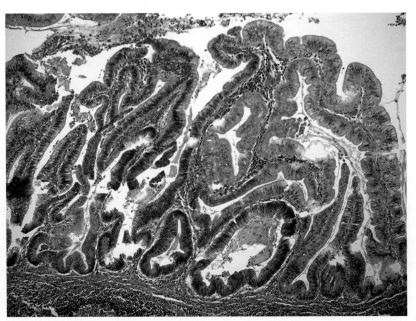

Fig. 7. Mucinous neoplasm of UMP. The tumor exhibits high-grade cytologic features and marked architectural complexity, but there was no invasive component or extra-appendiceal extension. However, the appendix was not submitted in its entirety for histologic examination (H&E, ×10).

Fig. 8. Low-grade mucinous adenocarcinoma. (*A*) The primary tumor exhibits no recognizable invasion (H&E, ×10). (*B*) An acellular mucin pool is present in the periappendiceal tissues in this section (H&E, ×10).

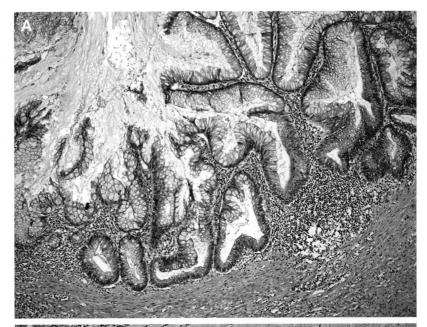

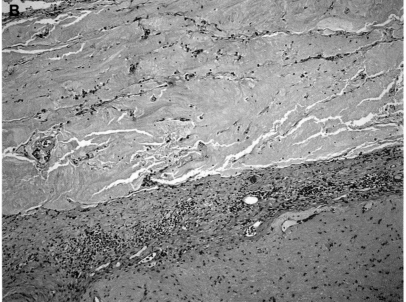

invasion and without peritoneal mucinous implants.[34]

- Mucinous cystadenoma with focal periappendiceal acellular mucin extravasation (see **Fig. 4**). This lesion corresponds to the group 2 lesions proposed by Pai and colleagues.[6] Some cases also have acellular mucin deposits outside of the right lower quadrant. The rationale for placing these lesions in the UMP category is that recurrent disease after resection has been reported in 3 of 64 patients from 2 separate reports.[6,36] However, it should be noted

that the entire appendix was not submitted for histologic examination from these patients. Therefore, it remains unknown whether local acellular mucin deposition really carries a risk of recurrent disease.

- Mucinous cystadenoma with high-grade cytologic atypia and/or architectural complexity but lacking unequivocal invasion and extra-appendiceal involvement (**Fig. 7**). In the study by Pai and colleagues,[6] all examples with these features also harbored invasive foci in the primary tumor, except for one, and all were

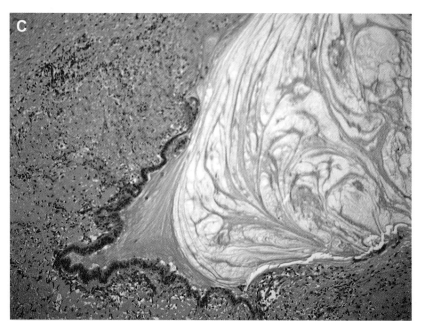

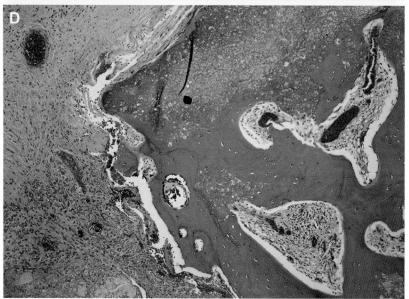

Fig. 8. (*C*) However, in another section from the mesoappendix, neoplastic epithelium is clearly present, diagnostic of low-grade adenocarcinoma (H&E, ×10). (*D*) Dystrophic bone formation is not uncommon in areas of mucin extravasation, which indicates the indolent progression of this type of tumor (H&E, ×4).

placed in group 4. It is possible that with complete submission of the entire appendix for histologic examination, focal invasion will be identified in every case. Nevertheless, it is difficult to justify the diagnosis of adenocarcinoma when high-grade dysplastic features are evident but no demonstrable invasion or extra-appendiceal spread is identified. However, given the unique unpredictability of the natural history of appendiceal mucinous cystadenomas, placing these lesions into the UMP group seems appropriate.

LOW-GRADE MUCINOUS ADENOCARCINOMA

In cases of low-grade mucinous adenocarcinomas, the appendiceal mucinous neoplasm exhibits low-grade cytologic atypia without frank invasion, but there are periappendiceal mucin pools containing neoplastic epithelium (**Fig. 8**). In many cases, paucicellular mucin implants are also present beyond the right lower quadrant, a condition referred to as disseminated peritoneal adenomucinosis (see earlier discussion). In the proposal by Pai's group, these cases are termed low-grade, high-risk mucinous neoplasms.

HIGH-GRADE MUCINOUS ADENOCARCINOMA

In cases of high-grade mucinous adenocarcinomas there is evidence of frank invasion, usually with associated high-grade cytologic atypia and complex glandular architecture (see **Fig. 5**). In addition, some cases exhibit signet-ring cell differentiation. When PMP is also present, it usually takes the form of PMCA.

PROGNOSIS

Adenomas or cystadenomas, defined as intramucosal mucinous tumors without evidence of invasion and not associated with periappendiceal mucin deposition, are clearly benign lesions that are cured by appendectomy. The prognosis of mucinous neoplasms of UMP is difficult to report accurately because the term for this intermediate category is used differently by various investigators. Mucinous tumors with localized periappendiceal acellular mucin deposition usually follow a nonaggressive clinical course, although rare cases have been reported to recur with wider peritoneal involvement. However, in the reported cases, the appendixes were not submitted entirely for microscopic examination.[33,36] The overall reported 5- and 10-year patient survival is nearly 100%.[6] In contrast, patients with low-grade mucinous adenocarcinoma and PMP have a disease-free 5- and 10-year survival of only 50% and 20%, respectively.[6] The reported overall 5-year survival for high-grade mucinous adenocarcinoma is dismal (28%).[6]

PMP is generally associated with a poor prognosis, with reported overall patient survival rates of around 50% to 75% at 5 years and 10% to 30% at 10 years.[37] A multidisciplinary approach to treatment combining cytoreductive surgery (subtotal peritonectomy or tumor debulking) with hyperthermic intraperitoneal chemotherapy (HIPEC) is now regarded as optimal, but recurrence occurs in at least 40% of patients.[38] In one study, disease-specific 3-year and 5-year survival rates of 71% and 60%, respectively, were reported. Factors associated with survival included histologic grade, completeness of cytoreduction, and degree and location of the tumor load.[38]

It had been suggested that p53 gene overexpression, nuclear factor κB expression, or β-catenin loss identified by immunohistochemistry might predict an adverse outcome in mucinous appendiceal adenocarcinomas.[39] In addition, some investigators advocated that an immunostain for Ki-67 be performed and a proliferative index be reported; however, these results have not been verified by other studies.

> ⓘ *Pitfalls*
> ### APPENDICEAL MUCINOUS TUMORS

- Periappendiceal acellular mucin deposition associated with rupture of a diverticulum should not be labeled as an appendiceal neoplasm.

- A mucinous cystadenoma with displacement of mucin pools and glandular elements into the appendiceal wall may mimic invasive adenocarcinoma.

- The cytologically bland, pushing front of a low-grade invasive appendiceal adenocarcinoma is difficult to distinguish from a mucinous cystadenoma with displacement of epithelial elements.

- Some low-grade invasive appendiceal adenocarcinomas are not recognized because the appendectomy specimen is not sampled thoroughly enough to identify neoplastic epithelium within periappendiceal mucin pools.

REFERENCES

1. Carr NJ, McCarthy WF, Sobin LH. Epithelial noncarcinoid tumors and tumor-like lesions of the appendix. A clinicopathologic study of 184 patients with a multivariate analysis of prognostic factors. Cancer 1995;75:757–68.
2. Smeenk RM, van Velthuysen ML, Verwaal VJ, et al. Appendiceal neoplasms and pseudomyxoma peritonei: a population based study. Eur J Surg Oncol 2008;34:196–201.
3. Lamps LW, Gray GF Jr, Dilday BR, et al. The coexistence of low-grade mucinous neoplasms of the appendix and appendiceal diverticula: a possible role in the pathogenesis of pseudomyxoma peritonei. Mod Pathol 2000;13:495–501.
4. Rubio CA. Serrated adenomas of the appendix. J Clin Pathol 2004;57:946–9.
5. Misdraji J, Yantiss RK, Graeme-Cook FM, et al. Appendiceal mucinous neoplasms: a clinicopathologic analysis of 107 cases. Am J Surg Pathol 2003;27:1089–103.

6. Pai RK, Beck AH, Norton JA, et al. Appendiceal mucinous neoplasms: clinicopathologic study of 116 cases with analysis of factors predicting recurrence. Am J Surg Pathol 2009;33:1425–39.

7. Young RH, Rosenberg AE, Clement PB. Mucin deposits within inguinal hernia sacs: a presenting finding of low-grade mucinous cystic tumors of the appendix. A report of two cases and a review of the literature. Mod Pathol 1997;10:1228–32.

8. Kuester D, Dalicho S, Monkemuller K, et al. Synchronous multifocal colorectal carcinoma in a patient with delayed diagnosis of ulcerative pancolitis. Pathol Res Pract 2008;204:905–10.

9. Orta L, Trindade AJ, Luo J, et al. Appendiceal mucinous cystadenoma is a neoplastic complication of IBD: case-control study of primary appendiceal neoplasms. Inflamm Bowel Dis 2009;15:415–21.

10. Khan MN, Moran BJ. Four percent of patients undergoing colorectal cancer surgery may have synchronous appendiceal neoplasia. Dis Colon Rectum 2007;50:1856–9.

11. Maru D, Wu TT, Canada A, et al. Loss of chromosome 18q and DPC4 (Smad4) mutations in appendiceal adenocarcinomas. Oncogene 2004;23:859–64.

12. Kabbani W, Houlihan PS, Luthra R, et al. Mucinous and nonmucinous appendiceal adenocarcinomas: different clinicopathological features but similar genetic alterations. Mod Pathol 2002;15:599–605.

13. Szych C, Staebler A, Connolly DC, et al. Molecular genetic evidence supporting the clonality and appendiceal origin of Pseudomyxoma peritonei in women. Am J Pathol 1999;154:1849–55.

14. Cuatrecasas M, Matias-Guiu X, Prat J. Synchronous mucinous tumors of the appendix and the ovary associated with pseudomyxoma peritonei. A clinicopathologic study of six cases with comparative analysis of c-Ki-ras mutations. Am J Surg Pathol 1996;20:739–46.

15. Dupre MP, Jadavji I, Matshes E, et al. Diverticular disease of the vermiform appendix: a diagnostic clue to underlying appendiceal neoplasm. Hum Pathol 2008;39:1823–6.

16. Hsu M, Young RH, Misdraji J. Ruptured appendiceal diverticula mimicking low-grade appendiceal mucinous neoplasms. Am J Surg Pathol 2009;33:1515–21.

17. Kanthan R, Saxena A, Kanthan SC. Goblet cell carcinoids of the appendix: immunophenotype and ultrastructural study. Arch Pathol Lab Med 2001;125:386–90.

18. Tang LH, Shia J, Soslow RA, et al. Pathologic classification and clinical behavior of the spectrum of goblet cell carcinoid tumors of the appendix. Am J Surg Pathol 2008;32:1429–43.

19. Wang HL, Dhall D. Goblet or signet ring cells: that is the question. Adv Anat Pathol 2009;16:247–54.

20. Hristov AC, Young RH, Vang R, et al. Ovarian metastases of appendiceal tumors with goblet cell carcinoidlike and signet ring cell patterns: a report of 30 cases. Am J Surg Pathol 2007;31:1502–11.

21. Ronnett BM, Zahn CM, Kurman RJ, et al. Disseminated peritoneal adenomucinosis and peritoneal mucinous carcinomatosis. A clinicopathologic analysis of 109 cases with emphasis on distinguishing pathologic features, site of origin, prognosis, and relationship to "pseudomyxoma peritonei". Am J Surg Pathol 1995;19:1390–408.

22. Hwang JH, So KA, Modi G, et al. Borderline-like mucinous tumor arising in mature cystic teratoma of the ovary associated with pseudomyxoma peritonei. Int J Gynecol Pathol 2009;28:376–80.

23. Stewart CJ, Tsukamoto T, Cooke B, et al. Ovarian mucinous tumour arising in mature cystic teratoma and associated with pseudomyxoma peritonei: report of two cases and comparison with ovarian involvement by low-grade appendiceal mucinous tumour. Pathology 2006;38:534–8.

24. O'Connell JT, Tomlinson JS, Roberts AA, et al. Pseudomyxoma peritonei is a disease of MUC2-expressing goblet cells. Am J Pathol 2002;161:551–64.

25. Yemelyanova AV, Vang R, Judson K, et al. Distinction of primary and metastatic mucinous tumors involving the ovary: analysis of size and laterality data by primary site with reevaluation of an algorithm for tumor classification. Am J Surg Pathol 2008;32:128–38.

26. McCluggage WG, Young RH. Primary ovarian mucinous tumors with signet ring cells: report of 3 cases with discussion of so-called primary Krukenberg tumor. Am J Surg Pathol 2008;32:1373–9.

27. Tornillo L, Moch H, Diener PA, et al. CDX-2 immunostaining in primary and secondary ovarian carcinomas. J Clin Pathol 2004;57:641–3.

28. Vang R, Gown AM, Wu LS, et al. Immunohistochemical expression of CDX2 in primary ovarian mucinous tumors and metastatic mucinous carcinomas involving the ovary: comparison with CK20 and correlation with coordinate expression of CK7. Mod Pathol 2006;19:1421–8.

29. Ciocca V, Bombonati A, Palazzo JP, et al. Guanylyl cyclase C is a specific marker for differentiating primary and metastatic ovarian mucinous neoplasms. Histopathology 2009;55:182–8.

30. Heinzelmann-Schwarz VA, Scolyer RA, Scurry JP, et al. Low meprin alpha expression differentiates primary ovarian mucinous carcinoma from gastrointestinal cancers that commonly metastasize to the ovaries. J Clin Pathol 2007;60:622–6.

31. Tran TA, Holloway RW, Finkler NJ. Metastatic appendiceal mucinous adenocarcinoma to well-differentiated diffuse mesothelioma of the peritoneal cavity: a mimicker of florid mesothelial hyperplasia in

association with neoplasms. Int J Gynecol Pathol 2008;27:526–30.

32. Rao P, Pinheiro N Jr, Franco M, et al. Pseudomyxoma peritonei associated with primary mucinous borderline tumor of the renal pelvicalyceal system. Arch Pathol Lab Med 2009;133:1472–6.

33. Pai RK, Longacre TA. Pseudomyxoma peritonei syndrome: classification of appendiceal mucinous tumours. Cancer Treat Res 2007;134:71–107.

34. Carr NJ, Sobin LH. Epithelial noncarcinoid tumors and tumor-like lesions of the appendix. Cancer 1995;76:2383–4.

35. Pai RK, Longacre TA. Appendiceal mucinous tumors and pseudomyxoma peritonei: histologic features, diagnostic problems, and proposed classification. Adv Anat Pathol 2005;12:291–311.

36. Yantiss RK, Shia J, Klimstra DS, et al. Prognostic significance of localized extra-appendiceal mucin deposition in appendiceal mucinous neoplasms. Am J Surg Pathol 2009;33:248–55.

37. Ronnett BM, Yan H, Kurman RJ, et al. Patients with pseudomyxoma peritonei associated with disseminated peritoneal adenomucinosis have a significantly more favorable prognosis than patients with peritoneal mucinous carcinomatosis. Cancer 2001;92: 85–91.

38. Smeenk RM, Verwaal VJ, Antonini N, et al. Survival analysis of pseudomyxoma peritonei patients treated by cytoreductive surgery and hyperthermic intraperitoneal chemotherapy [see comment]. Ann Surg 2007;245:104–9.

39. Yoon SO, Kim BH, Lee HS, et al. Differential protein immunoexpression profiles in appendiceal mucinous neoplasms: a special reference to classification and predictive factors. Mod Pathol 2009;22: 1102–12.

NEW ENDOSCOPIC TECHNIQUES: CHALLENGES AND OPPORTUNITIES FOR SURGICAL PATHOLOGISTS

Gregory Y. Lauwers, MD[a,b,*],
Kamran Badizadegan, MD[a,b,c]

KEYWORDS

- Endoscopic imaging • Endoscopic mucosal resection • Photodynamic therapy
- Gastrointestinal pathology

ABSTRACT

In recent years, significant clinical and technological advances have been made in endoscopic methods for diagnosis and treatment of early gastrointestinal neoplasms. However, essential information related to these novel techniques and their implications for practicing surgical pathologists have largely been missing in the general pathology literature. This article provides a general introduction to these novel therapeutic and diagnostic methods, and discusses their indications, contraindications, and potential limitations. The article aims to enable surgical pathologists to interact more efficiently with basic scientists and clinical colleagues to help implement and improve the existing clinical methods and to advance the new technologies.

NOVEL DIAGNOSTIC ENDOSCOPIC METHODS

ENDOSCOPIC IMAGING

Currently, full-spectrum white light imaging in the form of red-green-blue (RGB) video technology is the standard for endoscopic visualization of the gastrointestinal mucosa and its associated lesions. Although white light imaging is an attractive technology because of its similarity to the natural physiology of the human eye, it ignores and/or suppresses many potential sources of optical contrast, which may be invaluable in detection and diagnosis of mucosal lesions. In the past decade, several imaging alternatives have been introduced to enhance optical contrast, and many other promising technologies are under development. This section focuses on essential technologies that have shown promising results in enhanced detection of mucosal lesions using intrinsic sources of tissue contrast (**Fig. 1**).

Chromoendoscopy

Chromoendoscopy refers to the general principle of increasing tissue contrast by topical application of a dye or other chemical reagent before or during endoscopic visualization. Perhaps the most widely known clinical implementation of this technique is the application of acetic acid to highlight cervical intraepithelial lesions during colposcopy. Although

[a] Gastrointestinal Pathology Service, James Homer Wright Pathology Laboratories, 55 Fruit Street, WRN 219, Massachusetts General Hospital, Boston, MA 02114, USA
[b] Department of Pathology, Harvard Medical School, 25 Shattuck Street, Boston, MA 02115, USA
[c] Harvard-MIT Division of Health Sciences and Technology, 77 Massachusetts Avenue, Cambridge, MA 02139, USA
* Corresponding author. Department of Pathology, Massachusetts General Hospital, 55 Fruit Street, WRN 219, Boston, MA 02114.
E-mail address: glauwers@partners.org

Surgical Pathology 3 (2010) 411–428
doi:10.1016/j.path.2010.05.002
1875-9181/10/$ – see front matter © 2010 Elsevier Inc. All rights reserved.

Key Features
ENDOSCOPIC IMAGING FOR
THE PATHOLOGIST

- High-resolution chromoendoscopy is becoming the clinical standard in screening endoscopy such as surveillance for dysplasia in inflammatory bowel disease, and has proved effective in identification of gastric neoplastic lesions and dysplasia in Barrett esophagus (BE).

- Tissue fluorescence and reflectance can provide information about the biochemical and structural state of the tissue, which can in turn be used as a biomarker for changes that occur during disease development and progression.

- Confocal optics have the capability to collect only the photons that originate from a specific depth in the tissue, thus virtually sectioning the tissue in real time. Confocal techniques can be used in reflectance or fluorescence modes, enabling multimodal microscopic imaging. Confocal endomicroscopes are capable of submicron optical sectioning to a depth of 100 to 200 μm, ideal for identification and classification of early mucosal disease such as dysplasia or microvascular anatomy.

acetic acid has rarely proved effective in improving detectability of gastrointestinal lesions, several other chromogenic reagents, including Lugol solution, methylene blue, indigo carmine, and crystal violet, have been used with success for specific gastrointestinal applications (**Fig. 2**).[1] In addition, recent studies suggest that computer-assisted image processing may be considered a form of virtual chromoendoscopy for contrast enhancement in gastrointestinal endoscopy.[2,3]

Chromoendoscopy is perhaps most effective when combined with instrumentation enhancements such as high-magnification optics and high-density charge-coupled devices that increase the optical resolution of the endoscope, thus enabling high-magnification video imaging (magnification chromoendoscopy). With current optical components and detection devices, high-magnification video endoscopy provides enough resolving power to approach low-resolution microscopy, thus enabling visualization of critical morphologic features such as aberrant crypt patterns or abnormal vascular architecture. Although tedious and time-consuming, high-resolution chromoendoscopy is now rapidly becoming the clinical standard in screening endoscopy such as surveillance for dysplasia in inflammatory bowel disease,[4,5] and has proved highly effective in identification of gastric

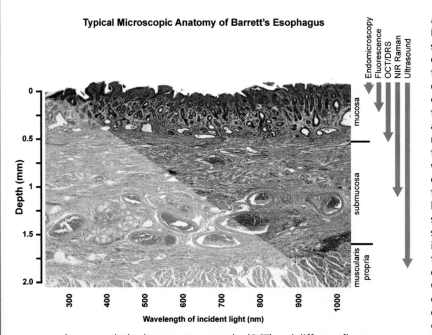

Fig. 1. Cross-section of Barrett esophagus (BE) showing the sampling depth of various imaging techniques. Penetration depth of the various optical methods is illustrated by the arrows and highlighted by the non-shaded portions of the tissue. Whereas the wavelength of the incident light determines the penetration depth, light-tissue interactions such as absorption and scattering determine the information content of the returning light collected by the detector. Consequently, endomicroscopy and fluorescence microscopy sample only the superficial mucosa, whereas optical coherence tomography (OCT) and diffuse reflectance spectroscopy (DRS) can potentially sample the full mucosal thickness. Near infrared (NIR) Raman spectroscopy is among the optical methods with the highest sampling depth (∼1 mm). In contrast to optical methods, common ultrasound methods can provide full-thickness mural images, albeit with limited resolution.

Fig. 2. Endoscopic appearance of a polypoid early gastric cancer after application of methylene blue. Notice how the chromogenic reagent increases the contrast of this lesion against the surrounding non-neoplastic mucosa.

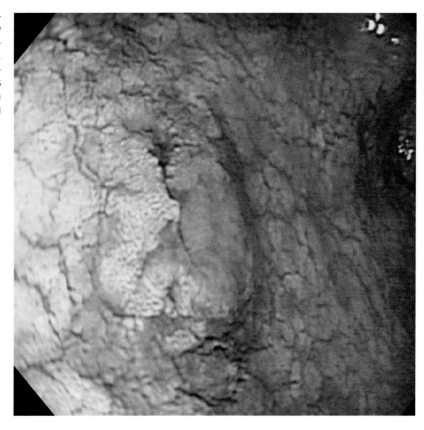

neoplastic lesions [6] and dysplasia in Barrett esophagus (BE).[7,8] As the quality of white light endoscopy alone continues to improve, however, added contrast from chromoendoscopy or narrow-band imaging (see later discussion) may not necessarily improve the diagnostic yield for endoscopic detection of neoplastic lesions.[9]

Narrow-band Imaging

Narrow band imaging (NBI) is a simple optical technology that takes particular advantage of hemoglobin as an intrinsic contrast agent for highlighting microvascular anatomy of the superficial mucosa. A strong absorption band (the Soret band) in the blue region of the absorption spectrum of heme proteins has been widely known. By narrowing the collection width of the white light spectrum using filter sets in the 400- to 500-nm region, NBI takes advantage of the strong hemoglobin absorption at approximately 415 nm to enhance the blood contrast in the endoscopic image (**Fig. 3**). Combined with a shallow penetration depth for the blue light (< ~250 nm), NBI provides a high-contrast image of the superficial microvasculature. This added contrast is often adequate for highlighting neoplastic lesions that

typically show an abnormal vascular pattern caused by angiogenesis and/or vascular remodeling. Additional narrow-band filters may be used in other regions of the visible spectrum, but the diagnostic usefulness of such additional and/or different filters has not been shown in gastrointestinal endoscopy.

NBI alone or in combination with magnification and/or chromoendoscopy has proved to be effective in detection and diagnosis of early neoplastic lesions in specific clinical scenarios such as screening in BE[10,11] or detection of small colorectal polyps (**Fig. 4**).[12] However, the efficacy of NBI in gastrointestinal endoscopy is not universally accepted, nor does it show a definitive improvement compared with high-resolution endoscopy or other established techniques.[9,13] Nevertheless, NBI remains a popular technique for contrast enhancement among gastrointestinal endoscopists.

Autofluorescence Imaging

Fluorescence imaging in the form of video fluorescence endoscopy is among the first true alternatives to standard white light endoscopy for providing optical contrast. Intrinsic tissue

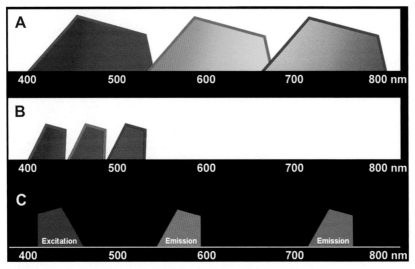

Fig. 3. (*A*) Common video endoscopy uses white light illumination and RGB filters to produce typical video endoscope images. (*B*) NBI also commonly uses white light illumination, but optical filters allow detection of only selected, small regions of the full spectrum. Here, 3 narrow-band filters are used to provide contrast in the blue region of the spectrum where hemoglobin absorption is dominant. Computer processing can assign arbitrary colors to data collected from each filter, producing pseudocolor RGB images. (*C*) In contrast to white light illumination methods, in fluorescence endoscopy the tissue is excited with a specific wavelength, and emitted light or spectra are collected by the detection system. Thus, fluorescence methods allow chemical imaging of the tissue based on the available tissue fluorophores and their excitation-emission characteristics.

fluorescence is associated with amino acids such as tryptophan, enzymes such as nicotinamide adenine dinucleotide reduced (NADH) and flavin adenine dinucleotide, and structural proteins such as collagen. Tissue fluorescence can therefore provide information about the biochemical and structural state of the tissue, which can in turn be used as a biomarker for changes that occur during disease development and progression.

Neoplastic progression in particular is associated with structural and biochemical changes in the epithelial lining and the extracellular matrix that collectively result in changes in intrinsic fluorescence of the bulk tissue. It is therefore not surprising that promising preliminary results were reported more than a decade ago using fluorescence imaging for diagnosis of neoplastic lesions in a variety of epithelial organs, including the gastrointestinal tract.[14–17] Clinical fluorescence imaging, however, required advances in instrumentation and methods that required several additional years.

Although a wide range of excitation-emission parameters are possible, currently available commercial instruments typically excite the tissue using a narrow source of blue light ($\sim$400–450 nm) and collect the emitted fluorescence in the green ($\sim$500–550 nm) and the red ($\sim$650–750 nm) regions of the visible spectrum. Although initial clinical studies showed little to no advantage compared with white light imaging in detection of

high-grade dysplasia in BE or colonic neoplasms,[18–22] more recent studies have consistently shown an improved detection rate for neoplastic lesions using autofluorescence imaging in conjunction with other endoscopic modalities.[21–24] Fluorescence imaging is likely to remain as a key capability in clinical endoscopes, and its applications are likely to become more widespread with the addition of extrinsic fluorescent markers and molecularly targeted fluorecent imaging.[25,26]

CONFOCAL ENDOMICROSCOPY

Although high-resolution magnification endoscopy can potentially provide subcellular images (5–7 μm resolution) of the tissue surface (5–10 μm deep), it lacks optical sectioning power that is essential for true endomicroscopy and three-dimensional morphologic reconstruction. To overcome this limitation, confocal optics, which are widely used in ex vivo microscopy, have recently been incorporated into endoscopic imaging devices, thus enabling true optical sectioning and real-time in vivo microscopy (**Fig. 5**). Confocal optics are able to collect only the photons that originate from a specific depth in the tissue, thus virtually sectioning the tissue in real time. Furthermore, confocal techniques can be used in reflectance or fluorescence modes, enabling multimodal

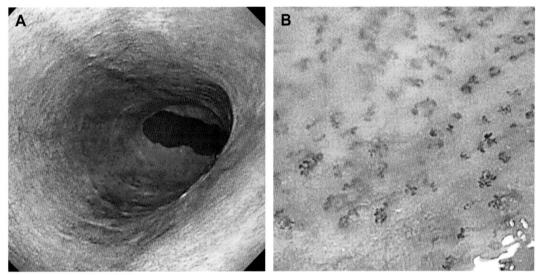

Fig. 4. NBI appearance of the normal squamous mucosa (*A*) and of dysplastic squamous epithelium characterized by an increased number of dilated, enlarged, and tortuous intrapapillary capillary vascular loops (*B*).

microscopic imaging. Commercially available confocal endomicroscopes are capable of submicron optical sectioning to a depth of 100 to 200 μm, ideal for identification and classification of early mucosal disease such as dysplasia or microvascular anatomy.[23,27] Although widespread clinical application is currently limited by the slow acquisition speed and lack of real-time three-dimensional analysis, technological advances should overcome these limitations in the near future.

Optical Coherence Tomography

Optical coherence tomography (OCT) is a micrometer-resolution optical imaging technique that produces cross-sectional images of the sample by measuring the amplitude and echo time delay of the backscattered light.[28] (Although there are fundamental differences between OCT and ultrasound, OCT data can be conceptually visualized as the optical equivalent of high-resolution ultrasound data.) Initial clinical applications of OCT in

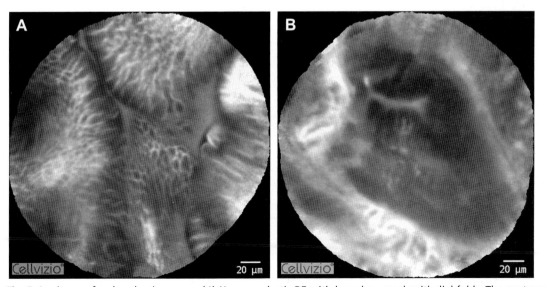

Fig. 5. In vivo confocal endomicroscopy. (*A*) Non-neoplastic BE with broad mucosal epithelial folds. The contour of the lining columnar cells is readily identified. (*B*) Neoplastic BE. The normal architecture is lost, with replacement of regularly-spaced normal cells by large clusters of irregularly arranged malignant cells. (*Courtesy of Michael B. Wallace, Mayo Clinic, Jacksonville, FL.*)

the gastrointestinal tract focused on point sampling (optical biopsy) that provided sufficient morphologic detail to allow classification and grading of mucosal lesions in well-defined clinical settings such as BE with promising sensitivity and specificity.[29–31] More recently, technological advances in OCT have introduced the possibility of high-resolution, wide-area imaging and three-dimensional reconstruction of the gastrointestinal mucosa.[32,33] These technological advances position OCT as a potential high-throughput endomicroscopy tool, although significant advances in instrumentation and software are needed to make high-resolution, wide-area OCT a clinical reality (**Fig. 6**).

Spectroscopic Imaging

With the exception of video fluorescence endoscopy, essentially all diagnostic modalities described earlier use light-tissue interaction as a basis for morphologic imaging of the tissue. Optical spectroscopy, on the other hand, has evolved as an important ancillary tool for tissue diagnosis based on structural and/or biochemical parameters that are often related to but analytically distinct from morphologic parameters.

Light propagating in biologic tissues interacts with various components of the tissue in a variety of ways. Elastic scattering (scattering without a change in the wavelength of incident light) is the predominant mode of light-tissue interaction, and results in familiar phenomena such as fluorescence and reflectance. Considering the incident light as a collection of photons, light can be scattered once (single scattering) or multiple times (diffusive scattering) before returning to the surface to be detected. Light can also be absorbed by chromophores such as hemoglobin without being re-emitted (absorption), or by fluorophores such as NADH and collagen, and be re-emitted at longer wavelengths (fluorescence) before being detected at the surface. In addition to elastic scattering, inelastic processes that shift the wavelength of incident light do occur and result in phenomena such as Raman scattering. In contrast to signals derived from elastic processes such as white light reflectance and fluorescence, Raman scattering is extremely weak, and its detection above background is challenging. In the past decade, essentially all of the spectroscopic modalities mentioned earlier have shown diagnostic potential in a variety of organ systems, including the gastrointestinal tract, specially for detection and diagnosis of dysplasia in BE (**Fig. 7**).[34–37]

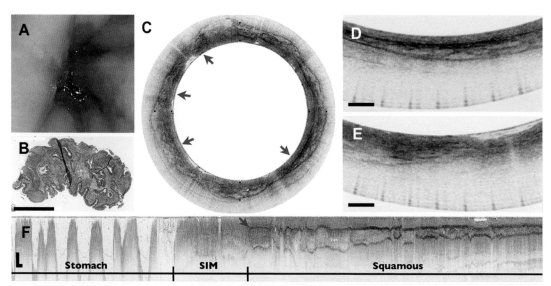

Fig. 6. OCT image of BE. (*A*) Irregular squamocolumnar junction (SCJ). (*B*) Biopsy specimen from the SCJ shows specialized columnar epithelium with-out dysplasia (hematoxylin and eosin, original magnification ×2). (*C*) Cross-sectional image reveals the normal layered appearance of squamous mucosa (*red arrow*, expanded in [*D*]) and tissue that satisfies the OCT criteria for specialized columnar epithelium (*blue arrows*, expanded in [*E*]). (*F*) Longitudinal section across the gastroesophageal junction shows the transition from squamous mucosa to specialized columnar epithelium to cardia. Scale bars and tick marks represent 1 mm. (*From* Suter MJ, Vakoc BJ, Yachimski PS, et al. Comprehensive microscopy of the esophagus in human patients with optical frequency domain imaging. Gastrointest Endosc 2008;68(4):750; with permission.)

Fig. 7. Quantitative spectroscopic imaging provides tissue structural and chemical information that is often complementary to morphology. Potential methods include intrinsic fluorescence spectroscopy (IFS) providing quantitative information about collagen, NADH, β-carotene, and other fluorophores and diffuse reflectance spec-

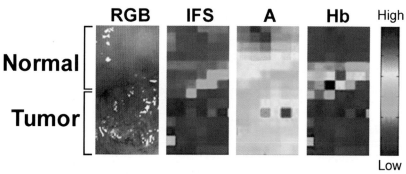

troscopy (DRS) providing information about tissue scattering and hemoglobin concentration and saturation. Shown here is an ex vivo colonic sample with normal and neoplastic regions, imaged using a raster scanning method. IFS panel shows collagen/NADH ratio, A is a measure of tissue scattering, and Hb is the total hemoglobin concentration.

Although most published studies of spectroscopic diagnosis have focused on point probe measurements of dysplasia (optical biopsy), efforts are under way for adaptation of various modalities for endoscopic imaging. In theory, essentially all spectroscopic diagnostic modalities can be used in the imaging mode, and several proof-of-principle studies have been published for imaging gastrointestinal lesions.[38,39] Nevertheless, significant technological research and development are required to develop clinically viable instrumentation for spectroscopic imaging. Recently developed enhanced backscattering spectroscopy techniques have shown the potential of optical spectroscopy as a noninvasive biomarker in screening for gastrointestinal neoplasia.[40,41] Although definite large-scale clinical results are still lacking, these novel techniques have the potential to significantly enhance the value of endospectroscopy in management of gastrointestinal neoplasia.

NOVEL THERAPEUTIC ENDOSCOPIC METHODS

PRINCIPLES OF ENDOSCOPIC RESECTION

Endoscopic resection (ER), either in the form of endoscopic mucosal resection (EMR) or endoscopic submucosal dissection (ESD), refers to minimally invasive procedures intended to remove superficial neoplastic lesions that exhibit minimal to no submucosal involvement. In addition to their diagnostic potential, these techniques are now widely accepted in the treatment of superficial gastrointestinal tract neoplasms, because they provide therapeutic success rates that are comparable to surgery, but without the morbidity and mortality that are typically associated with surgical resections. Furthermore, unlike the closely related

endoscopic ablation techniques, ERs enable complete microscopic examination of the diseased tissue, allowing postoperative histologic confirmation of the grade and depth of invasion (**Fig. 8**).

Originally popularized for resection of early gastric adenocarcinomas and esophageal squamous cell carcinomas in Japan and limited other clinical centers, ERs have now been widely adopted for the treatment of most superficial gastrointestinal lesions, including early esophageal neoplasms arising in BE, as well as superficial colonic and ampullary neoplasm.[42–44] There are many technical and clinical variations of ER, and a complete review of these methods is beyond the scope of this discussion. We briefly describe the techniques as practiced in North America and discuss pathologic issues related to handling and interpretation of ERs.

EMR Versus ESD

Originally described as strip-off biopsy, multiple techniques for ER of mucosal lesions have been developed over the years.[45] These methods are generally divided into EMR, in which electrocautery wire loops or similar cutting devices are used to excise superficial mucosal lesions without deliberate submucosa dissection, and ESD, in which electrocautery tools, knives, and/or scissors are used for en bloc resection of lesions through a circumferential mucosal incision followed by deep submucosa dissection. The overall goal in both techniques is to remove the mucosa and part or all of submucosa without penetrating the muscularis propria (see **Fig. 6**). Detailed description of these techniques can be found elsewhere.[45]

From a surgical pathology point of view, the fundamental difference between EMR and ESD specimens is that the latter is almost always performed with the intent for complete en bloc

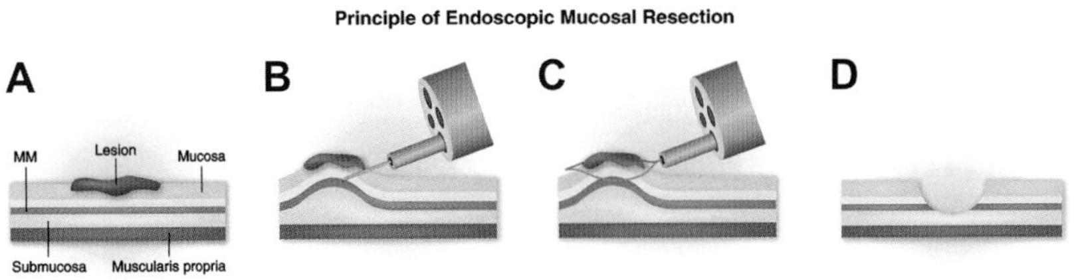

Principle of Endoscopic Mucosal Resection

A   B   C   D

MM   Lesion   Mucosa

Submucosa   Muscularis propria

Fig. 8. Principle of EMR. This technique is aimed at dissecting mucosal neoplasm (*A*). The endoscopist injects saline into the submucosa to form a bulla (*B*). Lifting the mucosal lesion from the submucosa allows the safe removal of the neoplasm without risk of perforation (*C*). After resection, the superficial mucosal ulceration heals rapidly (*D*).

excision of the lesion, and must therefore always be treated as a therapeutic surgical specimen with the need for complete evaluation of the lesion and the excision margins.

Handling of ER Specimens and Pathologic Evaluation

Proper histologic evaluation of ER specimens is cardinal, because it provides information about depth of infiltration and whether complete removal has been obtained. The specimens ought to be handled with the same thoroughness as surgical oncology specimens and should not be seen as big biopsies. Reporting of margins and depth of invasion is essential, because based on the information, additional therapeutic options may be decided, including repeat of ER or recourse to surgery.

In practice, ER specimens should be stretched gently and mounted on a firm surface such as paraffin before fixation. Photographing the specimen is a good practice not only to document fragmented specimens but also to help record and correlate the histologic mapping of the lesions. Inking of the deep and circumferential margins helps in assessing the overall completeness of the resection, particularly if proper orientation is difficult. After fixation, serial sectioning of the ER

is performed, optimally at 2-mm intervals (**Fig. 9**). If applicable, additional radial sections should be made at both ends of the specimen to further evaluate the status of the circumferential margin. If the specimen is small, however, both ends can be submitted en face. Piecemeal specimens are difficult to evaluate, because the fragments may be too small for stretching, and reconstructing the specimen for adequate evaluation of the excision margins may be impossible (**Fig. 10**). This problem is more common with the newly introduced band ligation technique, which allows resection of larger lesions, but usually yields several fragments.

In addition to the size of the specimen and the status of the margins (lateral and deep), important variables that should be reported include the grade of the lesion (low- and high-grade dysplasia, intramucosal, or invasive adenocarcinoma), degree of differentiation, and depth of invasion. The status of vascular invasion also should be noted, especially when submucosal extension is present, because it indicates a higher risk of recurrence.

THERAPEUTIC EFFICACY OF ER

The reported efficacy of ER has been variable, depending on the anatomic location within the gastrointestinal tract, the type of lesion being

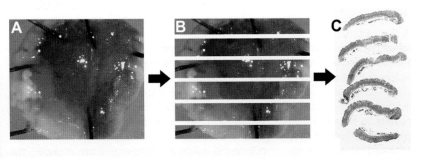

Fig. 9. EMR specimen fixated on a paraffin block (*A*). The tissue is fixed overnight and serially sectioned to allow proper reconstruction of the lesion and evaluation of the margins (*B*, *C*). Depending on the clinical circumstances, various ink markers and multiple cassettes may be necessary to achieve an adequate evaluation of the completeness of excision.

Fig. 10. Whole mount view of EMR. This specimen is well oriented. In this case, evaluation of the deep and lateral margins and, therefore, completeness of excision, is easily performed.

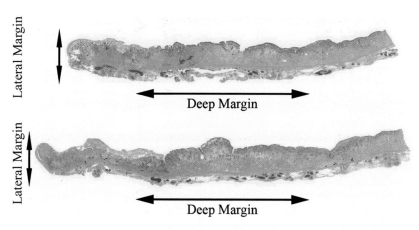

resected, and the protocol used for resection. We summarize the current status with regard to esophageal, gastric, ampullary, and colonic neoplasms, but again expand largely on EMRs for Barrett-related adenocarcinoma, because it is most commonly encountered in our practice and in North America in general.

ESOPHAGUS

EMR has been validated and largely accepted as a safe alternative to esophagectomy for early esophageal neoplasm. A recent prospective series of 100 patients with low-risk adenocarcinomas, defined as well- to moderately differentiated lesions 20 mm or less in diameter and confined to the mucosa without angiolymphatic invasion or ulceration, reported no death and an overall recurrence rate of 11% during a mean follow-up of 36.7 months (range 2–83 months).[46] Similar success rates have been reported for early squamous cell carcinomas of the esophagus treated by EMR.[47–49] Bleeding can be observed in up to 14% of patients treated by EMR, but most cases are successfully managed endoscopically in an outpatient setting. Perforation is rare (1.8% of the procedures) and treated effectively by medical therapy.[42,43,46,50] Esophageal stenoses may occur, but seem to be largely limited to circumferential resections.[51,52]

In ER of early esophageal carcinoma, depth of invasion, lesion size, and distribution seem to be the most significant determinant of therapeutic success as determined by completeness of excision and the rate of recurrence.[48,51–55] Specifically, mean specimen size and number of EMR specimens (both of which are a function of lesion size) are directly correlated with the success rate of complete en bloc resection and the rate of local recurrence. In addition, as expected, there is a direct correlation between depth of invasion and recurrence, with best outcomes for intraepithelial lesions (m1), followed by lamina propria invasion (m2), invasion into muscularis mucosae (m3), and submucosa (sm), respectively.[56–58]

Given the low risk of nodal metastasis for m1 and m2 lesions, EMR has become a favored therapeutic modality for lesions measuring less than 15 to 20 mm.[48,55,57] For larger or more deeply invasive lesions, ESD seems to be a promising approach for curative ER. In a direct comparison of ESD versus EMR, Ishihara and colleagues[48] recently reported a significantly better outcome with ESD for superficial squamous cell carcinomas measuring less than 20 mm. The difference in outcome was no longer apparent, however, when ESD was compared with EMR cap technique in lesions measuring less than 15 mm.[48] In a separate study, the same group reported a remarkably favorable outcome for larger (>20 mm) squamous cell carcinomas resected en bloc by ESD, with no recurrence after a median follow-up of 32 months.[47] However, complete en bloc resection for these larger lesions was achieved in only 34 of the 78 patients (43%), and there was a significant correlation between the number of pieces required for complete resection of lesions and disease-free survival.[47] These results seem less favorable than previously reported by Oyama and colleagues,[53] who reported 95% success rate in complete en bloc resection of superficial squamous cell carcinomas in 102 patients with a mean lesion size of 28 mm. It is likely, however, that the more favorable success rate reported by

Oyama and colleagues reflects the heterogeneity of their patient population, in which the lesion size varied from 4 to 64 mm. Nevertheless, both studies concur on high disease-free survival after 2 to 3 years of follow-up in patients with successful en bloc excision of lesions.

Designation of an ER as en bloc versus piecemeal is typically an endoscopic classification with clear prognostic consequences, as discussed earlier. The pathologic corollary of this classification, or the histologic status of excision margins, is an equally important prognostic indicator and a primary goal of the pathologic evaluation for EMR and ESD specimens. Unlike endoscopic success rates for en bloc excision, the high percentages of histologically positive margins (>75% of reported cases) can have a significant negative effect on patient outcome.[59–61] In one series, 86% of patients with positive deep margin had residual tumors in follow-up, despite the use of adjunct photodynamic therapy (PDT) in some cases.[61] Prasad and colleagues[59] also reported that in their series of 25 patients, none with negative mucosal margins had residual tumor at subsequent esophagectomy, whereas 50% of those with submucosal invasive adenocarcinoma had residual tumor, and 30% had nodal metastases. Both of these studies, however, are limited in statistical power and are restricted to glandular neoplastic lesions in the setting of BE only.

The experience with ER methods for excision of submucosal lesions such as mesenchymal tumors is limited and varied. Complete excision of submucosal lesions has been reported in 36% to 95% of the cases,[62–64] but definitive conclusions about the usefulness and effectiveness of EMR or ESD for management of submucosal lesions cannot be made.

DIAGNOSTIC EMR

In addition to its commonly accepted usefulness as a minimally invasive therapeutic modality, EMR also has been advocated as a superior staging and diagnostic tool.[50,61,65,66] In a 2006 study of 27 EMR specimens, reclassification of the original biopsies was required in 37% of the cases, with the biopsies underreporting the neoplastic grade in 21% of the cases and overreporting it in 16%.[61] In another series of 48 patients, 6 of 25 patients with an initial diagnosis of high-grade dysplasia were upgraded to intramucosal carcinoma (IMC) and 6 of 15 patients with a biopsy diagnosis of IMC were upstaged to invasive carcinoma.[65] As expected, discrepancies between original biopsies and subsequent EMRs are more common when the original lesions are large (>10

mm) and when less extensive biopsy sampling is performed.[66] Combination of EMR with optical diagnostic tools described in the previous section may soon become an invaluable tool not only in targeting biopsies in large lesions but also in guiding EMR by providing real-time diagnostic data.[67]

Reliable classification of grade and stage of neoplastic lesions is critical, because lymph node metastases are essentially absent in intraepithelial lesions, but can be observed in up to 4% of IMC and up to 27% of tumors invasive into the submucosa.[68–71] Tumor staging by endoscopic ultrasound (EUS) is widely used clinically, but EUS has only 72% to 95% accuracy in distinguishing between mucosal (m) and submucosal (sm) neoplasms, supporting the role of EMR as an adjunct staging method.[43,61,72] In our experience, a large vertical extent of the neoplasm in vivo and duplication of the muscularis mucosae are commonly associated with overstaging by EUS.[73]

EMR has also been noted to improve diagnostic consistency, with interobserver agreement significantly higher on EMR than on pre-EMR biopsy specimens.[61] This result likely relates to the larger tissue sampling and the ability to better evaluate mucosal landmarks such as duplicated muscularis mucosae. In our experience of 25 cases of combined biopsies and EMR, 100% interobserver agreement was never achieved on biopsies, whereas it was obtained in 16% of EMR.[61] Furthermore, diagnoses spanning 4 different grades were recorded in 12% of biopsies, but in only one EMR (4%).

STOMACH AND SMALL INTESTINE

ER has become the treatment of choice for superficial gastric and ampullary carcinomas. Originally, selection criteria for management of early gastric carcinoma by EMR were limiting and included several criteria regarding size and type of lesions, in addition to documentation of the absence of mural invasion and of lymph node metastases.[74,75] Recently, the criteria have been extended, largely reflecting better and more effective EMR methods and the slowly increasing popularity of ESD.[76–78] Although the experience with ESD for management of superficial gastric carcinomas has been largely limited to Japan, the positive experience with early adopters beyond Japan is suggestive that gastric ESD will likely become a mainstay of treatment of superficial gastric lesions worldwide.[79,80] Adding to this popularity are parallels between esophageal and gastric data regarding the diagnostic value of mucosal resections for reliable classification and staging of neoplasms,[81] likely resulting in an increasing share of gastric EMRs (instead of biopsies) as the initial diagnostic modality.

ERs have been attempted for a variety of small intestinal epithelial and submucosal lesions in an ad hoc fashion. For superficial ampullary neoplasms, however, endoscopic papillectomy is often the first line of treatment, and is considered curative if the margins are negative and microscopic examination excludes an invasive carcinoma.[82–84] Limited follow-up (6–12 months) is the norm for small, low-grade lesions with negative margins, although repeat examination (1–3 months) is advised for fragmented, high-grade dysplastic lesions or early invasive carcinoma.[85] However, recurrence is more common in patients with familial adenomatous polyposis compared with sporadic lesions. [86] Invasive ampullary lesions may necessitate surgical resection for definitive treatment.

COLON AND RECTUM

Although traditional polypectomy is useful for most small or early colonic neoplasms (eg, early-stage colorectal cancer, flat tubular adenoma, and carcinoid or low-grade neuroendocrine neoplasm), large lesions (>3 cm) involving more than one-third of the circumference or exhibiting a flat or depressed appearance are challenging to remove with standard polypectomy techniques. Such lesions are amenable to ER methods, which can provide en bloc excision and allow histologic evaluation of the middle to deep submucosa, which is not available after standard polypectomy. Specifically, EMR is recommended for treatment of large and/or flat adenomas and small, well-differentiated adenocarcinomas confined to the mucosa, or invasive carcinomas with superficial invasion into the submucosa, without known lymphovascular or nodal involvement. Under such circumstances, a simple inject-and-cut EMR approach proved effective in complete histologic excision of 87% of 224 colonic lesions, with a less than 3% overall complication rate, including bleeding (2.2%) and perforation (0.4%).[87] These recent data are similar to some of the earliest series of colorectal EMRs, in which complete removal was achieved in 87% of 337 cases, with 0.7% and 0.4% rates of perforation and bleeding, respectively,[88] suggesting little effect from new technological improvements on the overall management of colorectal neoplasms by EMR.

The experience with ESD for excision of large lesions in the colorectum is limited, but it is rapidly gaining popularity.[89] Comparable with the esophageal experience, the size of the colonic lesion usually dictates the proportion of piecemeal versus en bloc resection. In a series of 59 colorectal lesions larger than 20 mm, Katsinelos and colleagues[90] reported an en bloc resection rate of 70% for cases measuring less than 20 to 29 mm, compared with none of the 26 lesions measuring greater than 29 mm. Overall, however, the en bloc resection rates for colorectal ESD seem to be favorable, ranging from 84% to 98% in large series,[91–93] including disease-free (histologically complete) en bloc excision in more than 70% of lesions.[91] The most common complications of colorectal ESD are bleeding (0%–2%) and perforations (0%–5%).[90,91,93]

ENDOSCOPIC MUCOSAL ABLATIVE THERAPY

PHOTODYNAMIC THERAPY

Photodynamic therapy (PDT) has been extensively investigated for the ablation of superficial neoplasms associated with BE. The method is based on the use of an inactive photosensitive drug that accumulates within the epithelium. As the drug selectively absorbs the energy of an endoscopically delivered light of appropriate wavelength, the drug is activated, resulting in a photoreaction that generates high-energy cytotoxic singlet oxygen molecules that damage the tissue (**Fig. 11**).[94]

Two photosensitizing agents have been widely evaluated in clinical studies of BE: 5-aminolevulinic acid (5-ALA) and porfimer sodium (Photofrin, Axcan Pharma Inc, Birmingham, AL, USA). The advantages of 5-ALA include oral administration, rapid onset of photosensitivity (4–6 hours), and short duration of photosensitivity (days); however, the depth of mucosal destruction is more superficial than with porfimer sodium, which is administered intravenously. After PDT, dysplasia and/or superficial adenocarcinomas have been noted to disappear in 67% to 100% of cases.[95–97] A recent 5-year follow-up study reported typical results of PDT with overall eradication of high-grade dysplasia in 77% of patients compared with 39% treated with omeprazole alone.[96] Furthermore, PDT resulted in a decreased risk of metachronous adenocarcinomas compared with the control group.[96]

HISTOLOGIC CHANGES AFTER PDT

Squamous re-epithelialization is common after PDT, with islands of neosquamous epithelium noted in 77.5% of biopsies after PDT (vs 36.7% before PDT) (**Fig. 12**).[98] Mild reactive atypia of the columnar epithelium and crypt regenerative activity is noted after PDT, but these changes are

A

Photodynamic therapy (PDT)

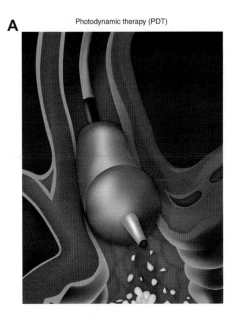

Fig. 11. PDT. The photosensitizing agent accumulates preferentially into the neoplastic epithelium. After activation by endoscopic delivery of light of appropriate wavelength (*A*), the cytotoxic singlet oxygen generated destroys the neoplastic cells (*B*).

B

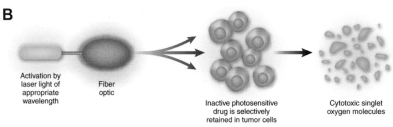

Activation by laser light of appropriate wavelength

Fiber optic

Inactive photosensitive drug is selectively retained in tumor cells

Cytotoxic singlet oxygen molecules

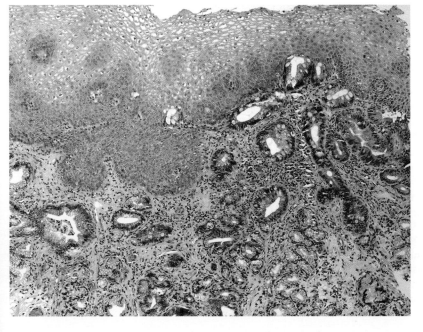

Fig. 12. Following PDT, the restored squamous epithelium replaces the Barrett epithelium and grows along the Barrett gland. In this case, residual buried Barrett epithelium is present, putting this patient at risk for unsuspected neoplastic proliferation.

usually are not diagnostically challenging.[99,100] Distally located neoplastic lesions and multifocal lesions are more likely to persist after PDT, although their histologic grade is commonly unchanged compared with before PDT.[98] Esophageal stricture requiring dilatation is a common non-neoplastic complication of PDT, and seems to be directly related to the extent of BE and number of cycles of treatment.[101]

POST-PDT BURIED NEOPLASIA

A significant long-term consequence of PDT is the follow-up of buried metaplastic and potentially neoplastic mucosal, which is concealed by an overgrowth of neosquamous epithelium (see **Fig. 12**). So-called buried BE may be associated with subsurface neoplastic transformation, not readily detectable by routine endoscopic surveillance.[99,102,103] In our experience, 7.4% of post-PDT neoplasms were completely concealed by neosquamous epithelium, and in most cases, represented the highest grade and usually the sole residual neoplastic focus.[99] The concern for increased incidence of concealed neoplasms in patients after PDT has been contended in a recent publication,[104] although differences in PDT protocol and exclusion of intramucosal and superficially invasive carcinomas in this report preclude a definitive comparison between this and earlier studies. Regardless of the contentious role of PDT in the pathogenesis of buried lesions, there is general consensus that neoplastic glandular epithelium may be concealed by islands of benign squamous epithelium, thus necessitating thorough endoscopic surveillance with deep biopsies in islands or regions of squamous epithelium in the background of BE.

OTHER ABLATIVE THERAPIES

Novel endoscopic techniques seeking to complement some of the main shortcomings of PDT, including incomplete ablation efficacy and post-procedure photosensitivity and stricturing, have been developed. Radiofrequency ablation has been used for the ablation of BE and various grades of dysplasia with reasonable success.[105–107] Cryospray ablation techniques have also been used in the esophagus, especially in treating superficial squamous cell carcinomas.[108,109] Both of these techniques are potential alternatives to PDT, although definitive conclusions cannot be made, given limited controlled data about the effectiveness of these techniques versus PDT, and limited pathologic data in the context of these alternative techniques.

SUMMARY

Recent technological advances in endoscopic tools and methods have created a wealth of new challenges and opportunities for gastrointestinal pathology. As a commonly accepted gold standard, surgical pathology remains a cornerstone of new technology development and clinical validation, thus requiring the surgical pathologist to maintain a basic understanding of the underlying science and technology. In a recent consensus

Pitfalls
ENDOSCOPIC IMAGING FOR
THE PATHOLOGIST

! White light imaging ignores and/or suppresses many potential sources of optical contrast, which may be invaluable in detection and diagnosis of mucosal lesions.

! Added contrast from chromoendoscopy or narrow-band imaging may not necessarily improve the diagnostic yield for detection of mucosal lesions but remains a popular technique for contrast enhancement among gastrointestinal endoscopists.

! From a surgical pathology point of view, the fundamental difference between EMR and ESD specimens is that the latter is almost always performed with the intent for complete en bloc excision of the lesion, and must therefore always be treated as a therapeutic surgical specimen with the need for complete evaluation of the lesion and the excision margins.

! Proper histologic evaluation of ER specimens is cardinal, because it provides information about depth of infiltration and whether complete removal has been obtained. The specimens ought to be handled with the same thoroughness as surgical oncology specimens and should not be seen as big biopsies. Reporting of margins and depth of invasion is essential, because based on the information, additional therapeutic options may be decided.

! Piecemeal specimens from ER are difficult to evaluate, because the fragments may be too small for stretching, and reconstructing the specimen for adequate evaluation of the excision margins may be impossible.

! Band ligation technique allows resection of larger lesions, but usually yields several fragments that are difficult to evaluate for the reasons noted in the preceding point.

report, the Pathology Working Group of the Network for Translational Research in Optical Imaging emphasized the critical role of pathology and pathologists in technology validation, biomarker discovery, and clinical translation at the National Cancer Institute.[110] For the practicing gastrointestinal pathologist, however, this mandate goes beyond the small number of studies supported by the National Cancer Institute, and includes virtually every diagnostic specimen obtained through a new or incompletely characterized clinical tool such as optical imaging, ER, or ablative therapy. It is therefore our hope that this article provides the foundation on which every gastrointestinal pathologist will build a fundamental knowledge of modern endoscopic techniques for diagnosis and therapy.

REFERENCES

1. Wong Kee Song LM, Adler DG, Chand B, et al. Chromoendoscopy. Gastrointest Endosc 2007; 66(4):639.
2. Pohl J, Nguyen-Tat M, Pech O, et al. Computed virtual chromoendoscopy for classification of small colorectal lesions: a prospective comparative study. Am J Gastroenterol 2008;103(3):562.
3. Coriat R, Chryssostalis A, Zeitoun JD, et al. Computed virtual chromoendoscopy system (FICE): a new tool for upper endoscopy? Gastroenterol Clin Biol 2008;32(4):363.
4. Kiesslich R, Goetz M, Lammersdorf K, et al. Chromoscopy-guided endomicroscopy increases the diagnostic yield of intraepithelial neoplasia in ulcerative colitis. Gastroenterology 2007;132(3): 874.
5. Marion JF, Waye JD, Present DH, et al. Chromoendoscopy-targeted biopsies are superior to standard colonoscopic surveillance for detecting dysplasia in inflammatory bowel disease patients: a prospective endoscopic trial. Am J Gastroenterol 2008;103(9):2342.
6. Areia M, Amaro P, Dinis-Ribeiro M, et al. External validation of a classification for methylene blue magnification chromoendoscopy in premalignant gastric lesions. Gastrointest Endosc 2008;67(7):1011.
7. Pohl J, May A, Rabenstein T, et al. Comparison of computed virtual chromoendoscopy and conventional chromoendoscopy with acetic acid for detection of neoplasia in Barrett's esophagus. Endoscopy 2007;39(7):594.
8. Ormeci N, Savas B, Coban S, et al. The usefulness of chromoendoscopy with methylene blue in Barrett's metaplasia and early esophageal carcinoma. Surg Endosc 2008;22(3):693.
9. Curvers W, Baak L, Kiesslich R, et al. Chromoendoscopy and narrow-band imaging compared with high-resolution magnification endoscopy in Barrett's esophagus. Gastroenterology 2008;134(3):670.
10. Wolfsen HC, Crook JE, Krishna M, et al. Prospective, controlled tandem endoscopy study of narrow band imaging for dysplasia detection in Barrett's Esophagus. Gastroenterology 2008;135(1):24.
11. Singh R, Karageorgiou H, Owen V, et al. Comparison of high-resolution magnification narrow-band imaging and white-light endoscopy in the prediction of histology in Barrett's oesophagus. Scand J Gastroenterol 2009;44(1):1.
12. East JE, Suzuki N, Bassett P, et al. Narrow band imaging with magnification for the characterization of small and diminutive colonic polyps: pit pattern and vascular pattern intensity. Endoscopy 2008; 40(10):811.
13. Adler A, Aschenbeck J, Yenerim T, et al. Narrow-band versus white-light high definition television endoscopic imaging for screening colonoscopy: a prospective randomized trial. Gastroenterology 2009;136(2):410.
14. Cothren RM, Sivak MV Jr, Van Dam J, et al. Detection of dysplasia at colonoscopy using laser-induced fluorescence: a blinded study. Gastrointest Endosc 1996;44(2):168.
15. Mycek MA, Schomacker KT, Nishioka NS. Colonic polyp differentiation using time-resolved autofluorescence spectroscopy. Gastrointest Endosc 1998;48(4):390.
16. Panjehpour M, Overholt BF, Vo-Dinh T, et al. Endoscopic fluorescence detection of high-grade dysplasia in Barrett's esophagus. Gastroenterology 1996;111(1):93.
17. Schomacker KT, Frisoli JK, Compton CC, et al. Ultraviolet laser-induced fluorescence of colonic polyps. Gastroenterology 1992;102(4 Pt 1):1155.
18. Niepsuj K, Niepsuj G, Cebula W, et al. Autofluorescence endoscopy for detection of high-grade dysplasia in short-segment Barrett's esophagus. Gastrointest Endosc 2003;58(5):715.
19. Kara MA, Smits ME, Rosmolen WD, et al. A randomized crossover study comparing light-induced fluorescence endoscopy with standard videoendoscopy for the detection of early neoplasia in Barrett's esophagus. Gastrointest Endosc 2005;61(6):671.
20. Kara MA, Peters FP, Ten Kate FJ, et al. Endoscopic video autofluorescence imaging may improve the detection of early neoplasia in patients with Barrett's esophagus. Gastrointest Endosc 2005;61(6): 679.
21. Matsuda T, Saito Y, Fu KI, et al. Does autofluorescence imaging videoendoscopy system improve the colonoscopic polyp detection rate?–a pilot study. Am J Gastroenterol 2008;103(8):1926.
22. McCallum AL, Jenkins JT, Gillen D, et al. Evaluation of autofluorescence colonoscopy for the detection

and diagnosis of colonic polyps. Gastrointest Endosc 2008;68(2):283.

23. Becker V, Vieth M, Bajbouj M, et al. Confocal laser scanning fluorescence microscopy for in vivo determination of microvessel density in Barrett's esophagus. Endoscopy 2008;40(11):888.

24. van den Broek FJ, Fockens P, van Eeden S, et al. Endoscopic tri-modal imaging for surveillance in ulcerative colitis: randomised comparison of high-resolution endoscopy and autofluorescence imaging for neoplasia detection; and evaluation of narrow-band imaging for classification of lesions. Gut 2008;57(8):1083.

25. Muguruma N, Ito S. Labeled anti-mucin antibody detectable by infrared-fluorescence endoscopy. Cancer Biomark 2008;4(6):321.

26. Pierce MC, Javier DJ, Richards-Kortum R. Optical contrast agents and imaging systems for detection and diagnosis of cancer. Int J Cancer 2008;123(9):1979.

27. Kara MA, DaCosta RS, Streutker CJ, et al. Characterization of tissue autofluorescence in Barrett's esophagus by confocal fluorescence microscopy. Dis Esophagus 2007;20(2):141.

28. Fujimoto JG, Brezinski ME, Tearney GJ, et al. Optical biopsy and imaging using optical coherence tomography. Nat Med 1995;1(9):970.

29. Chen Y, Aguirre AD, Hsiung PL, et al. Ultrahigh resolution optical coherence tomography of Barrett's esophagus: preliminary descriptive clinical study correlating images with histology. Endoscopy 2007;39(7):599.

30. Evans JA, Nishioka NS. The use of optical coherence tomography in screening and surveillance of Barrett's esophagus. Clin Gastroenterol Hepatol 2005;3(7 Suppl 1):S8.

31. Li XD, Boppart SA, Van Dam J, et al. Optical coherence tomography: advanced technology for the endoscopic imaging of Barrett's esophagus. Endoscopy 2000;32(12):921.

32. Adler DC, Zhou C, Tsai TH, et al. Three-dimensional endomicroscopy of the human colon using optical coherence tomography. Opt Express 2009;17(2):784.

33. Suter MJ, Vakoc BJ, Yachimski PS, et al. Comprehensive microscopy of the esophagus in human patients with optical frequency domain imaging. Gastrointest Endosc 2008;68(4):745.

34. Wilson BC. Detection and treatment of dysplasia in Barrett's esophagus: a pivotal challenge in translating biophotonics from bench to bedside. J Biomed Opt 2007;12(5):051401.

35. Georgakoudi I, Feld MS. The combined use of fluorescence, reflectance, and light-scattering spectroscopy for evaluating dysplasia in Barrett's esophagus. Gastrointest Endosc Clin N Am 2004;14(3):519.

36. Wong Kee Song M, Molckovsky A, Wang KK, et al. Diagnostic potential of Raman spectroscopy in Barrett's esophagus. In Proceedings of SPIE, Bellingham (WA), 2005. p. 140.

37. Badizadegan K, Backman V, Boone CW, et al. Spectroscopic diagnosis and imaging of invisible pre-cancer. Faraday Discuss 2004;126:265.

38. Gurjar RS, Backman V, Perelman LT, et al. Imaging human epithelial properties with polarized light-scattering spectroscopy. Nat Med 2001;7(11):1245.

39. Yu CC, Lau C, O'Donoghue G, et al. Quantitative spectroscopic imaging for non-invasive early cancer detection. Opt Express 2008;16(20):16227.

40. Roy HK, Gomes A, Turzhitsky V, et al. Spectroscopic microvascular blood detection from the endoscopically normal colonic mucosa: biomarker for neoplasia risk. Gastroenterology 2008;135(4):1069.

41. Roy HK, Turzhitsky V, Kim YL, et al. Spectral slope from the endoscopically-normal mucosa predicts concurrent colonic neoplasia: a pilot ex-vivo clinical study. Dis Colon Rectum 2008;51(9):1381.

42. May A, Gossner L, Behrens A, et al. A prospective randomized trial of two different endoscopic resection techniques for early stage cancer of the esophagus. Gastrointest Endosc 2003;58(2):167.

43. Nijhawan PK, Wang KK. Endoscopic mucosal resection for lesions with endoscopic features suggestive of malignancy and high-grade dysplasia within Barrett's esophagus. Gastrointest Endosc 2000;52(3):328.

44. Ell C, May A, Gossner L, et al. Endoscopic mucosal resection of early cancer and high-grade dysplasia in Barrett's esophagus. Gastroenterology 2000;118(4):670.

45. Kantsevoy SV, Adler DG, Conway JD, et al. Endoscopic mucosal resection and endoscopic submucosal dissection. Gastrointest Endosc 2008;68(1):11.

46. Ell C, May A, Pech O, et al. Curative endoscopic resection of early esophageal adenocarcinomas (Barrett's cancer). Gastrointest Endosc 2007;65(1):3.

47. Ishihara R, Iishi H, Takeuchi Y, et al. Local recurrence of large squamous-cell carcinoma of the esophagus after endoscopic resection. Gastrointest Endosc 2008;67(6):799.

48. Ishihara R, Iishi H, Uedo N, et al. Comparison of EMR and endoscopic submucosal dissection for en bloc resection of early esophageal cancers in Japan. Gastrointest Endosc 2008;68(6):1066.

49. Katada C, Muto M, Momma K, et al. Clinical outcome after endoscopic mucosal resection for esophageal squamous cell carcinoma invading the muscularis mucosae–a multicenter retrospective cohort study. Endoscopy 2007;39(9):779.

50. Ahmad NA, Kochman ML, Long WB, et al. Efficacy, safety, and clinical outcomes of endoscopic mucosal resection: a study of 101 cases. Gastrointest Endosc 2002;55(3):390.

51. Takeo Y, Yoshida T, Shigemitu T, et al. Endoscopic mucosal resection for early esophageal cancer and esophageal dysplasia. Hepatogastroenterology 2001;48(38):453.

52. Ciocirlan M, Lapalus MG, Hervieu V, et al. Endoscopic mucosal resection for squamous premalignant and early malignant lesions of the esophagus. Endoscopy 2007;39(1):24.

53. Oyama T, Tomori A, Hotta K, et al. Endoscopic submucosal dissection of early esophageal cancer. Clin Gastroenterol Hepatol 2005;3(7 Suppl 1): S67.

54. Nomura T, Boku N, Ohtsu A, et al. Recurrence after endoscopic mucosal resection for superficial esophageal cancer. Endoscopy 2000;32(4):277.

55. Esaki M, Matsumoto T, Hirakawa K, et al. Risk factors for local recurrence of superficial esophageal cancer after treatment by endoscopic mucosal resection. Endoscopy 2007;39(1):41.

56. Shimizu Y, Kato M, Yamamoto J, et al. Histologic results of EMR for esophageal lesions diagnosed as high-grade intraepithelial squamous neoplasia by endoscopic biopsy. Gastrointest Endosc 2006; 63(1):16.

57. Higuchi K, Tanabe S, Koizumi W, et al. Expansion of the indications for endoscopic mucosal resection in patients with superficial esophageal carcinoma. Endoscopy 2007;39(1):36.

58. Shimizu Y, Tsukagoshi H, Fujita M, et al. Long-term outcome after endoscopic mucosal resection in patients with esophageal squamous cell carcinoma invading the muscularis mucosae or deeper. Gastrointest Endosc 2002;56(3):387.

59. Prasad GA, Buttar NS, Wongkeesong LM, et al. Significance of neoplastic involvement of margins obtained by endoscopic mucosal resection in Barrett's esophagus. Am J Gastroenterol 2007; 102(11):2380.

60. Vieth M, Ell C, Gossner L, et al. Histological analysis of endoscopic resection specimens from 326 patients with Barrett's esophagus and early neoplasia. Endoscopy 2004;36(9):776.

61. Mino-Kenudson M, Brugge WR, Puricelli WP, et al. Management of superficial Barrett's epithelium-related neoplasms by endoscopic mucosal resection: clinicopathologic analysis of 27 cases. Am J Surg Pathol 2005;29(5):680.

62. Battaglia G, Rampado S, Bocus P, et al. Single-band mucosectomy for granular cell tumor of the esophagus: safe and easy technique. Surg Endosc 2006;20(8):1296.

63. Park YS, Park SW, Kim TI, et al. Endoscopic enucleation of upper-GI submucosal tumors by using an insulated-tip electrosurgical knife. Gastrointest Endosc 2004;59(3):409.

64. Rosch T, Sarbia M, Schumacher B, et al. Attempted endoscopic en bloc resection of mucosal and submucosal tumors using insulated-tip knives: a pilot series. Endoscopy 2004;36(9):788.

65. Lauwers GY, Ban S, Mino M, et al. Endoscopic mucosal resection for gastric epithelial neoplasms: a study of 39 cases with emphasis on the evaluation of specimens and recommendations for optimal pathologic analysis. Mod Pathol 2004; 17(1):2.

66. Hull MJ, Mino-Kenudson M, Nishioka NS, et al. Endoscopic mucosal resection: an improved diagnostic procedure for early gastroesophageal epithelial neoplasms. Am J Surg Pathol 2006; 30(1):114.

67. Leung KK, Maru D, Abraham S, et al. Confocal endomicroscopy-targeted EMR of focal high-grade dysplasia in Barrett's esophagus. Gastrointest Endosc 2009;69(1):170.

68. Westerterp M, Koppert LB, Buskens CJ, et al. Outcome of surgical treatment for early adenocarcinoma of the esophagus or gastro-esophageal junction. Virchows Arch 2005;446(5):497.

69. Stein HJ, Feith M, Bruecher BL, et al. Early esophageal cancer: pattern of lymphatic spread and prognostic factors for long-term survival after surgical resection. Ann Surg 2005;242(4):566.

70. Oh DS, Hagen JA, Chandrasoma PT, et al. Clinical biology and surgical therapy of intramucosal adenocarcinoma of the esophagus. J Am Coll Surg 2006;203(2):152.

71. Liu L, Hofstetter WL, Rashid A, et al. Significance of the depth of tumor invasion and lymph node metastasis in superficially invasive (T1) esophageal adenocarcinoma. Am J Surg Pathol 2005;29(8):1079.

72. Scotiniotis IA, Kochman ML, Lewis JD, et al. Accuracy of EUS in the evaluation of Barrett's esophagus and high-grade dysplasia or intramucosal carcinoma. Gastrointest Endosc 2001; 54(6):689.

73. Mandal RV, Forcione DG, Brugge WR, et al. Effect of tumor characteristics and duplication of the muscularis mucosae on the endoscopic staging of superficial Barrett esophagus-related neoplasia. Am J Surg Pathol 2009;33(4):620.

74. Noda M, Kodama T, Atsumi M, et al. Possibilities and limitations of endoscopic resection for early gastric cancer. Endoscopy 1997;29(5):361.

75. Ono H, Kondo H, Gotoda T, et al. Endoscopic mucosal resection for treatment of early gastric cancer. Gut 2001;48(2):225.

76. Chen PJ, Chu HC, Chang WK, et al. Endoscopic submucosal dissection with internal traction for early gastric cancer (with video). Gastrointest Endosc 2008;67(1):128.

77. Tanaka M, Ono H, Hasuike N, et al. Endoscopic submucosal dissection of early gastric cancer. Digestion 2008;77(Suppl 1):23.

78. Kume K, Yamasaki M, Tashiro M, et al. Endoscopic mucosal resection for early gastric cancer: comparison of two modifications of the cap method. Endoscopy 2008;40(4):280.

79. Kim JJ, Lee JH, Jung HY, et al. EMR for early gastric cancer in Korea: a multicenter retrospective study. Gastrointest Endosc 2007;66(4):693.

80. Lee IL, Wu CS, Tung SY, et al. Endoscopic submucosal dissection for early gastric cancers: experience from a new endoscopic center in Taiwan. J Clin Gastroenterol 2008;42(1):42.

81. Szaloki T, Toth V, Nemeth I, et al. Endoscopic mucosal resection: not only therapeutic, but a diagnostic procedure for sessile gastric polyps. J Gastroenterol Hepatol 2008;23(4):551.

82. Lee SY, Jang KT, Lee KT, et al. Can endoscopic resection be applied for early stage ampulla of Vater cancer? Gastrointest Endosc 2006;63(6):783.

83. Yoon SM, Kim MH, Kim MJ, et al. Focal early stage cancer in ampullary adenoma: surgery or endoscopic papillectomy? Gastrointest Endosc 2007; 66(4):701.

84. Boix J, Lorenzo-Zuniga V, Moreno de Vega V, et al. Endoscopic resection of ampullary tumors: 12-year review of 21 cases. Surg Endosc 2009; 23(1):45.

85. Hernandez LV, Catalano MF. Endoscopic papillectomy. Curr Opin Gastroenterol 2008;24(5):617.

86. Catalano MF, Linder JD, Chak A, et al. Endoscopic management of adenoma of the major duodenal papilla. Gastrointest Endosc 2004;59(2):225.

87. Mahadeva S, Rembacken BJ. Standard "inject and cut" endoscopic mucosal resection technique is practical and effective in the management of superficial colorectal neoplasms. Surg Endosc 2009;23(2):417.

88. Yokota T, Sugihara K, Yoshida S. Endoscopic mucosal resection for colorectal neoplastic lesions. Dis Colon Rectum 1994;37(11):1108.

89. Tanaka S, Oka S, Chayama K. Colorectal endoscopic submucosal dissection: present status and future perspective, including its differentiation from endoscopic mucosal resection. J Gastroenterol 2008;43(9):641.

90. Katsinelos P, Kountouras J, Paroutoglou G, et al. Endoscopic mucosal resection of large sessile colorectal polyps with submucosal injection of hypertonic 50 percent dextrose-epinephrine solution. Dis Colon Rectum 2006;49(9):1384.

91. Fujishiro M, Yahagi N, Kakushima N, et al. Outcomes of endoscopic submucosal dissection for colorectal epithelial neoplasms in 200 consecutive cases. Clin Gastroenterol Hepatol 2007; 5(6):678.

92. Tamegai Y, Saito Y, Masaki N, et al. Endoscopic submucosal dissection: a safe technique for colorectal tumors. Endoscopy 2007;39(5):418.

93. Saito Y, Uraoka T, Matsuda T, et al. Endoscopic treatment of large superficial colorectal tumors: a case series of 200 endoscopic submucosal dissections (with video). Gastrointest Endosc 2007;66(5):966.

94. Pass HI. Photodynamic therapy in oncology: mechanisms and clinical use. J Natl Cancer Inst 1993; 85(6):443.

95. Pech O, Gossner L, May A, et al. Long-term results of photodynamic therapy with 5-aminolevulinic acid for superficial Barrett's cancer and high-grade intraepithelial neoplasia. Gastrointest Endosc 2005; 62(1):24.

96. Overholt BF, Lightdale CJ, Wang KK, et al. Photodynamic therapy with porfimer sodium for ablation of high-grade dysplasia in Barrett's esophagus: international, partially blinded, randomized phase III trial. Gastrointest Endosc 2005;62(4):488.

97. Gossner L, Stolte M, Sroka R, et al. Photodynamic ablation of high-grade dysplasia and early cancer in Barrett's esophagus by means of 5-aminolevulinic acid. Gastroenterology 1998;114(3):448.

98. Ban S, Mino M, Nishioka NS, et al. Histopathologic aspects of photodynamic therapy for dysplasia and early adenocarcinoma arising in Barrett's esophagus. Am J Surg Pathol 2004;28(11):1466.

99. Mino-Kenudson M, Ban S, Ohana M, et al. Buried dysplasia and early adenocarcinoma arising in Barrett esophagus after porfimer-photodynamic therapy. Am J Surg Pathol 2007;31(3):403.

100. Hornick JL, Mino-Kenudson M, Lauwers GY, et al. Buried Barrett's epithelium following photodynamic therapy shows reduced crypt proliferation and absence of DNA content abnormalities. Am J Gastroenterol 2008;103(1):38.

101. Yachimski P, Puricelli WP, Nishioka NS. Patient predictors of esophageal stricture development after photodynamic therapy. Clin Gastroenterol Hepatol 2008;6(3):302.

102. Van Laethem JL, Peny MO, Salmon I, et al. Intramucosal adenocarcinoma arising under squamous re-epithelialisation of Barrett's oesophagus. Gut 2000; 46(4):574.

103. Overholt BF, Panjehpour M, Halberg DL. Photodynamic therapy for Barrett's esophagus with dysplasia and/or early stage carcinoma: long-term results. Gastrointest Endosc 2003;58(2):183.

104. Bronner MP, Overholt BF, Taylor SL, et al. Squamous overgrowth is not a safety concern for photodynamic therapy for Barrett's esophagus with high-grade dysplasia. Gastroenterology 2009;136(1):56.

105. Sharma VK, Wang KK, Overholt BF, et al. Balloon-based, circumferential, endoscopic radiofrequency ablation of Barrett's esophagus: 1-year

follow-up of 100 patients. Gastrointest Endosc 2007;65(2):185.

106. Pouw RE, Sharma VK, Bergman JJ, et al. Radiofrequency ablation for total Barrett's eradication: a description of the endoscopic technique, its clinical results and future prospects. Endoscopy 2008; 40(12):1033.

107. Ganz RA, Overholt BF, Sharma VK, et al. Circumferential ablation of Barrett's esophagus that contains high-grade dysplasia: a U.S. Multicenter Registry. Gastrointest Endosc 2008;68(1):35.

108. Cash BD, Johnston LR, Johnston MH. Cryospray ablation (CSA) in the palliative treatment of squamous cell carcinoma of the esophagus. World J Surg Oncol 2007;5:34.

109. Raju GS, Ahmed I, Xiao SY, et al. Graded esophageal mucosal ablation with cryotherapy, and the protective effects of submucosal saline. Endoscopy 2005;37(6):523.

110. Wells WA, Barker PE, MacAulay C, et al. Validation of novel optical imaging technologies: the pathologists' view. J Biomed Opt 2007;12(5):051801.

MOLECULAR TESTING IN COLORECTAL CARCINOMA

Reetesh K. Pai, MD[a], Rish K. Pai, MD, PhD[b],*

KEYWORDS
- Colorectal carcinoma • Molecular testing • Lynch syndrome • KRAS

ABSTRACT

An estimated 150,000 individuals are diagnosed with colorectal carcinoma (CRC) each year, and approximately 50,000 will die from this disease, making CRC the third leading cause of cancer deaths in the United States. For this reason, an enormous amount of effort has been spent to understand the molecular pathogenesis of this disease and to develop screening tests and prognostic markers. In the last 10 years, there has been a revolution in the understanding of CRC due to the identification of multiple distinct molecular pathways. With the introduction of biologic agents that target particular subtypes of CRC, molecular analysis of CRC is becoming standard of care in surgical pathology. In this context, the authors first describe the multiple molecular pathways leading to CRC and then discuss the role of molecular testing in the diagnosis of Lynch syndrome (formerly hereditary nonpolyposis colorectal carcinoma), prognosis, and therapy.

OVERVIEW

Classically, colorectal carcinoma (CRC) has been divided into cancers that exhibit chromosomal instability (CIN) and those that exhibit microsatellite instability (MSI). More recently, CRCs that exhibit high levels of promoter methylation of CpG islands have been identified. Classifying CRC based on these three molecular features is useful in terms of prognosis and therapy (**Table 1**).

CIN PATHWAY

Chromosomal instability tumors are defined by the presence of alterations in chromosome number, chromosomal rearrangements, or gene amplifications. CIN accounts for between 50% and 80% of CRCs.[1–4] The reason for this substantial variation in incidence is due to the tremendous diversity within CIN tumors that makes screening for genomic instability difficult. Furthermore, diagnostic criteria to identify CIN tumors have not been developed.

The understanding of the CIN pathway is in large part due to analysis of patients with familial adenomatous polyposis (FAP). FAP patients have germline mutations in the tumor suppressor gene adenomatous polyposis coli (APC) and develop tumors with extensive genomic instability.[5] APC also is commonly mutated in sporadic CIN tumors and occurs early in tumor development. APC is involved in various cellular functions including cell adhesion, migration, chromosome segregation, and signal transduction.[6–9] Inactivation of APC, by itself, may result in CIN,[6] but most likely creates a permissive environment for CIN to develop.[2] Numerous other genes have been implicated in CIN including genes that encode mitotic checkpoint proteins (BUB1 and BUB1b),[10] cell cycle regulatory genes (TP53 and Aurora kinase A),[11] and genes involved in regulating repair of damaged DNA.[2]

[a] Department of Pathology, Stanford University Medical Center, Stanford University School of Medicine, 300 Pasteur Drive, L235 MC 5324, Stanford, CA 94305, USA
[b] Division of Anatomic and Molecular Pathology, Department of Pathology and Immunology, Washington University School of Medicine, 660 South Euclid Avenue, Box 8118, St Louis, MO 63110, USA
* Corresponding author.
E-mail address: rishkpai@gmail.com

Surgical Pathology 3 (2010) 429–445
doi:10.1016/j.path.2010.05.005

Table 1
Classification of CRC based on MSI, CIMP, KRAS, and BRAF

Feature	Group 1	Group 2[a]	Group 3	Group 4	Group 5
CIMP	High	Negative	High	Low	Negative
MSI	High	High	Stable	Stable/low	Stable/low
RAS/RAF mutation	BRAF	Wild-type	Variable BRAF	KRAS	Variable BRAF and KRAS
Precursor lesion	SSA	TA	SSA	Unclear	TA
Ploidy	Dip >> An	Dip >> An	Dip >> An	Dip > An	An >> Dip
Location	Right >> left	Right >> left	Right >> left	Left >> right	Left >> right
Histology	Poor differentiation, mucinous, serration, circumscribed, tumor-infiltrating lymphocytes	Poor differentiation, mucinous, serration, circumscribed, tumor-infiltrating lymphocytes	Not well defined but likely poor differentiation and mucinous	Not well defined	Dirty necrosis, tumor budding
Gender	F > M	M = F	F > M	M > F	M = F
Incidence	10%	3%–5%	5%–15%	30%–35%	Approximately 40%
Response to 5-FU	Poor	Poor	Variable	Variable	Variable
Response to anti-EGFR therapy	Poor	Unclear	Variable	Poor	Variable
Clinical outcome	Improved prognosis	Improved prognosis	Improved prognosis	Unclear, likely worse prognosis	Variable, mostly worse prognosis

Abbreviations: An, aneuploid; CIMP, CpG island methylator phenotype; CRC, colorectal carcinoma; Dip, diploid; MSI, microsatellite instability; SSA, sessile serrated polyp; TA, tubular adenoma.

[a] Group 2 is comprised of Lynch syndrome patients.

MSI PATHWAY

In the MSI pathway, the primary alteration is the loss of mismatch repair (MMR) gene function. MMR genes include MLH1, MSH2, MSH6, and PMS2. Loss of MMR function can occur through germline mutations as seen in patients with Lynch syndrome (HNPCC) or though somatic inactivation. As MMR proteins repair DNA mismatches made during replication, loss of function results in a high rate of replicative error. In particular, short one to six DNA nucleotide repeats or microsatellites are highly prone to mismatches during replication. Without intact DNA MMR machinery microsatellites become unstable resulting in high levels of MSI (MSI-H). Although microsatellites are found commonly within noncoding regions of the genome, some genes have them within exons. If a mismatch occurs in the setting of defective MMR activity, the resulting mutation can lead to alteration in protein function. Genes that are commonly mutated in MSI-H tumors include TGFBR2, BAX, ACVR2, and E2F4.[2] Tumors that exhibit low levels of MSI (MSI-L) also have been identified, but it remains unclear if these tumors represent a distinct subgroup of CRC.

CPG ISLAND METHYLATOR PHENOTYPE

More recently it has become clear that simply dividing CRC into CIN or MSI-H does not accurately reflect the molecular diversity in these tumors. In particular, the role of epigenetic alterations through methylation of CpG islands and the contribution of mutations in the RAS/RAF/MAP kinase pathway have not been emphasized. The RAS/RAF/MAP kinase pathway is an intracellular signaling pathway downstream of various cell surface receptors, including the epidermal growth factor receptor (EGF-R).[12] Subdividing tumors based on CpG island methylation, mutations in the RAS/RAF/MAP kinase pathway, and MSI may prove the most useful to the clinicians in terms of prognosis and potentially treatment (see **Table 1**).[3,4]

CpG islands are regions of the genome present in promoters of numerous genes. When these islands are methylated, gene transcription is silenced. In 15% of sporadic CRCs, there is extensive methylation of CpG islands in the promoters of various genes.[3,4,13–15] For this reason, these tumors have been called CIMP-H tumors (CpG island methylator phenotype-high). Although consensus criteria to classify CIMP-H tumors have not been established, recent publications have identified a list of five genes that are commonly methylated in these tumors: RUNX3,

NEUROG1, SOCS1, IGF2, and CACNA1G.[16–18] Approximately 60% to 80% of CIMP-H tumors also harbor mutations in BRAF, a serine threonine kinase in the RAS/RAF/MAPK pathway.[14,15,19–21] These particular CRCs are also often characterized by MSI-H due to the presence of a CpG island in the promoter region of the MMR gene, MLH1.[1,15,20] Up to 30% of CIMP-H tumors, however, are microsatellite stable (MSS).

Before the identification of a panel of methylated genes highly specific for CIMP, there were some conflicting reports regarding the association of CIMP and KRAS mutations.[14,22,23] Subsequent analysis revealed that some CRCs have low levels of CpG island methylation (CIMP-L) often characterized by a random methylation pattern of CIMP markers.[17,22,24–26] CIMP-L tumors now are recognized as a distinct subset of CRCs that are not associated with BRAF mutations, but rather with mutations in KRAS, a serine threonine kinase upstream of BRAF.[3,22,25] CIMP-L tumors are not associated with MSI-H.

CLINICOPATHOLOGIC FEATURES OF CRC AND PROGNOSIS

The earliest precursor of CIN tumors is the dysplastic aberrant crypt focus (ACF). Dysplastic ACFs often have mutations in APC and progress to conventional tubular adenomas. As more mutations and DNA abnormalities accumulate, tubular adenomas progress to an advanced adenoma characterized by large size (>1 cm) and high-grade dysplasia. Advanced adenomas have a high risk of progressing to frank invasive carcinoma. The presence of an advanced adenoma is also a strong predictor of subsequent adenomas.[27] Invasive CIN carcinomas are more likely to be left sided, contain dirty necrosis, and have foci of tumor budding.

MSI-H CRCs occurring in HNPCC also progress through conventional adenomas. On the other hand, sporadic MSI-H/CIMP-H tumors arise through a newly described precursor lesion, sessile serrated adenoma (SSA).[28,29] SSAs have a serrated architecture similar to a hyperplastic polyp, but have dilated crypts at the base that tend to expand laterally along the muscularis mucosae, have increased mitotic activity, have serrations throughout the crypt, and exhibit subtle cytologic atypia (dysmaturation) (**Fig. 1**). SSAs can become overtly dysplastic (SSAs with dysplasia) and progress to invasive carcinoma. Like the tumors they give rise to, SSAs demonstrate extensive CpG island methylation and often harbor mutations in BRAF.[1,30–32]

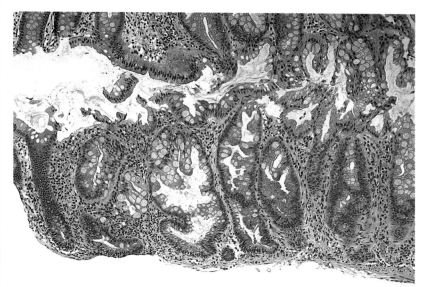

Fig. 1. This serrated polyp was located in the right colon and measured 1.5 cm. Unlike a hyperplastic polyp, the serrations extend to the base of the crypts. In addition, some of the crypts are dilated at the base and extend laterally along the muscularis mucosae. Although there is mild cytologic atypia, nuclear changes seen in conventional tubular adenomas are not present.

MSI-H CRCs, whether associated with CIMP-H or with HNPCC, have similar histologic features. These tumors tend to be located in the proximal colon and are often exophytic and well circumscribed with pushing borders. Histologically they are characterized by poor differentiation, mucin production, tumor-infiltrating lymphocytes, and peritumoral lymphoid aggregates. Sporadic CIMP-H tumors are also more common in elderly women and smokers.[3,33,34] The precursor lesion of CIMP-L tumors is not well defined but may arise from traditional serrated adenomas and tubular adenomas with some features of traditional serrated adenoma.[35] In contrast with CIMP-H tumors, CIMP-L tumors are associated with the male sex.[25]

Numerous studies have shown that sporadic or syndromic MSI-H tumors are associated with a relatively good prognosis compared with MSS/CIN tumors.[20,36–39] There are some conflicting data regarding the prognosis of CIMP-H tumors that are MSS[40]; however, the most recent and comprehensive analysis indicates an improved prognosis.[20] The relationship between BRAF mutations and prognosis is less clear. BRAF mutated tumors that are also CIMP-H do have an improved prognosis; however, the small percentage of tumors that have BRAF mutations in the absence of CIMP-H or MSI-H may have a worse prognosis.[20] The prognosis of CIMP-L tumors has not been well defined.

MOLECULAR TESTING IN HNPCC

In the mid-1960s, Henry Lynch described a family from Nebraska with an unusually high prevalence of early CRC characterized by an absence of polyposis and raised the possibility of a new form of hereditary CRC.[41] Currently, HNPCC is the most commonly diagnosed form of hereditary CRC, accounting for 3% to 5% of all CRCs. In the early 1990s, germline mutations giving rise to HNPCC were identified in MLH1 and MSH2, genes

Key Features
In Molecular Testing in HNPCC

- HNPCC is an autosomal dominant hereditary syndrome that predisposes to colorectal carcinoma among others.

- Patients fulfilling Bethesda criteria should be tested for HNPCC.

- Practically, pathologists should perform reflex testing on all patients with CRC under the age of 50 and those under the age of 60 with CRC that has histologic features (eg, mucinous, poorly differentiated, tumor infiltrating lymphocytes) compatible with HNPCC.

- MSI testing and immunohistochemical testing for MMR proteins are both excellent first-line screening tests for HNPCC.

- A definitive diagnosis of HNPCC requires germline mutational analysis. Immunohistochemical analysis of MMR proteins can be helpful in determining which gene to target for sequencing.

involved in DNA MMR.[42–45] Mutations in four DNA MMR genes are thought to occur in HNPCC patients: MLH1 (40% to 45% of cases), MSH2 (40% to 45%), MSH6 (5% to 10%), and PMS2 (1%).[46–48] Currently, in about 5% of cases, a germline mutation in a known DNA MMR gene cannot be identified.[41] Affected persons with HNPCC carry one mutated copy of the gene in all of their tissues, and the second normal allele is either lost or undergoes somatic mutation, leading to profound impairment of MMR function. Over many cell divisions, mutations accumulate and tumors form, predominately in the colon but also in the upper gastrointestinal tract, pancreas, biliary tract, endometrium, ovaries, and upper urinary tract. The onset of these tumors is usually between age 40 and 60 years.

PATHOLOGIC FEATURES

As mentioned above, both HNPCC CRCs and sporadic MSI-H CRCs have similar histologic features; thus histologic distinction between sporadic and HNPCC tumors is not possible.[49,50] However, sporadic CRCs with MMR protein abnormalities commonly develop within serrated lesions, are solitary, and are even more likely to demonstrate mucinous histology.[49,51] Although age and positive family history can be useful in distinguishing between these two entities, the age of presentation in HNPCC overlaps considerably with sporadic CRCs.

The role of the pathologist in the diagnosis of HNPCC is to help determine which patients should be screened for and undergo analysis for mutations in DNA MMR genes. The revised Bethesda criteria provide a sensitive tool to determine which patients should undergo testing (**Table 2**).[52] Once clinical/pathologic suspicion of HNPCC exists (ie, fulfills the Bethesda criteria), tumor samples should be screened by MSI testing, MMR protein immunohistochemistry, or both. No specific guidelines for testing have been proposed, and some institutions screen all colon cancers for MSI. A proposed guideline for HNPCC screening is shown in **Fig. 2**.

MOLECULAR FINDINGS

Detection of the causative germline mutation in a MMR gene is the ultimate diagnostic criterion for HNPCC. However, screening for a germline mutation is both costly and time-consuming and will not detect the small number (approximately 5%) of cases in which a germline mutation in a known DNA MMR gene cannot be identified.[41] Surrogate tests have been developed to analyze

Table 2
Revised Bethesda criteria for HNPCC screening
Revised Bethesda: One of the Following Criteria Need to be Met:
Diagnosed with colorectal carcinoma (CRC) before the age of 50 years
Synchronous or metachronous CRC or other Lynch syndrome (HNPCC)-related tumors (stomach, bladder, ureter, renal pelvis, biliary tract, brain (glioblastoma), sebeceous gland adenomas, keratoacanthomas, and small bowel carcinoma, regardless of age.
CRC with a high-microsatellite instability morphology (tumor infiltrating lymphocytes, Crohn-like reaction, mucinous/signet ring differentation, or medullary growth pattern) that was diagnosed before the age of 60 years
CRC with one or more first-degree relative with CRC or other HNPCC-related tumors with one of the cancers being diagnosed under age 50 years (or adenoma under age 40 years)
CRC with two or more relatives with CRC or other HNPCC-related tumors, regardless of age

for defects in DNA MMR based on MSI and to detect the absence of MMR protein expression by immunohistochemistry.

MSI TESTING

In 1997, the National Cancer Institute recommended use of a panel of five microsatellites, referred to as the Bethesda panel, which included two mononucleotide repeats (BAT-25 and BAT-26) and three dinucleotide repeats (D2S-123, D5S-346, and D17S250) to detect MSI by polymerase chain reaction (PCR).

Over the last decade, many investigators have found mononucleotide markers to be more sensitive and more specific than dinucleotide markers for the detection of MSI. The revised Bethesda guidelines suggest testing a secondary panel of mononucleotide markers to exclude MSI-L in cases in which only dinucleotide repeats are mutated.[52] Many laboratories are now only performing MSI testing with a panel of five mononucleotide markers (BAT-25, BAT-26, NR-21, MONO-27, and BAT-40) and two pentanucleotide repeats (Penta C and Penta D) incorporated into a multiplex fluorescence assay—the Promega MSI Analysis System (Promega, Madison, WI, USA) (**Fig. 3**).[53] The five mononucleotide repeats are quasi-monomorphic, with almost all individuals being homozygous for the same common allele for a given marker. The pentanucleotide

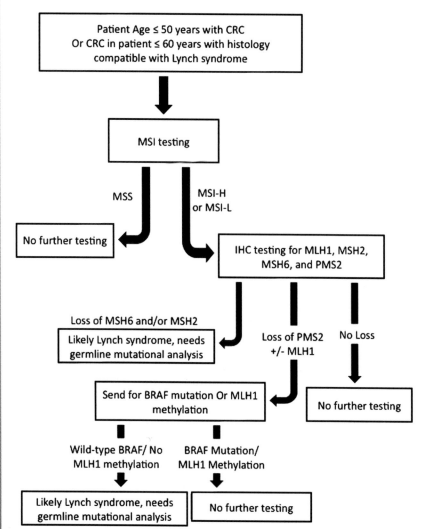

Fig. 2. A proposed reflex testing protocol to identify Lynch syndrome patients.

repeat markers are selected for their high level of polymorphism and low degree of MSI and serve as an internal control to ensure that the tumor and matching normal specimens are from the same patient. This multiplex PCR approach for MSI screening is performed in a single reaction, thus significantly reducing cost. Testing typically is performed on colonic tumors from patients with suspected HNPCC, although extracolonic sites, particularly the gynecologic tract[54] and skin sebaceous neoplasms,[55] increasingly are being tested for MSI. Formalin-fixed paraffin-embedded tissue is an adequate source of DNA. Typically DNA is extracted from the tumor and compared with the extracted DNA from surrounding uninvolved tissue. Testing usually is not performed on adenomas because of the low likelihood of MSI even in HNPCC patients.

If none of the microsatellites show evidence of a mutation, then the tumor is termed MSS.

MSI-H tumors are defined as those demonstrating two or more (more than 40%) unstable microsatellites. A poorly defined category of MSI-L tumors with only one (<20%) unstable microsatellite also has been proposed. HNPCC patients with a germline mutation in MSH6 often exhibit MSI-L,[56,57] and these patients typically have a selective instability for mononucleotide repeats. Recent clinical data suggest that most MSI-L tumors behave similarly to MSS tumors,[20] although more studies are necessary to further define the clinical behavior of MSI-L CRCs.

MMR PROTEIN IMMUNOHISTOCHEMISTRY

Immunohistochemical staining for MMR proteins is complementary to the MSI PCR studies. Early reports initially suggested that MMR protein immunohistochemistry was inferior to MSI as a screening tool for HNPCC. These early studies,

Fig. 3. Microsatellite instability analysis by multiplex polymerase chain reaction (PCR). The two panels illustrate the size of the PCR products from a multiplex reaction that amplifies the five mononucleotide repeats (BAT-

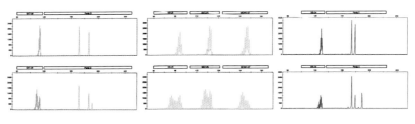

25, BAT-26, NR-21, MONO-27, and BAT-40) and two pentanucleotide repeats (Penta C and Penta D). The top panel shows the size of the PCR fragments amplified from nontumoral DNA, and the bottom panel shows the PCR products amplified from tumoral DNA. There is substantial variation in the size of the PCR products for all five microsatellites between the two DNA samples indicative of high levels of MSI.

however, primarily assessed MLH1 and MSH2 immunohistochemistry without using antibodies directed against MSH6 and PMS2. More recent literature suggests that the use of all four antibodies (MLH1, MSH2, MSH6, and PMS2) is as sensitive in predicting germline MMR protein mutations as MSI testing.[58–60] Moreover, a recent study proposes that immunohistochemistry for MSH6 and PMS2 as a two-antibody panel may be as sensitive as the four-antibody panel in identifying potential MSI-H cases.[61] Loss of MMR protein expression by immunohistochemistry is defined as complete absence of nuclear staining within all tumor cells in a given tissue section in the face of concurrent positive nuclear labeling in internal non-neoplastic tissues (**Fig. 4**). Cytoplasmic staining has no known significance.

Knowledge of the basic biology of MMR proteins helps to better understand the immunohistochemical staining patterns often observed in MMR-deficient CRCs. In their functional state within a cell, MLH1 dimerizes with PMS2, and MSH2 dimerizes with MSH6. MLH1 and MSH2 are the obligatory partners for their respective heterodimers. In general, germline mutations in the obligatory partners MLH1 and MSH2 most often will result in degradation of the heterodimer and the consequent proteolytic degradation of their respective secondary partners, PMS2 and MSH6. For example, germline mutations in MLH1 or MSH2 most often will result in concurrent loss of immunohistochemical expression of MLH1/PMS2 or MSH2/MSH6, respectively.[47] In contrast, germline mutations in the secondary partners MSH6 and PMS2 may not result in proteolytic degradation of its obligatory partner, as the function of the secondary protein may be compensated by other proteins. Thus, a germline mutation of PMS2 or MSH6 may result in isolated loss of immunohistochemical expression of these proteins. Importantly, immunohistochemistry with

MLH1 alone has a low sensitivity in detecting mutation in MLH1. This is primarily due to the fact that up to one third of MLH1 mutations are missense mutations resulting in functionally inactive but antigenically intact MLH1 mutant protein.[48,62] For such tumors, a false-normal staining pattern with MLH1 will be observed; however, immunohistochemical expression of its secondary partner PMS2 will be absent.

Limitations of MMR immunohistochemistry mostly relate to staining quality, which may render interpretation of the staining difficult.[47] Tissue preservation, including cautery artifact, and tissue hypoxia affect MMR protein expression and often give rise to regional staining within a tumor. Occasionally, both tumor and internal non-neoplastic control tissues will lack MMR protein expression. Such cases are best interpreted as equivocal and should be correlated with concurrent MSI PCR studies. Advantages of MMR protein immunohistochemistry include that it may help to distinguish between sporadic and HNPCC MSI-H CRCs, as loss of expression of mismatch repair genes other than MLH1 is highly suggestive of HNPCC. In addition, MMR protein immunohistochemistry is useful in directing germline mutation testing efforts in MSI-H samples.

GERMLINE MUTATION TESTING

If the initial screen with MSI and MMR protein immunohistochemistry is negative, no further testing should be performed; however, MSI-H tumor samples should be screened for germline mutations. MMR protein immunohistochemistry is extremely useful in helping to direct gene sequencing efforts in patients with MSI-H tumor samples.[46,60,63] The approximate success of finding a disease-causing mutation is only 50% to 70% in current clinical genetic testing laboratories.[60] Once a disease-causing mutation is found,

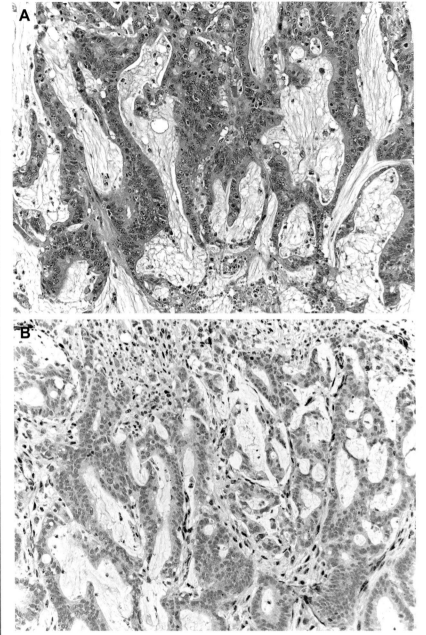

Fig. 4. Mucinous colorectal adenocarcinoma (*A*) in a young patient located in the cecum highly suspicious for Lynch syndrome. MLH1 (*B*) protein expression is lost in the tumor cells but retained in the supporting stroma and lymphocytes.

subsequent testing for family members can detect the mutation with close to 100% accuracy.

MOLECULAR TESTING IN SPORADIC COLORECTAL CANCER

The definitive treatment of CRC is surgical resection of the tumor and draining lymph nodes. Stage 1 tumors are cured by this approach. Some stage 2 and most stage 3 stage tumors, however, are treated with adjuvant chemotherapy with a regimen consisting of 5-FU/oxaliplatin/leucovorin (FOLFOX) or 5-FU/leucovorin/irinotecan (FOLFIRI) due to a high rate of disease progression if left untreated.[64] Nevertheless, approximately 30% to 40% of patients treated with this regimen will progress and develop distant metastatic disease. Molecular tests that can help predict those stage

Fig. 4. PMS2 (*C*) protein expression is lost in the tumor cells but retained in the supporting stroma and lymphocytes. Expression of MSH2 (*D*) is retained in the tumor. Further testing is needed to confirm Lynch syndrome (see **Fig. 2**).

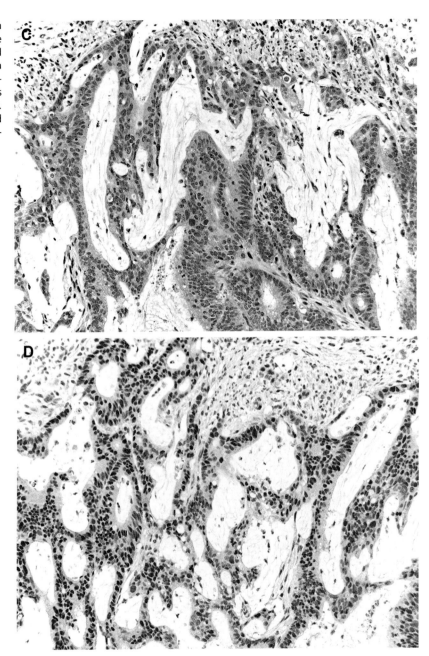

2/3 patients who will benefit from adjuvant chemotherapy and those who will progress despite chemotherapy would be invaluable.

In addition to these patients who progress on first-line therapy, 20% will present with metastatic disease. In the distant metastatic setting, oncologic options are limited. In 2004, cetuximab, an anti-EGF-R antibody, was approved for second-line therapy in metastatic CRC. In 2007, another anti-EGF-R antibody, panitumumab was approved.

Recent studies also have highlighted the role for these antibodies in addition to standard chemotherapy for first-line therapy in metastatic CRC.

EGF-R is a member of the erbB family of receptor tyrosine kinases that also include erbB2 (HER/2neu), erbB3 (HER3), and erbB4 (HER4).[12] The EGF-R is expressed in various epithelial tissues and promotes cell growth, differentiation, survival, cell cycle progression, and angiogenesis. The ligands for EGF-R

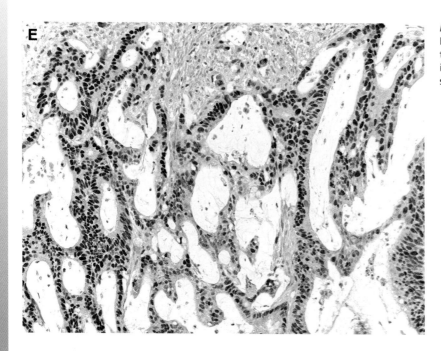

Fig. 4. Expression of MSH6 (*E*) is retained in the tumor. Further testing is needed to confirm Lynch syndrome (see **Fig. 2**).

Potential Pitfalls
IN IMMUNOHISTOCHEMICAL
ANALYSIS FOR HNPCC INCLUDE

- MMR protein expression is highly dependent on adequate tissue preservation. Cautery artifact, tissue hypoxia and poor fixation affect MMR protein expression and may give rise to regional staining within a tumor.

- True loss of MMR expression only results when nuclear protein expression is loss in all tumor cells on a given slide with concomitant staining in some stromal cell and lymphocytes.

- Occasionally expression will be absent in both tumor and supporting stroma. Repeat immunohistochemical staining should be performed, and the results should be correlated with MSI analysis.

- Expression of MLH1/PMS2 and MSH2/MSH6 are linked. A mutation in MLH1 commonly results in loss of both MLH1 and PMS2 expression. A mutation in MSH2 and MSH6 commonly results in loss of both MSH2 and MSH6 expression.

- Germline mutations in MSH6 and PMS2 result in isolated loss of these proteins. Some mutations in MLH1, however, result in retention of MLH1 expression but isolated loss of PMS2.

include the EGF, transforming growth factor alpha, and amphiregulin. In the presence ligand, EGF-R dimerizes with other erbB receptors, resulting in phosphorylation of the intracellular portion of the receptor and activation of three main signaling pathways, the RAS/RAF/MAPK pathway, the PI3 kinase (PI3 K) pathway, and the JAK/STAT pathway (**Fig. 5**).[12] The final target of the RAS/RAF/MAPK pathway is MEK and ERK1/2. These targets control cellular events such as apoptosis and proliferation.[65] The downstream targets of the PI3 K pathway are Akt and GSK3.[66] These effectors also are involved in cell survival and growth. The PI3 K pathway is negatively regulated by phosphatase protein homolog to tensin (PTEN). EGF-R has been implicated in various solid tumors such as lung, breast, pancreas, and CRC.[12] Knowledge of the role that EGF-R plays in epithelial cancers provided the rationale for the development of antibodies that target and block activity of this receptor. These antibodies, however, are costly and associated with clinically significant adverse effects.[67] In addition, the initial studies have shown that only 10% of patients with metastatic CRC respond to anti-EGFR therapy.[68] Again, molecular testing that can predict response to these biologic agents is essential. This section discusses molecular testing in CRC as it relates to prognosis and treatment.

> ### Key Features
> #### IN MOLECULAR TESTING IN
> #### SPORADIC COLORECTAL CANCER INCLUDE
>
> - KRAS and BRAF are serine threonine kinases downstream of the EGF-R and are involved in various cellular functions including cell growth and survival.
>
> - KRAS mutations occur in approximately 40% of CRCs, and mutations in KRAS confer resistance to therapies with anti-EGF-R antibodies, cetuximab, and panitumumab.
>
> - The sensitivity of PCR and pyrosequencing assays is higher than traditional Sanger sequencing methods, although all three show a high concordance rate with regards to detecting KRAS mutations.
>
> - It is essential that surgical pathologists select appropriate blocks with abundant tumor to guide manual microdissection. Ideally, blocks with more than 50% tumor should be selected for analysis.
>
> - Preliminary data also indicated that V600E mutations in BRAF confer resistance to anti-EGF-R therapy.

MOLECULAR FINDINGS

KRAS MUTATIONAL STATUS

KRAS is a member of the RAS family of serine threonine kinases that transduces signals from cell surface receptors to numerous intracellular targets. KRAS is active when bound by GTP, and deactivation of KRAS occurs through its inherent GTPase activity and is facilitated by guanine nucleotide exchange factors and GTPase activating proteins.[69] Oncogenic mutations in KRAS alter GTPase function, resulting in constitutive activation, which occurs in approximately 40% of CRCs. Over 95% of the activating mutations in KRAS occur in codons 12 and 13 of exons 2, and less than 5% occur in codons 61 and 146.[69–71] As KRAS is downstream of the EGF-R, activating mutations in KRAS theoretically would render treatment with anti-EGFR antibodies, cetuximab, and panitumumab, ineffective. This hypothesis has been tested and confirmed over the last few years.

The efficacy of anti-EGFR antibodies has been studied extensively in patients with metastatic CRC who have progressed on first-line chemotherapy. In these studies, the number of patients ranged from 27 to 113, and the percentage of tumors with KRAS mutations ranged from 13% to 42%.[72–78] Although direct comparison between these studies it not entirely accurate, a rough analysis of their composite data revealed an objective remission rate (ORR) of only 4% in KRAS -mutated tumors (7 of 171 tumors). In contrast, the objective remission rate was 38% (105 of 278 tumors) for KRAS wild-type tumors. The progression-free survival (PFS) also was increased between 1 and 5 months for KRAS wild-type tumors. In addition, three of four studies demonstrated a significant increase in overall survival upon the addition of cetuximab in KRAS wild-type tumors.[72,73,77]

Given the cited results, it is not surprising that cetuximab also has proven effective as a component of first-line therapy in metastatic CRC in combination with either FOLFOX or FOLFIRI. Bokemeyer and colleagues[79] evaluated 233 patients with metastatic CRC, 134 of whom had wild-type KRAS tumors. In the FOLFOX plus cetuximab arm, the ORR was 61% for KRAS wild-type tumors compared with 33% of KRAS-mutated tumors. The PFS also was improved by 2.2 months upon the addition of cetuximab in KRAS wild-type tumors. In a larger study of 540 tumors by Van Cutsem and colleagues,[80] the PFS also was improved in KRAS wild-type tumors treated with FOLFIRI plus cetuximab by 2.3 months. Based on these results, the American Society of Clinical Oncology recommend that all tumors with metastases should be tested for mutations in codons 12 and 13 of exon 2 of the KRAS gene before the institution of anti-EGF-R therapy.[81]

The concordance rate of KRAS mutational status between the metastatic and primary tumor is quite high.[82–85] Thus testing can be performed on the initial resection specimen or biopsy. Furthermore, chemotherapy does not seem to affect KRAS mutational status, although definitive proof is lacking. Formalin-fixed paraffin-embedded tissue is sufficient for testing, and no particular testing method has been recommended for screening.[81] Although a discussion of all the available tests is beyond the scope of this article, the authors provide an overview of three basic technologies that are routinely employed:

1. Sanger dideoxy sequencing
2. PCR
3. Pyrosequencing.

In addition, numerous commercial kits exist that employ proprietary technology and reagents (**Fig. 6**). The sensitivity of these technologies varies considerably. Sanger sequencing is highly specific, although the sensitivity is quite low in

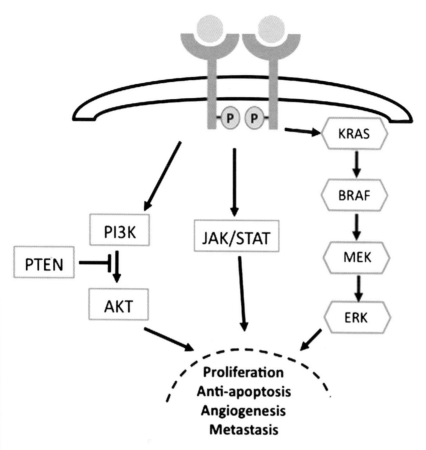

Fig. 5. Schematic diagram of the epidermal growth factor receptor (EGF-R) signaling pathway. Once EGF-R is bound by ligand, the intracellular portion of the receptor becomes phosphorylated and activates the downstream signaling pathways including the PI3 K pathway, the JAK/STAT pathway, and the MAPK pathway. The downstream effectors of these pathways results in transcriptional activation of a wide variety of genes involved in cell growth and survival, anti-apoptosis, metastasis, and angiogenesis.

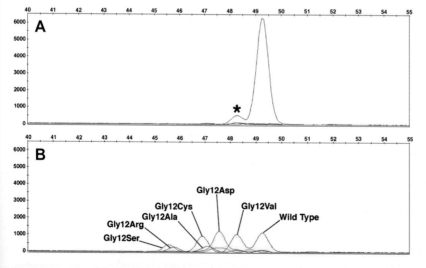

Fig. 6. KRAS mutational analysis employing shifted termination assay technology from TrimGen (Mutector II KRAS mutation kit, Sparks, MD, USA). In this assay there are specific primers that recognize twelve mutations in codons 12 and 13. Once one of these specific primers anneals to a particular DNA sequence, there is selective extension of the polymerase chain reaction (PCR). Capillary electrophoresis is then used to separate the PCR products for detection of mutations. The top panel (*A*) shows a colorectal carcinoma with two PCR products for a reaction amplifying codon 12. Comparison of these two peaks with a control reaction containing six codon 12 mutations; (*B*) demonstrates that the larger peak corresponds to a wild-type signal and the smaller peak corresponds to the Gly12Val KRAS mutation.

unenriched samples.[71] In contrast, PCR and pyrosequencing methods can detect a KRAS mutation in samples containing very small populations of mutated cells (approximately 5% to 10%).[86,87] Before testing, the surgical pathologist plays a critical role in selecting a block with an appropriate percentage of viable tumor cells. Furthermore, the hematoxylin and eosin slide can be used as a guide for manual microdissection to enrich the sample even further. Laser capture microdissection is employed only in rare cases in which only very small foci of tumor are present such as in treated rectal cancer.

There have been only a few studies comparing these various assays; however, the studies that have been performed show that many of the assays detect KRAS mutations at a comparable rate. Whitehall and colleagues[88] evaluated six different assays at seven different centers. Using the five best performing assays, a concordance rate of 96% was observed.[88] Weichert and colleagues[89] tested 263 CRCs for KRAS mutations using the Sanger method, real-time PCR, array analysis, and pyrosequencing. Forty percent of tumors contained mutations in KRAS, and the different methods reported concordant results with a kappa score of more than 0.9, which is almost perfect agreement.[89] In the study by Weichert and colleagues,[89] no mutations were detected in samples in which the percent tumor was less than 10%. This result confirms the need for dialog between the surgical and molecular pathologist in selecting the appropriate block and to guide manual microdissection for enrichment.

BRAF MUTATIONAL STATUS

BRAF is a serine threonine kinase that is downstream of KRAS and EGF-R, and activating mutations are found in approximately 10% to 15% of sporadic CRCs.[3,4] Unlike KRAS, the overwhelming number of mutations occur in exon 15 at codon 600 and involves a point mutation resulting in a substitution of valine for glutamate (V600E). Given its involvement in the EGF-R pathway, activating mutations in BRAF also may reduce the effectiveness of treatment with cetuximab or panitumumab. Recent studies in the past year have confirmed this hypothesis. Di Nicolantonio and colleagues[90] analyzed 79 patients with wild-type KRAS for BRAF mutations. Eleven mutations were found, and none of these patients responded to anti-EGFR therapy. Souglakos and colleagues[91] also found a lack of response to cetuximab in BRAF mutated metastatic CRC. Other studies,

however, have shown only a borderline effect of BRAF mutational status on response to anti-EGFR therapy.[92,93] Currently, no recommendations regarding screening for BRAF exist, although it is likely in the near future that knowledge of BRAF mutational status will be required before institution of anti-EGF-R therapy. Similar to KRAS, numerous methods have been employed to screen for the V600E BRAF mutation, and all seem equally valid.

MSI TESTING

Sporadic MSI-H cancers account for approximately 15% of CRCs and almost invariably arise due to hypermethylation of CpG islands in the MLH1 promoter.[94] As mentioned previously, these CIMP-H tumors display methylation of various tumor suppressor gene promoters, including cell cycle control genes (CDKN2A and INK4A), DNA repair genes (MGMT), DNA MMR genes (MLH1), and genes involved in cell signaling (APC, SOCS1, and LKB1), rendering them inactive. MLH1 promoter methylation leads to MLH1 gene silencing, giving rise to high MSI and concurrent loss of MLH1 and PMS2 expression by immunohistochemistry.[47,94] Thus, the demonstration of MSI-H in any given CRC is not diagnostic of HNPCC, and additional testing must be performed to exclude the possibility of a sporadic MSI-H CRC related to CIMP. In fact, analysis of CIMP, and in particular MLH1 promoter methylation, is used to exclude HNPCC among patients who exhibit MSI-H, since HNPCC CRCs seldom exhibit MLH1 promoter hypermethylation.[95] The V600E BRAF mutation is also strongly associated with CIMP; screening for V600E BRAF mutations by PCR may be a simple way to exclude HNPCC among patients who exhibit MSI-H, since Lynch colorectal carcinomas seldom contain BRAF mutations.[95,96]

MSI testing may provide important prognostic and therapeutic information in CRC. As mentioned, numerous studies, including recent large meta-analyses, have shown that sporadic or syndromic MSI-H tumors are associated with a relatively good prognosis compared with MSS tumors.[97,98] In addition, most studies have shown that patients with stage 2 or 4 MSI-H CRCs do not appear to benefit from adjuvant therapy with 5-FU.[99] One retrospective analysis, however, did not find MSI-H status to predict response to adjuvant chemotherapy.[38] The impact of MSI status on the response to new chemotherapeutic regimens that include oxaliplatin is unclear. Although clinical guidelines have not been standardized, many institutions are using MSI status to guide decision making in stage 2 CRC. In particular, stage 2 MSI-H CRC may not need adjuvant chemotherapy given its relatively good prognosis and the chemoresistance to 5-FU.[39] In stage 3 MSI-H CRC, the data are much less clear, and MSI status may not be helpful in making treatment decisions.

SUMMARY

CRC was once considered a relatively homogenous entity; however, work in the past decade has revolutionized the understanding of this complex disease. Along with improved knowledge of the molecular pathogenesis of CRC came new biologic therapies and molecular prognostic markers. KRAS, BRAF, and testing for HNPCC testing are likely only the beginning of molecular testing in CRC. Indeed, recent studies have implicated PIK3CA as a possible candidate for future testing.[91,100,101] It is clear that surgical pathologists play a key role in molecular testing in CRC as they serve as key intermediaries between oncologists and the molecular diagnostics laboratories.

REFERENCES

1. Kambara T, Simms LA, Whitehall VL, et al. BRAF mutation is associated with DNA methylation in serrated polyps and cancers of the colorectum. Gut 2004;53(8):1137–44.
2. Grady WM, Carethers JM. Genomic and epigenetic instability in colorectal cancer pathogenesis. Gastroenterology 2008;135(4):1079–99.
3. Ogino S, Goel A. Molecular classification and correlates in colorectal cancer. J Mol Diagn 2008; 10(1):13–27.
4. Jass JR. Classification of colorectal cancer based on correlation of clinical, morphological and molecular features. Histopathology 2007;50(1):113–30.
5. Fearon ER, Vogelstein B. A genetic model for colorectal tumorigenesis. Cell 1990;61(5):759–67.
6. Fodde R, Kuipers J, Rosenberg C, et al. Mutations in the APC tumour suppressor gene cause chromosomal instability. Nat Cell Biol 2001;3(4):433–8.
7. Alberici P, Fodde R. The role of the APC tumor suppressor in chromosomal instability. Genome Dyn 2006;1:149–70.
8. Kaplan KB, Burds AA, Swedlow JR, et al. A role for the adenomatous polyposis coli protein in chromosome segregation. Nat Cell Biol 2001; 3(4):429–32.
9. Nathke I. Cytoskeleton out of the cupboard: colon cancer and cytoskeletal changes induced by loss of APC. Nat Rev Cancer 2006;6(12):967–74.
10. Cahill DP, Lengauer C, Yu J, et al. Mutations of mitotic checkpoint genes in human cancers. Nature 1998;392(6673):300–3.
11. Bischoff JR, Anderson L, Zhu Y, et al. A homologue of Drosophila aurora kinase is oncogenic and amplified in human colorectal cancers. EMBO J 1998;17(11):3052–65.
12. Hynes NE, Lane HA. ERBB receptors and cancer: the complexity of targeted inhibitors. Nat Rev Cancer 2005;5(5):341–54.
13. Issa JP. CpG island methylator phenotype in cancer. Natl Rev 2004;4(12):988–93.
14. Samowitz WS, Albertsen H, Herrick J, et al. Evaluation of a large, population-based sample supports a CpG island methylator phenotype in colon cancer. Gastroenterology 2005;129(3):837–45.
15. Goel A, Nagasaka T, Arnold CN, et al. The CpG island methylator phenotype and chromosomal instability are inversely correlated in sporadic colorectal cancer. Gastroenterology 2007;132(1):127–38.
16. Weisenberger DJ, Siegmund KD, Campan M, et al. CpG island methylator phenotype underlies sporadic microsatellite instability and is tightly associated with BRAF mutation in colorectal cancer. Nat Genet 2006;38(7):787–93.
17. Nosho K, Irahara N, Shima K, et al. Comprehensive biostatistical analysis of CpG island methylator phenotype in colorectal cancer using a large population-based sample. PLoS One 2008;3(11):e3698.
18. Ogino S, Kawasaki T, Kirkner GJ, et al. Evaluation of markers for CpG island methylator phenotype (CIMP) in colorectal cancer by a large population-based sample. J Mol Diagn 2007;9(3):305–14.
19. Tanaka H, Deng G, Matsuzaki K, et al. BRAF mutation, CpG island methylator phenotype and microsatellite instability occur more frequently and concordantly in mucinous than nonmucinous colorectal cancer. Int J Cancer 2006;118(11): 2765–71.
20. Ogino S, Nosho K, Kirkner GJ, et al. CpG island methylator phenotype, microsatellite instability, BRAF mutation, and clinical outcome in colon cancer. Gut 2009;58(1):90–6.
21. Young J, Barker MA, Simms LA, et al. Evidence for BRAF mutation and variable levels of microsatellite instability in a syndrome of familial colorectal cancer. Clin Gastroenterol Hepatol 2005;3(3): 254–63.
22. Nagasaka T, Koi M, Kloor M, et al. Mutations in both KRAS and BRAF may contribute to the methylator phenotype in colon cancer. Gastroenterology 2008;134(7):1950–60, 1960.e1.
23. Ogino S, Cantor M, Kawasaki T, et al. CpG island methylator phenotype (CIMP) of colorectal cancer is best characterised by quantitative DNA methylation analysis and prospective cohort studies. Gut 2006;55(7):1000–6.
24. Shen L, Toyota M, Kondo Y, et al. Integrated genetic and epigenetic analysis identifies three

different subclasses of colon cancer. Proc Natl Acad Sci U S A 2007;104(47):18654–9.

25. Ogino S, Kawasaki T, Kirkner GJ, et al. CpG island methylator phenotype-low (CIMP-low) in colorectal cancer: possible associations with male sex and KRAS mutations. J Mol Diagn 2006;8(5):582–8.

26. Kawasaki T, Ohnishi M, Nosho K, et al. CpG island methylator phenotype-low (CIMP-low) colorectal cancer shows not only few methylated CIMP-high-specific CpG islands, but also low-level methylation at individual loci. Mod Pathol 2008;21(3):245–55.

27. Winawer SJ, Zauber AG, Fletcher RH, et al. Guidelines for colonoscopy surveillance after polypectomy: a consensus update by the US Multi-Society Task Force on Colorectal Cancer and the American Cancer Society. Gastroenterology 2006; 130(6):1872–85.

28. Torlakovic E, Skovlund E, Snover DC, et al. Morphologic reappraisal of serrated colorectal polyps. Am J Surg Pathol 2003;27(1):65–81.

29. Goldstein NS, Bhanot P, Odish E, et al. Hyperplastic-like colon polyps that preceded microsatellite-unstable adenocarcinomas. Am J Clin Pathol 2003; 119(6):778–96.

30. Spring KJ, Zhao ZZ, Karamatic R, et al. High prevalence of sessile serrated adenomas with BRAF mutations: a prospective study of patients undergoing colonoscopy. Gastroenterology 2006;131(5):1400–7.

31. O'Brien MJ, Yang S, Mack C, et al. Comparison of microsatellite instability, CpG island methylation phenotype, BRAF and KRAS status in serrated polyps and traditional adenomas indicates separate pathways to distinct colorectal carcinoma end points. Am J Surg Pathol 2006;30(12):1491–501.

32. Kim YH, Kakar S, Cun L, et al. Distinct CpG island methylation profiles and BRAF mutation status in serrated and adenomatous colorectal polyps. Int J Cancer 2008;123(11):2587–93.

33. Samowitz WS, Albertsen H, Sweeney C, et al. Association of smoking, CpG island methylator phenotype, and V600E BRAF mutations in colon cancer. J Natl Cancer Inst 2006;98(23):1731–8.

34. Slattery ML, Curtin K, Sweeney C, et al. Diet and lifestyle factor associations with CpG island methylator phenotype and BRAF mutations in colon cancer. Int J Cancer 2007;120(3):656–63.

35. Jass JR, Baker K, Zlobec I, et al. Advanced colorectal polyps with the molecular and morphological features of serrated polyps and adenomas: concept of a 'fusion' pathway to colorectal cancer. Histopathology 2006;49(2):121–31.

36. Pawlik TM, Raut CP, Rodriguez-Bigas MA. Colorectal carcinogenesis: MSI-H versus MSI-L. Dis Markers 2004;20(4–5):199–206.

37. Soreide K, Janssen EA, Soiland H, et al. Microsatellite instability in colorectal cancer. Br J Surg 2006; 93(4):395–406.

38. Kim GP, Colangelo LH, Wieand HS, et al. Prognostic and predictive roles of high-degree microsatellite instability in colon cancer: a National Cancer Institute–National Surgical Adjuvant Breast and Bowel Project Collaborative Study. J Clin Oncol 2007;25(7):767–72.

39. Sinicrope FA, Sargent DJ. Clinical implications of microsatellite instability in sporadic colon cancers. Curr Opin Oncol 2009;21(4):369–73.

40. Ward RL, Cheong K, Ku S, et al. Adverse prognostic effect of methylation in colorectal cancer is reversed by microsatellite instability. J Clin Oncol 2003;21(20):3729–36.

41. Lynch HT, Lynch JF. Lynch syndrome: history and current status. Dis Markers 2004;20:181–98.

42. Fishel R, Lescoe MK, Rao MR, et al. The human mutator gene homolog MSH2 and its association with hereditary nonpolyposis colon cancer. Cell 1993;75(5):1027–38.

43. Papadopoulos N, Nicolaides NC, Wei YF, et al. Mutation of a mutL homolog in hereditary colon cancer. Science 1994;263(5153):1625–9.

44. Leach FS, Nicolaides NC, Papadopoulos N, et al. Mutations of a mutS homolog in hereditary nonpolyposis colorectal cancer. Cell 1993;75(6):1215–25.

45. Bronner CE, Baker SM, Morrison PT, et al. Mutation in the DNA mismatch repair gene homologue hMLH1 is associated with hereditary nonpolyposis colon cancer. Nature 1994;368(6468): 258–61.

46. Burgart LJ. Testing for defective DNA mismatch repair in colorectal carcinoma: a practical guide. Arch Pathol Lab Med 2005;129(11):1385–9.

47. Shia J. Immunohistochemistry versus microsatellite instability testing for screening colorectal cancer patients at risk for hereditary nonpolyposis colorectal cancer syndrome. Part I. The utility of immunohistochemistry. J Mol Diagn 2008;10(4): 293–300.

48. Peltomaki P, Vasen H. Mutations associated with HNPCC predisposition – update of ICG-HNPCC/INSiGHT mutation database. Dis Markers 2004; 20(4–5):269–76.

49. Jass JR. Role of the pathologist in the diagnosis of hereditary non-polyposis colorectal cancer. Dis Markers 2004;20(4–5):215–24.

50. Jenkins MA, Hayashi S, O'Shea A, et al. Pathology features in Bethesda guidelines predict colorectal cancer microsatellite instability: a population-based study. Gastroenterology 2007;133(1):48–56.

51. Young J, Simms LA, Biden KG, et al. Features of colorectal cancers with high-level microsatellite instability occurring in familial and sporadic settings: parallel pathways of tumorigenesis. Am J Pathol 2001;159(6):2107–16.

52. Umar A, Boland CR, Terdiman JP, et al. Revised Bethesda Guidelines for hereditary nonpolyposis

colorectal cancer (Lynch syndrome) and microsatellite instability. J Natl Cancer Inst 2004;96(4):261–8.

53. Suraweera N, Duval A, Reperant M, et al. Evaluation of tumor microsatellite instability using five quasimonomorphic mononucleotide repeats and pentaplex PCR. Gastroenterology 2002;123(6): 1804–11.

54. Garg K, Shih K, Barakat R, et al. Endometrial carcinomas in women aged 40 years and younger: tumors associated with loss of DNA mismatch repair proteins comprise a distinct clinicopathologic subset. Am J Surg Pathol 2009;33(12): 1869–77.

55. Orta L, Klimstra DS, Qin J, et al. Towards identification of hereditary DNA mismatch repair deficiency: sebaceous neoplasm warrants routine immunohistochemical screening regardless of patient's age or other clinical characteristics. Am J Surg Pathol 2009;33(6):934–44.

56. Berends MJ, Wu Y, Sijmons RH, et al. Molecular and clinical characteristics of MSH6 variants: an analysis of 25 index carriers of a germline variant. Am J Hum Genet 2002;70(1):26–37.

57. Buttin BM, Powell MA, Mutch DG, et al. Penetrance and expressivity of MSH6 germline mutations in seven kindreds not ascertained by family history. Am J Hum Genet 2004;74(6):1262–9.

58. Hampel H, Frankel WL, Martin E, et al. Screening for the Lynch syndrome (hereditary nonpolyposis colorectal cancer). N Engl J Med 2005;352(18): 1851–60.

59. Southey MC, Jenkins MA, Mead L, et al. Use of molecular tumor characteristics to prioritize mismatch repair gene testing in early onset colorectal cancer. J Clin Oncol 2005;23(27):6524–32.

60. Lagerstedt Robinson K, Liu T, Vandrovcova J, et al. Lynch syndrome (hereditary nonpolyposis colorectal cancer) diagnostics. J Natl Cancer Inst 2007;99(4):291–9.

61. Shia J, Tang LH, Vakiani E, et al. Immunohistochemistry as first-line screening for detecting colorectal cancer patients at risk for hereditary nonpolyposis colorectal cancer syndrome: a 2-antibody panel may be as predictive as a 4-antibody panel. Am J Surg Pathol 2009;33(11): 1639–45.

62. Salahshor S, Koelble K, Rubio C, et al. Microsatellite Instability and hMLH1 and hMSH2 expression analysis in familial and sporadic colorectal cancer. Lab Invest 2001;81(4):535–41.

63. Barnetson RA, Tenesa A, Farrington SM, et al. Identification and survival of carriers of mutations in DNA mismatch-repair genes in colon cancer. N Engl J Med 2006;354(26):2751–63.

64. Mano M, Duhoux F. Colon cancer: update on adjuvant therapy. Clin Colorectal Cancer 2008;7(3): 178–83.

65. Roberts PJ, Der CJ. Targeting the Raf-MEK-ERK mitogen-activated protein kinase cascade for the treatment of cancer. Oncogene 2007;26(22): 3291–310.

66. Engelman JA. Targeting PI3K signalling in cancer: opportunities, challenges and limitations. Nat Rev Cancer 2009;9(8):550–62.

67. Dalle S, Thieblemont C, Thomas L, et al. Monoclonal antibodies in clinical oncology. Anticancer Agents Med Chem 2008;8(5):523–32.

68. Cunningham D, Humblet Y, Siena S, et al. Cetuximab monotherapy and cetuximab plus irinotecan in irinotecan-refractory metastatic colorectal cancer. N Engl J Med 2004;351(4):337–45.

69. Walther A, Johnstone E, Swanton C, et al. Genetic prognostic and predictive markers in colorectal cancer. Nat Rev Cancer 2009;9(7):489–99.

70. Plesec TP, Hunt JL. KRAS mutation testing in colorectal cancer. Adv Anat Pathol 2009;16(4):196–203.

71. Wang HL, Lopategui J, Amin MB, et al. KRAS Mutation Testing in Human Cancers: the pathologist's role in the era of personalized medicine. Adv Anat Pathol 2010;17(1):23–32.

72. Lièvre A, Bachet J, Le Corre D, et al. KRAS mutation status is predictive of response to cetuximab therapy in colorectal cancer. Cancer Res 2006; 66(8):3992–5.

73. Lièvre A, Bachet J, Boige V, et al. KRAS mutations as an independent prognostic factor in patients with advanced colorectal cancer treated with cetuximab. J Clin Oncol 2008;26(3):374–9.

74. Benvenuti S, Sartore-Bianchi A, Di Nicolantonio F, et al. Oncogenic activation of the RAS/RAF signaling pathway impairs the response of metastatic colorectal cancers to anti-epidermal growth factor receptor antibody therapies. Cancer Res 2007;67(6):2643–8.

75. Frattini M, Saletti P, Romagnani E, et al. PTEN loss of expression predicts cetuximab efficacy in metastatic colorectal cancer patients. Br J Cancer 2007; 97(8):1139–45.

76. Di Fiore F, Blanchard F, Charbonnier F, et al. Clinical relevance of KRAS mutation detection in metastatic colorectal cancer treated by Cetuximab plus chemotherapy. Br J Cancer 2007; 96(8):1166–9.

77. De Roock W, Piessevaux H, De Schutter J, et al. KRAS wild-type state predicts survival and is associated to early radiological response in metastatic colorectal cancer treated with cetuximab. Ann Oncol 2008;19(3):508–15.

78. Cappuzzo F, Varella-Garcia M, Finocchiaro G, et al. Primary resistance to cetuximab therapy in EGFR FISH-positive colorectal cancer patients. Br J Cancer 2008;99(1):83–9.

79. Bokemeyer C, Bondarenko I, Makhson A, et al. Fluorouracil, leucovorin, and oxaliplatin with and

without cetuximab in the first-line treatment of metastatic colorectal cancer. J Clin Oncol 2009; 27(5):663–71.

80. Van Cutsem E, Köhne C, Hitre E, et al. Cetuximab and chemotherapy as initial treatment for metastatic colorectal cancer. N Engl J Med 2009; 360(14):1408–17.

81. Allegra CJ, Jessup JM, Somerfield MR, et al. American Society of Clinical Oncology provisional clinical opinion: testing for KRAS gene mutations in patients with metastatic colorectal carcinoma to predict response to anti-epidermal growth factor receptor monoclonal antibody therapy. J Clin Oncol 2009;27(12):2091–6.

82. Artale S, Sartore-Bianchi A, Veronese SM, et al. Mutations of KRAS and BRAF in primary and matched metastatic sites of colorectal cancer. J Clin Oncol 2008;26(25):4217–9.

83. Santini D, Loupakis F, Vincenzi B, et al. High concordance of KRAS status between primary colorectal tumors and related metastatic sites: implications for clinical practice. Oncologist 2008; 13(12):1270–5.

84. Zauber P, Sabbath-Solitare M, Marotta SP, et al. Molecular changes in the Ki-ras and APC genes in primary colorectal carcinoma and synchronous metastases compared with the findings in accompanying adenomas. Mol Pathol 2003;56(3):137–40.

85. Losi L, Benhattar J, Costa J. Stability of K-ras mutations throughout the natural history of human colorectal cancer. Eur J Cancer 1992;28(6–7): 1115–20.

86. Dufort S, Richard M, de Fraipont F. Pyrosequencing method to detect KRAS mutation in formalin-fixed and paraffin-embedded tumor tissues. Anal Biochem 2009;391(2):166–8.

87. Krypuy M, Newnham GM, Thomas DM, et al. High-resolution melting analysis for the rapid and sensitive detection of mutations in clinical samples: KRAS codon 12 and 13 mutations in nonsmall cell lung cancer. BMC Cancer 2006;6:295.

88. Whitehall V, Tran K, Umapathy A, et al. A multicenter blinded study to evaluate KRAS mutation testing methodologies in the clinical setting. J Mol Diagn 2009;11(6):543–52.

89. Weichert W, Schewe C, Lehmann A, et al. KRAS genotyping of paraffin-embedded colorectal cancer tissue in routine diagnostics: comparison of methods and impact of histology. J Mol Diagn 2010;12(1):35–42.

90. Di Nicolantonio F, Martini M, Molinari F, et al. Wild-type BRAF is required for response to panitumumab

or cetuximab in metastatic colorectal cancer. J Clin Oncol 2008;26(35):5705–12.

91. Souglakos J, Philips J, Wang R, et al. Prognostic and predictive value of common mutations for treatment response and survival in patients with metastatic colorectal cancer. Br J Cancer 2009; 101(3):465–72.

92. Laurent-Puig P, Cayre A, Manceau G, et al. Analysis of PTEN, BRAF, and EGFR status in determining benefit from cetuximab therapy in wild-type KRAS metastatic colon cancer. J Clin Oncol 2009. Available at: http://www.ncbi.nlm.nih.gov/pubmed/19884556. Accessed December 7, 2009.

93. Sartore-Bianchi A, Di Nicolantonio F, Nichelatti M, et al. Multideterminants analysis of molecular alterations for predicting clinical benefit to EGFR-targeted monoclonal antibodies in colorectal cancer. PLoS One 2009;4(10):e7287.

94. Herman JG, Umar A, Polyak K, et al. Incidence and functional consequences of hMLH1 promoter hypermethylation in colorectal carcinoma. Proc Natl Acad Sci U S A 1998;95(12):6870–5.

95. Wang L, Cunningham JM, Winters JL, et al. BRAF mutations in colon cancer are not likely attributable to defective DNA mismatch repair. Cancer Res 2003;63(17):5209–12.

96. Domingo E, Laiho P, Ollikainen M, et al. BRAF screening as a low-cost effective strategy for simplifying HNPCC genetic testing. J Med Genet 2004;41(9):664–8.

97. Popat S, Hubner R, Houlston RS. Systematic review of microsatellite instability and colorectal cancer prognosis. J Clin Oncol 2005;23(3):609–18.

98. Walther A, Houlston R, Tomlinson I. Association between chromosomal instability and prognosis in colorectal cancer: a meta-analysis. Gut 2008; 57(7):941–50.

99. Ribic CM, Sargent DJ, Moore MJ, et al. Tumor microsatellite-instability status as a predictor of benefit from fluorouracil-based adjuvant chemotherapy for colon cancer. N Engl J Med 2003; 349(3):247–57.

100. Sartore-Bianchi A, Martini M, Molinari F, et al. PIK3CA mutations in colorectal cancer are associated with clinical resistance to EGFR-targeted monoclonal antibodies. Cancer Res 2009;69(5): 1851–7.

101. Jhawer M, Goel S, Wilson AJ, et al. PIK3CA mutation/PTEN expression status predicts response of colon cancer cells to the epidermal growth factor receptor inhibitor cetuximab. Cancer Res 2008; 68(6):1953–61.

INDEX

Note: Page numbers of article titles are in **boldface** type.

A

Ablative therapy, endoscopic mucosal, 421–422
  cryospray, 423
  photodynamic therapy, 421–423
  radiofrequency, 423
Adenocarcinoma, gastrointestinal neuroendocrine
  tumor vs., 332
Age, eosinophilic esophagitis and, 277
Amoebiasis, complications of, 322, 324
  diagnosis of, 322
  dysentery in, 319
  flask-shaped lesions in, 320
  microscopic features of, amoebae, 321, 323
    distinction of trophozoietes from
      macrophages, 321, 324
    invasive amoeba, 321–322
    necrotic debris, 319, 320
    neutrophilic infiltrate, 319–320
    ulcers, 320–321
  prevalence of, 319
  risk factors for, 319
Anthraquinone laxatives, neural damage from,
  385–386
Antimicrobial drug injury, *Candida* esophagitis, 377
  diagnosis of, 379
  esophagitis, pill-induced, 377
  from penicillins, 377
  gastrointestinal, 377
  microscopic features of, 377, 379
Appendiceal mucinous tumors, diagnosis of,
  adenoma, 404
    cystadenoma of uncertain malignant potential,
      404–406
    high-grade adenocarcinoma, 407
    low-grade neoplasm, 403–404, 403–406
    neoplasms of uncertain malignant potential
      in, 403
    pseudomyxoma peritonei in, 403–404
  diagnostic categories of, 395
  differential diagnosis of, 401–402
  gross features of, mucocele, 396–397
    pseudomyxoma peritonei-associated, 397
  low-grade, 397–398, 403–404
  metastatic to ovary, 401–402
  microscopic features of, 397–401
    acellular mucin extravasation in, 397, 400
    atrophy of lymphoid tissue, 397, 399
    concurrent diverticulum, 397

    flattening of neoplastic epithelium in mucinous
      cysadenoma, 397, 399
    goblet cell carcinoid component, 400
    immunohistochemistry of, 400
    in adenocarcinomas, 398, 401
    periappendiceal mucin extravasation, 397, 400
    villus adenoma architecture, 398
  morphology of, tubular or villous, 395
  nomenclature for, 396
  pathologic features of, 395
  presentation mimicking acute appendicitis,
    395–396
  risk factors for, 396
  survival rates for, 406–407
Appendiceal neuroendocrine tumors (NETs),
  340–341
  enterochromaffin cell, 340
  goblet cell carcinoids in, 342–343
  infiltration into muscularis propria, 341
  metastatic disease in, 341–342
  morphology of, carcinoid, 342
  tubular carcinoid, 343

B

Bisphosphonates, GI injury from, 384
BRAF mutational status, effect on cetuximab and
  panitumumab theray, 441

C

C. difficile-related pseudomembranous colitis,
  amoebiasis vs., 321
Cetuximab, 437, 439, 441
Chemotherapeutic agents, GI effects of, 366–367
  GI injury from, differential diagnosis of, 373–374
    gross and endoscopic features of, 369–370
    microscopic features of, 370–373
  GI side effects of, damage to nerves, 369
    direct damage, 368
    indirect damage, 368–369
    pathophysiology of, 368–369
Children, enterohemorrhagic *E. coli* in, prognosis
  of, 319
Chondrosarcoma, GISTs resembling, 246, 257
  GIST vs., 257–258, 262–263
Chordoma, GISTs resembling, 246, 257
Chordomas, GIST vs., 257–258, 262–263

doi:10.1016/S1875-9181(10)00071-1
1875-9181/10/$ – see front matter © 2010 Elsevier Inc. All rights reserved.

surgpath.theclinics.com

Moving?

Make sure your subscription moves with you!

To notify us of your new address, find your **Clinics Account Number** (located on your mailing label above your name), and contact customer service at:

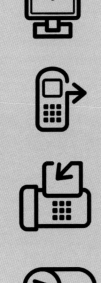

Email: journalscustomerservice-usa@elsevier.com

800-654-2452 (subscribers in the U.S. & Canada)
314-447-8871 (subscribers outside of the U.S. & Canada)

Fax number: 314-447-8029

Elsevier Health Sciences Division
Subscription Customer Service
3251 Riverport Lane
Maryland Heights, MO 63043

*To ensure uninterrupted delivery of your subscription, please notify us at least 4 weeks in advance of move.

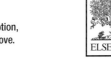